/

ADVANCE REVIEWS

"This book should be read by anyone wondering what's wrong with our medical system. Dr. Maykel reminds us that doctors must first learn to listen and to watch their patients so that they can treat the whole person as a single system rather than their artificially separated chronic ailments. Through well-researched and entertaining case reports, Dr. Maykel opens our eyes to the critically defective components of medical care today."

DEVRA DAVIS, PHD MPH Fellow American College of Epidemiology, President Environmental Health Trust – Assoc. Editor, Frontiers in Radiation and Health, Author of *Disconnect: the truth about cell phone radiation* and *The Secret History of the War on Cancer*

"I simply do not see how anyone, healthcare practitioner or otherwise who is interested in natural health can get by without reading this wonderful piece of work. *The Tune Up* is easy to read and understand as well as incredibly well-referenced and researched."

RICHARD A. BELLI, DC, DACNB, FABNN, CFMP

"I am blessed to know Dr. Bill Maykel as a kinesiologist and health healing pioneer for 50+ years. Bill's passion, knowledge, persistence, and determination for healing, nurturing, and improving the health of patients are legend. Using non-invasive natural procedures, Bill provides a pathway to healing. Also, by providing guidance relative to proper exercise and diet, he truly gives people the tools to heal. *The Tune Up—Hot Medicine for Everyone* is a must read for all who wish to cultivate, enhance and preserve their health."

JIM COGHLIN SR. Founder, 15-40 Connection

"I feel very fortunate to have met Bill Maykel at a YPO conference over 30 years ago and have been the beneficiary of the magic of his functional medicine therapies and practices ever since. His book *The Tune Up* combines a profound prospective on the current positioning of the U.S. Healthcare system and the promise that functional medicine holds by chronicling an important array of first hand clinical experiences and case outcomes over a wide range of conditions and issues. It should be required reading for both patients and practitioners."

TOM N. DAVIDSON Past International Chairman of YPO (Young Presidents Organization) and WPO (World Presidents Organization)

"*The Tune Up* represents timeless health principles that every doctor should know and every patient could benefit from. Tune Up is a phrase that should become as much a part of our health vernacular as the term 'yearly physical.' I applaud Dr. William Maykel's tireless work and triumph in expounding the virtues of Professional Applied Kinesiology and Functional Medicine."

EUGENE CHARLES, D.C., D.I.B.A.K. Diplomate, International Board of Applied Kinesiology, Director of the Applied Kinesiology Center of New York

The Tune Up

HOT MEDICINE™ FOR EVERYONE

HIPPOCRATIC ORDER OF TREATMENT LEAST INVASIVE FIRST

The Tune Up

HOT MEDICINE™ FOR EVERYONE

HIPPOCRATIC ORDER OF TREATMENT LEAST INVASIVE FIRST

William M. Maykel

D.C., D.I.B.A.K.

WELLNESS MEDICINE

The Tune Up: Hot Medicine™ for Everyone
William M. Maykel, D.C., D.I.B.A.K.

ISBN: 978-1-942545-63-7
Library of Congress Control Number: 2016911143

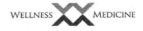

Published by Wellness Medicine
An imprint of Wyatt-MacKenzie

Foreword

Dr. William Maykel has accomplished what many people have thought to be "impossible," that is to make the concepts and application of Functional Medicine understandable and actionable for the non-medical reader. He has done it by allowing the story to be told through the success stories of his patients. It is a compelling book that incorporates real examples of the power of the Functional Medicine model that is a patient-centered approach to identifying and treating the cause and not just the symptoms of illness. When I founded the Institute for Functional Medicine in 2001 in order to develop the model more fully and to train health practitioners in its application I hoped that it would attract dedicated and talented professionals to it. Dr. Maykel represents the realization of my hopes. He has taken the Functional Medicine approach to health and healing and made it accessible to patients with chronic health problems. His book "The Tune-Up" takes the reader on a magnificent journey through the Functional Medicine system of healing and provides the "news to use" that makes it more than an abstract concept, but rather a tool that can be applied by anyone in need.

The origin of Functional Medicine grew out of the frustration that I and many colleagues had that medicine was not focused on the treatment of chronic illness. The drugs and surgeries used in medicine were finely tuned to treat acute diseases, but were not successful in safely and effectively managing chronic illness. A new approach was needed to deal with the ever-increasing burden of chronic illness. As is often the case, when there is a need the solution appeared in the form of new research and understanding about the cause of chronic illnesses. From this emerging revolution of new ideas came the recognition that we could group the root causes for the chronic diseases into disturbances among seven core physiological processes. Imbalances in one or more of these seven processes was associated with a functional physiological, cognitive, or physical dysfunction that was called a specific illness or disease. Understanding the specific imbalance in the person and then directing the therapy to resolve the imbalance was the focus on the Functional Medicine practitioner.

Dr. Maykel is a clinical expert in the application of this approach to health and healing. In his book he describes through the experiences of his patients how to identify the imbalances and then what to do to rectify the problems. It is a classic example of making the difficult seem easy that only comes about as a result of Dr. Maykel's deep understanding of how to make Functional Medicine a tool for improving patient health outcomes.

I take some vicarious pride in seeing how the Functional Medicine approach to health and healing has been successfully applied by Dr. Maykel and how many people's health will be positively influenced by reading his book. I am pleased to call Dr. Maykel a colleague and friend, and know that this book will guide many people aspiring to improve their health to achieve their objectives.

Jeffrey Bland, Ph.D., FACN, FACB
Co-Founder, Institute for Functional Medicine
President, Personalized Lifestyle Medicine Institute

Dedicated to my family.

ACKNOWLEDGEMENTS

As with all things of importance there are many hearts, minds and hands that have contributed to the creation of this book. The adage that it takes a village to raise a child rings true with this book as well.

First I would like to thank the late Dr. George Goodheart, who was not only the founder and developer of Professional Applied Kinesiology, but also a friend. This includes his wife JoAnne, whose love and support provided the basis for his insatiable creativity to grow and mature. The same holds true for the late Dr. David Walther and his wife Jean, whose textbooks created the fundamental teaching tools needed for this new approach in healthcare. Thank you to my first PAK teachers, Drs. David Leaf and John Campbell, as well as all the contributions from my brothers and sisters throughout the world joined by the family of the International College of Applied Kinesiology.

On the shoulders of giants we all stand and I would be remiss not to mention those of Dr. Major Bertarand Dejarnette, founder of the Sacro-Occipital Technique (SOT) and his student Dr. Marc Pick. The pioneering research, writing and teaching work of Dr. John Upledger represents another giant milestone. Thanks go to Drs. Jonathan Wright and Alan Gaby for their courses on evidence-based clinical nutrition.

I applaud the work of the following teachers: Dr. Sherry Rogers, William Falloon, Dr. Julian Whitaker, Dr. Steve Sinatra, Dr. John Diamond, Dr. Joseph Mercola, Ron Cummings, Atty. Steve Druker, Jeff Smith, Joseph Chilton Pearce and Dr. Russell Blaylock. They represent true foot soldiers in the march towards better world health.

Next is the work of the systems-based approach of the Institute for Functional Medicine founded by Drs. Jeffrey Bland and David Jones. I feel truly blessed to have had the privilege of learning from thirty plus years the truly prescient news from Dr. Bland and his unbelievable cohort of professional teachers. These include Drs. Robert Rakowski, Joel Furhman, Dean Ornish. Joe Pizzorno Jr., David Perlmutter, Datis Kharrazian and many others.

I would like to thank all of the people who have and do entrust their healthcare to my heart and soul. Thank you so much for teaching me humility and patience and opening up my mind to the greater good.

I am indebted to all of my clinical staff members, both past and present for all of your help: Paul Reith, Lyn Foster, Rosemary Flynn, Dr. Donn Paul Rademacher and Michael McLaughlin. Thank you for your support. It has been truly great.

Thanks go to my cousin, Al Maykel, and his wife Maggy for their terrific support and friendship. A very special thanks goes to his sister Nancy and her husband Jim Coghlin Sr, who invited me to participate as a resource/speaker for the Young Presidents Organization. This opportunity has allowed me to create a global family of patients and friends.

There are two core professional team members that I've worked side by side with for over thirty years. First is Bernice Morrisette, whose work is providing Therese Pfrimmer's deep muscle therapy. Your treatment on myself and my patients has been truly awesome. Second, is Dr. Gary Wetriech, prosthodontist extraordinaire, whose skill set in restorative dentistry and occlusal equilibration is truly unsurpassed.

I owe thanks to the great staff at the UMass Medical School library for their outstanding research services. It has truly been a pleasure to work with Mr. Steve Moskowitz. His patience and professionalism as a medical illustrator are only surpassed by his work.

My family and friends have been right there providing inestimable support and love. My hat is off to Greg Zlotnick for bringing Mr. Paul Tournaquindici in as a new patient, many years ago. As it turns out, Paul has selflessly laid this book out in Adobe InDesign™ and has been a guiding light in this book's maturity. Thank you.

I regret that my mother Helen, who just recently passed, is not alive to see this book completed as she was my major cheerleader. My four sisters, Linda, Elaine, Diane, Michelle, as well as my brother Mitchel have provided great feedback. My two daughters Tiffany and Vanessa have patiently supported me as well.

My deepest thanks by far goes to my partner Deb Gayner for her ongoing support at every level, without whose help this book would not have materialized.

THE TUNE-UP
Creating Health Consciously

Table of Contents

I.   Foreword By Jeffrey S. Bland, PhD   v.

II. Acknowledgements   ix.

III. Preface   xviii.

IV. Introduction: Healthy Stories   ixx.

    Why Using Common Sense is the Only Way   1
    to Create More Effective Medicine

    Functional Medicine: A Systems-Based Approach to the   30
    Web of Wellness

    Professional Applied Kinesiology-Browser for the Web of Wellness   45

IV. The Stories

    A. Chapter I: Newborn (0-six months)

        1) Failure to Thrive   77

        2) Neonatal Bloody Stools   85

        3) Un-Descended Testicle (Cryptorchidism)   88

    B. Chapter II: Infants and Toddlers (six months-5 years old)

        4) Autism   89

        5) Drug-Resistant Clostridium Difficile Infection,
        Severe Abdominal Pain and Diarrhea   99

        6) Severe Asthma   101

7) Recurrent Otitis Media   106

8) Blocked Naso-Lacrimal Canal   108

C. Chapter III: Children (6-12 years old)

9) ADD/ADHD (Attention Deficit Disorder, Attention Deficit
Hyperactivity Disorder)   109

10) Constipation   112

11) Encopresis (Loss of Bowel Control) and Eczema   115

12) Fainting   117

13) Chronic Drug-Resistant Throat Infection   118

14) Allergies/Asthma   119

15) Habitual Stress Cough   122

16) Chronic Juvenile Migraines   122

CI. Chapter IV: Teens (13-19 years old)

17) Drug-Resistant Hives   125

18) Arm Paralysis Post-Cervical Fracture   126

19) Recurrent Sinus Infection, Drug-Resistant   129

20) Severe Mercury Poisoning   133

21) Post-Extraction Trismus, Lockjaw   138

CII. Chapter V: Young Adults (20-40 years old)

22) Crippling PreMenstrual Syndrome (PMS)   141

23) Amennorhea   143

24) GERD (Gastro-Esophageal Reflux Disorder)   144

25) Cervical Herniated Disc with Severe Left Arm Pain   149

26) Anemia, Allergies, Asthma; Chronic Back, Chest and Low Back
Pain; Recurrent Yeast Infections, Anxiety, Insomnia, Polycystic
Ovary Disease, Bilateral Plantar Fascitis, Hiatal Hernia and
Heartburn, Moderate PMS   152

27) Severe Dry Heaves and Endometriosis   155

28) Mononucleosis and Sciatica   157

29) Chronic Recurrent Torticollis   160

30) Recurrent Vaginal Yeast Infections and   162
Chronic Left Subscapular Pain

31) Rheumatoid Arthritis and Electric Blankets   164

32) Chronic Insomnia/Tension Headaches   166

33) Carpal Tunnel Syndrome   169

F. Chapter VI: Mid-Adults (41-60 years old)

34) Alopecia Arreata   171

35) Car Seat Heaters and Full Body Pain   175

36) Thoracic Outlet Syndrome (TOS)   177

37) Vertigo and Sub-Occipital Headaches   182

38) Bell's Palsy   184

39) Gallstones and Right Upper Abdominal   187
Pain

40) Torn Medial Meniscus   190

41) Profuse Sweating   192

42) Post-Surgical Foot Drop and Low Back Pain   195

43) Irritable Bowel Syndrome (IBS), Abdominal Pain, Cervical Dysplasia   198

44) Fibromyalgia, Chronic Fatigue Syndrome (CFS), Irritable Bowel Syndrome (IBS)   202

45) Exhaustion, Severe Depression, Chronic Cervico-Thoracic Pain   207

46) Shingles, and Spine and Shoulder Pain   209

47) Empty Nest Syndrome and Sciatica   211

48) Incontinence   212

49) Severe Abdominal Pain   214

50) Severe Epicondylitis with Two Torn Rotator Cuffs   216

G. Chapter VII: Advancing Adults (61-69 years old)

51) Post Coronary Artery Bypass Graft (CABG), Singulitis (Hiccups)   218

52) A Twenty-Year Cluster Headache   219

53) Chronic Testicular Pain (Orchitis)   224

54) Erectile Dysfunction   226

55) Vocal Cord Paralysis, Spasmodic Dysphonia   227

H. Chapter VIII: Advanced Adults (70+ years old)

56) Lumbar Disc Herniation, Bulging Degenerative Discs with Severe Leg Pain   230

57) Severe 10-year Leg Itching, Recurrent Bronchitis, Allergies 231

58) Incapacitating Foot Pain 233

59) High Blood Pressure, Blocked Naso-Lacrimal Duct, Vertigo 235

60) Global Body Pain/Osteoarthritis 237

I. Appendices

1) The One System Tensegrity Body 239
2) Your Health Means Balance: Are you Anabolic or Catabolic? 239
3) PAK™ Functional Neurological Tools 241
4) Understanding the Cranial Complex 242
   a) Normal Cranial Complex Motion- *Illustration (Illu)* 244
   b) The Spinal Dural Membrane (Meninges)-*Illu* 245
5) Understanding the Pelvic-Spinal Complex 245
   a) Normal Pelvic-Spinal Complex Motion-*Illu* 247
   b) The Fluid Dynamics of Human Motion-*Illu* 248
6) The Normal Vertebral Complex 249
   a) The Normal Vertebral Complex-*Illu* 250
7) Understanding the Tarsal Tunnel Complex 250
   a) The Tarsal Tunnel Complex- *Illu* 252
8) Cranial Complex Stress MAPs 253
   a) A Cranial Stress Map—RRR- *Illu* 255
9) Pelvic-Spinal Complex MAPs 255
   a) Pelvic-Spinal Complex Stress MAPs- *Illu* 257
10) A Prescient Point of View on Balance by Dr. Barry Wyke 258
11) The Composition of Intervertebral Discs 259
   a) The Intervertebral Disc: Structural Facts, Pro-Active
Thoughts, Degenerative Changes and Related Terminology-*Illus* 263
   b) Using PAK Challenge to Diagnose IVD Problems-*Illu* 264
12) Tarsal Tunnel Complex:The Most Common Stress MAP-*Illu* 265
13) Stay Tuned Up: What's the Evidence? 266
14) Good Posture Promotes Good Health 267
15) Spinal Decay Phases Chart 270
16) Cervical Intervertebral Disc Exercises 271
17) Thoracic Spine Stretches 272
18) Lumbar Disc Exercises 273
19) Mattress Matters 274

20) Pillow Talk: Some Good News 276

21) The Importance of Having A Body Therapy Team 277

22) The Correct Use of Moist Cold 278

23) Where to find FM and PAK Providers for Your Health Team 279

24) The Medical Symptoms Questionnaire 280

25) Key Gastrointestinal and Immune Function Areas 281

26) The Meridians and Their Emotions, by John Diamond MD 282

27) The Wonders of Medical Food 283

28) Tricks to Keep a Positive Magnesium Status 285

29) A Short List of Technologies to be Wary of 288

30) FYI : Related Books 293

31) Some CDs of Interest 296

32) TED.com 297

J. Glossary 298

K. References 326

*"The best way to predict the future is to create it.
Imagination is the only key to the future. Without it none exists—with it
all things are possible."*

Ida Tarbell (1857-1944)

II. Preface

The Institute of Medicine was established in 1970 by the National Academy of Sciences to secure the services of eminent members of appropriate professions in the examination of policy matters pertaining to the health of the public. The Institute acts under the responsibility given to the National Academy of Sciences by its congressional charter to be an advisor to the federal government and upon its own initiative, to identify issues of medical care, research and education.

In 2001, the Institute of Medicine prepared a report called, *Crossing the Quality Chasm—A New Health System for the 21st Century.* In the Executive Summary of this report, they said, "Quality problems are everywhere, affecting many patients. Between the healthcare we have and the healthcare we could have, lies not just a gap, but a chasm."

In 1855, the great Niagara Suspension Bridge was built by flying a child's kite across the 855-foot chasm. Attached to this kite was a string, attached to the string was a cord, attached to the cord was a rope, and attached to the rope was a cable—sure and strong.

Sixteen years following the Institute's report, it is my hope that this book may be that kite, our citizen readers the string, our political leaders the cord, our healthcare institutions the rope, and global consensus the cable, to erect the bridge crossing the quality chasm in healthcare once and for all.

Fast forward ten years from that initial report, to 2011 when the Institute of Medicine published their new report, *Relieving Pain in America: A Blueprint for Transforming Prevention, Care, Education and Research.* One of their directives is that federal agencies and other stakeholders should redesign educational programs to address gaps in knowledge. Implicit in this directive is the need for interdisciplinary recognition, cooperation and respect: "Given the overwhelming burden of pain in human lives, dollars and social consequence, relieving pain should be a national priority." Here's how we can do it and more.

*"Keeping the public well informed is an essential component
of a vibrant democracy."*
Jefferson and Madison

"Knowledge is the most Democratic source of power."
Alvin Toffler

III. Introduction—Healthy Stories

Many years ago I thought I was headed for a career as a general surgeon. One day in my third year of pre-med studies, something happened that forever changed my life. Looking back, I describe the event as a cosmic take down. After finishing a chemistry class one Friday morning, I experienced sharp, severe right lower quadrant abdominal pain that dropped me to my knees. Several doctors at the University of Massachusetts Infirmary thought it was appendicitis, so I was whisked away by ambulance to the nearby Cooley-Dickinson Hospital in North Hampton, Massachusetts. A surgeon there diagnosed an acute "retro-cecal appendicitis" (the appendix was bent up behind the intestine, explaining why the pain was not lower in my groin). He convinced my father that he needed to remove the appendix immediately. My father wanted his medical friends to take a look at me 50 miles away in Worcester, Massachusetts. The surgeon convinced him that a drive like that could cause the appendix to rupture, infecting the entire abdomen with a life-threatening condition called peritonitis. My father reluctantly gave him the go-ahead. The surgeon found the appendix to be normal, so he removed it and performed an "exploratory procedure to feel for tumors or other reasons for my pain."

I went home the next day, Saturday, and was told I should be able to return to class on the following Tuesday. By Tuesday, things were not going well for me, as peritonitis had set in with severe abdominal pain that made me rigid. I was taken to St. Vincent's Hospital in Worcester, Massachusetts. I spent one month on intravenous antibiotics, near death, as the infection had spread throughout my entire body. I was septic. The infection had transcended the peritoneal barrier and was now spread throughout the entire 62,000 miles of my blood vessels. Somehow I lived through that near-death experience and got out of the hospital alive. The only problem was that I still had the same right lower abdominal pain, now chronic instead of acute.

My mother, a registered nurse, always had her "ear to the ground" with respect to break-through treatments. She suggested that I visit a chiropractic kinesiologist whom she had heard good things about. I made an appointment with Dr. Ken Harling and told him my story. He listened, asked me to hold out my arm, and in the next instant pushed on my abdomen causing my arm to weaken. He told me I had a spasm of my ileo-cecal valve, the valve separating the small intestine from the large intestine, like the door between the kitchen and the pantry. He had me lie on my side while he adjusted my third lumbar vertebra. Then I stood up, and to my utter amazement, the pain that had nearly killed me had vanished!

When I finally retracted my jaw from the floor to articulate, I asked him if he had ever had any similar cases. He told the following two stories: A fifteen-year-old girl was experiencing severe visual problems — blind in one eye, losing sight in her other eye, as well as headaches. He examined her, X-rayed her neck and then adjusted her neck.

"Odds of you being born in this particular time, place and circumstance: About 1 in 400,000,000,000."

ONE, by Kobi Yamada and Dan Zadra

The following week, she was supposed to come in for a report of findings. When she did not show up he called her mother, who said her daughter's headaches were gone, and she could see perfectly again out of both eyes. While she didn't believe she needed any further care, Dr. Harling had her come in for a complementary re-exam. Her vision tested a perfect 20/20 in both eyes.

The second story was that of a 22-year-old paraplegic male who came to Dr. Harling for the treatment of neck pain and headaches. This young man had never walked, and had been confined to a wheelchair his entire life. His medical history revealed that he had been a "high-forceps" delivery, which means he was forcefully extracted from his mother's womb with a pair of tongs. After several months of chiropractic care, coupled with physical therapy, this young man was able to walk, then run for the first time in his life. After hearing these stories, I knew what I wanted to do, to bring healing to patients using this kind of integrative medicine.

"Nature applies common assembly rules, recurring patterns–the body is organized hierarchically as tiers of systems within systems. Humans and other creatures are constructed using a common form of architecture known as tensegrity. The term refers to a system that stabilizes itself mechanically because of the way in which tensional and compressive forces are distributed and balanced within the structure."
Donald Ingber, MD, PhD
"The Architecture of Life," *Scientific American,* Jan 1998

I am currently in my 39th year of the practice of Professional Applied Kinesiology (PAK™) and Functional Medicine (FM). These two new innovative integrative medical specialties were born out of the intellectual and cultural diversity that is the United States. American-born innovations are the future of humanity's health. As Americans we can be proud of this. Once fully integrated, their impact will advance medicine and human health on a scale equal to or greater than the impact of the automobile for transportation. In this book I hope to educate and excite you about these healthcare advances, by not only describing them, but also by telling you true stories of their application. They are the future of healthcare. By becoming aware of these innovations, you can spread the word, creating a greater demand for them and leveling the playing field to accelerate them to "business as usual" status.

It's your world and it's your responsibility to make it better. The best news is that it's already happening!

"One of the penalties of not participating in politics is that you will be governed by your inferiors."

Plato

"In the final analysis, voters who make their wishes unmistakably clear to Congress in overwhelming numbers have the best chance to defeat the special interest lobbies. That's the way our system works."
Barbara Kennedy

President and CEO of the National Committee to preserve Social Security and Medicare

During my years in practice, I have come to recognize specific core patterns the body takes on in an attempt to adapt to stress and trauma. Bruce McEwen,

PhD, called "the leading living scholar of stress" by professor Robert Sapolsky, PhD, has updated the whole body response to stress with the term **allostasis**. He notes that this begins in the brain with our hypothalamic-pituitary-adrenal (HPA) axis and when the stress response system turns against us, the term is **allostatic load**. The physical body is one closed kinematic chain, or web if you will, the functional mechano-biological house we call home. This means that everything is interconnected, with every single part having a known effect on every other single part. Another term for the "one closed system" concept is **tensegrity**. You can think of this as body geometry. If you alter one tension, the entire structure rearranges to accommodate. Intact geometry upregulates all systems or has "a systemic effect."

The patterns of life stresses and traumas are both predictable and correctable with the new technologies we now have in hand. Our medical diagnostic acumen has lurched light years ahead with the ability to assess functional changes in the Web of Wellness. From the structural viewpoint to facilitate ease of understanding, I call them stress maps or **mal–adaptation patterns (MAPS)**. There are four areas that are the body's geometrical set points–the head, pelvic-spine, and upper and lower extremities. Stress MAPs in these areas create systemic effects, laying the functional groundwork that leads to loss of function, reduced quality of life and later disease.

> *"It is a part of the American character to consider nothing as desperate; to surmount every difficulty by resolution and contrivance."*
>
> Thomas Jefferson

> *"Enthusiasm is one of the most powerful engines of success. Nothing great was ever achieved without enthusiasm."*
>
> Ralph Waldo Emerson

I have attempted to clearly delineate these patterns, with the sincere hope that this will become the "common knowledge" of the people serving to leverage their health acumen. It is only with this kind of clear insight that we may invoke the correct critical healthcare choices and changes both for ourselves and our loved ones. The current fifteen-year-wait, from scientific publication to mainstream medical awareness, followed by a further thirty-year plus wait for incorporation, can now be consumer-driven to extinction.

The recognition of these patterns, together with a dynamic team approach (as supported in recent medical literature)[1-3] to their resolution throughout our entire lifespan, offers a huge opportunity for us to fix what ails us. It is entirely possible to cut our national healthcare bill in half within five to ten years, and reduce GNP spending on health by 10%. There is no reason that this country should not be the world leader in healthcare.

In effect, this information is slanted towards the women of the world since they often manage their family's health, and in general take better care of their health than men do. Seventy-five to eighty percent of all healthcare practices are treating women. This is perhaps one of the main reasons that women live, on average, longer than men. They take better care of themselves.

At the end of the Institute of Medicine's text, *Crossing the Quality Chasm, A New Health System for the 21st Century,* is Appendix B - "Redesigning Healthcare with Insights from the Science of Complex Adaptive Systems." Here the author, Paul Plesk, states, "Therefore, rather than agonizing over plans, the goal is to generate a 'good enough plan' and begin to observe what happens." The plan should be guided by a few simple rules that allow innovation to emerge. This book lays the groundwork for one "good enough plan," elucidated in my upcoming book, *The Beacon, Making the United States First in Global Healthcare.*

The idea that structural alignment is one of the eight fundamental biological processes common to all body systems, and therefore all disease processes, may come as a surprise to some. With this fundamental position comes direct effects on the other seven components of the Web of Wellness, including: attitude (body-mind balance), diet, digestion, immunity, detoxification, cellular communication and energetics. Our improved understanding of neuroanatomy has taught us that neck dysfunction, mediated through sympathetic nerves, has been associated with a number of disorders, which include 20 kinds of diseases or symptom-groups, such as hyper-tension, cardiac arrhythmias, dizziness, eyesight malfunction and gastrointestinal dysfunction. [4] The use of ongoing physical medicine in the form of chiropractic, deep muscle therapy, acupuncture and physical therapy together with functional medical know-how called "First line Lifestyle" counseling teams will pave the way to the future.

The seamless integration of soft tissue injury clinics (STICS) into hospitals alongside emergency rooms with freestanding community-based healthcare centers (CBHCs) is a key second step. The rationale for these steps becomes more clear with the following information. Consider the fact that the latest final data (2007) showed that unintentional injuries continue to be the fifth leading cause of death.[5] On top of this, "every hour there are 4,440 medically consulted injuries in this country." [6]

One in eight, or 38.9 million Americans, sought medical attention in 2009[7] for non-fatal injuries. This wouldn't be a problem if treated appropriately, but sadly this is not the case. At a mean of 15.5 years post-whiplash trauma, 70% of patients continue to complain of symptoms referable to the original accident (neck pain in 65% and LBP in 48%)[8]. These are systemic, whole body complaints[9]. Even worse is that 60% of symptomatic patients have not seen a doctor in the previous five years because the doctors were unable to help. [10]

According to the U.S. Bureau of Labor Statistics, "Sprains and strains were the most common types of injury involving days away from work in 2008, accounting for 39% of the total 1.07 million injuries in private industry. Soreness and pain was the second most common type of injury."[11]

Physical medicine complaints are a huge problem. "The most costly lost time worker's compensation claims, by cause of injury, according to the NCCI's (National Council on Compensation Insurance Company) data are those resulting from motor vehicle crashes. These injuries averaged $65,875 per worker's comp claim filed in 2007 and 2008." In 2007 and 2008, 70% of the worker's comp cases involved injuries directly creating stress MAPs related to the key areas of discussion in this book.

"How many people does it take to make a difference? ONE."
Dan Zadra and Kobi Yamata

"We have only this moment, sparkling like a star in our hand and melting like a snowflake."
Marie Byron Ray

"Besides the estimated 693.5 billion dollars in economic losses from unintentional injuries in 2009, lost quality of life from these injuries was valued at an additional 3.4 trillion dollars, making the comprehensive cost 4.1 trillion dollars in 2009." [12]

Recent scientific studies [13-17] help us to appreciate the complexity of structure and its relation to function. Every cell in the body requires just the right amount of motion to function optimally. Structure interfaces with function and vice versa. Structure affects both metabolism and neuro-physiology. Fascia is part of the extra-cellular matrix that affects function and metabolism. Pressure in the right place alters tissue and organ function via mechanical transduction. The existence of a connective tissue signaling network profoundly influences our understanding of health and disease. The body's extracellular matrix (ECM) is a newly recognized electromagnetic signaling system that attaches directly to the skin of our cells that controls our genetic expression. The ECM also helps to circulate nutrients and remove cellular waste products. The ECM is a huge contributor to our exposome, the sum total of our environmental, dietary and lifestyle exposure directly affecting our genetic expression.

The key takeaway here is that healing requires movement. The connection of our cells to their external environments, through their membranes or windows, directs the nuclear material to create proteins. Positive body stress[18] is the end result of a therapeutic healing regimen that optimally may include hands-on-healing adjustments, massage, full body stretching and relaxation, and long deep breathing (diaphragmatic breathing), together with yoga, exercise (both cardio and resistance) and acupuncture. Knowing and understanding the benefits of the full health choice menu creates informed health consumerism.

Simply understanding how we are hardwired in a web, and how stress distorts this web (from our nervous system's point of view) is an important insight. In a nutshell, at any one moment in our life, 90% of our ability to function is carried out subconsciously by our autonomic (automatic) nervous system. This system is composed of two parts: the parasympathetic and the sympathetic nervous systems. The other 10%, referred to as the somatic nervous system, is under our conscious control.

The parasympathetic nervous system exits from both ends of the spine—the top (the cranial nerves: 3, 7, 9 and 10) and the bottom (sacral nerves: 2, 3). It is responsible for the daily activities in the lives of our cells. It allows our cells to be open and relaxed, capable of imbibing nutrients and digesting them, as well as detoxifying and eliminating toxins. When you add cellular healing and reproduction you truly have the "rest and repair" mode that provides the architecture of health and life for our body. The vagus nerve (cranial nerve 10), exiting the cranium and descending into the thoracic and abdominal cavities, are responsible for 75% of the parasympathetic nervous system's function and are therefore often referred to by physiologists when speaking of the parasympathetic nervous system. The vagus nerves along with their nuclei form a complex that supplies parasympathetic nerves to the lungs, heart, esophagus, stomach, entire small intestine, liver, gallbladder, pancreas, proximal half of the colon and upper portions of the ureters (tubes from the kidneys to the bladder). The word "vagus" stems from the root meaning "great wanderer," due to its extensive effect. The Polyvagal Theory of Dr. Stephen Porgess provides exciting new insights into the way our autonomic nervous system unconsciously mediates social engagement, trust and intimacy.

"Our generation has been called to create a passionate and sustainable world community. We are co-creators, each with unique gifts and expertise, sharing a responsibility to individually do what we can to usher in the new civilization."

Ruth Hanavans, Communications Director, Kosmos Journal.

"The greatness of America lies not in being more enlightened than any other nation, but rather her ability to repair her faults."

Alexis de Tocqueville

The sympathetic nervous system exits into our chest and abdomen from the thoracic spine and is in charge of survival mode. It overrides the parasympathetic functions, shutting them down so that we can run or fight. When we don't or can't move to burn off their chemical messengers, they sit around and disrupt our internal physiology. An excellent example may be cortisol, the major stress hormone, which causes the membrane receptors in the hippocampus, the information integration way station of the brain, to become misshapen thereby causing cognitive dysfunction. Another example is noradrenalin, a major by-product of chronic stress fight-or-flight, which builds up in the brain, causing fear, hate and a plethora of mental health disorders.[19]

The two arms of the nervous system together form a powerful team that allows our body to deal with 10^{23} things every moment. This is a huge number called a septillion representing more planets than there are in nine universes! Given this vast job, one can appreciate why we only have a mere 10% of our nervous system in our conscious or volitional control. Living in today's world, sets the stage for chronic disease, due in a large part to a continuous sympathetic stress response. This causes a feed forward "locking in" of the accelerator part of our autonomic nervous system. This functional disturbance of the HPA axis is a great contributor to the creation of allostatic load.

Thomas Hanna, in his book *Somatics: Reawakening the Mind's Control of Movement, Flexibility and Health*, clearly describes the musculoskeletal response to stress. He calls the neuromuscular adaptation to sustained negative stress ("distress," which is fear) the withdrawal response or the "Red Light" reflex. He notes that it occurs primarily in the front of the body. The muscle contraction pattern starts with the jaw muscles and then insidiously moves to torso flexion and contracture. He notes that chronic stress responses, are mistakenly blamed on "a fictitious disease called 'aging'."

Things run smoothly as long as the sympathetic fight or flight mode functions in "bursts." Problems crop up when this system becomes chronically overactive, depleting and exhausting itself. It's like trying to control your car with the accelerator stuck to the floor. This pattern sets the stage not only for chronic structural pain and loss of function, but also negatively affects the other web components, resulting in varying degrees of anxiety or depression, maldigestion, poor dietary choices, malnutrition, poor immune function, toxicity, fatigue and inflammation. The body is put in a pro-aging state, where just standing in an idle state consumes energy.

The unstable body exists in a state of compression where, according to Dr. Jeff Spencer, "It creates magnetic fields that lay down bone like concrete and muscles like leather." This leads to a loss of ability to actively participate in life.

The balance between these two systems plays a significant role in maintaining allostasis in our body. The autonomic nervous system is intimately related to the immune system. Body temperature will drop when the sympathetic nervous system takes over. When body temperature drops by one degree, there is a 36% decline in immune function, a 12% decline in base metabolism, and a 50% reduction in enzyme activation. [20] Over time, these fundamental imbalances contribute substantially to all chronic complex diseases.

Our latest knowledge, with respect to how the nervous system functions, lends vast credibility and evidence to guide our increased use of the cutting edge, evidence guided, non-invasive, cost-effective healing tools of integrative medicine. It helps us understand why the ongoing use of touch-based healing modalities is absolutely required for optimal health and thus is a key building block of health and wellness. We live in a receptor-based nervous system. The largest "pipes" or sources of information arriving at the base of our brain (the cerebellum) come from the specialized nerve endings in our muscles. These mechanoreceptors are called muscle spindles and golgi tendon receptors. When these are fired off by chiropractic adjustment, deep tissue massage, acupuncture, stretching/yoga, long deep breathing or exercise, the signals activate the cerebellum.

> "The book resolves long-standing confusions about the significance
> of holistic and complementary therapies. The collagenous matrix and
> ground substance of the human body form a totally pervasive system,
> a major organ, that reaches into every part and whose properties are
> absolutely vital to the operation of the whole."
>
> James Oschman, PhD
>
> The Extracellular Matrix and Ground Regulation
>
> Introduction to the English Edition

This triggers the cerebellum to send signals to the upper midbrain (the mesencephalon) located in the upper neck, which turns off the sympathetic stress signals. Autonomic nervous system balance is then restored. This sets the stage for healing as the parasympathetic nervous system can now carry on its life-sustaining tasks of rest, relax, regenerate and repair.

It is my belief that by quickly instituting a massive program of physician educational reform and oversight, to ensure the broad implementation of Professional Applied Kinesiology and Functional Medicine, that we can cross our healthcare quality chasm. With input from citizen action groups and cooperation from our leaders in government and business we can make America first in health within the next decade, to act as the global model for medical integration. We can do this together.

> *"All organized structures that were developed in the industrial era have been commodified and are now stuck in for-maximum-profit materialism."*[21]
>
> Nancy Roof

I offer these true stories depicting the systems effect throughout life of functional stress MAPs as well as some bold and concrete steps we can take to promote the health of our nation and the world at large. We have the intelligence and the wealth to envision and create a peaceful, abundant garden planet for our children and grandchildren. Now is the time to turn crisis into opportunity. We need to change what we have been doing at light speed to not just become fiscally responsible but to stop our species' downward spiral. We all need to join together to create one healthy world now.

LeadingMedicine.com is a website being designed to help educate everyone about key issues that directly affect our health and our children's well-being. This is a place to engage our collective consciousness to create consensus, design and build the relevant legal framework for positive change. In moving healthcare from Wall Street to Main Street, the concept of the world as full of endless frontiers, changes to one of a spaceship[22] with the core approach of a civil society embracing stewardship.

Your sincere input and active participation is invaluable.

> *"The doctor of the future will give no medicine, but will interest her or his patients in the care of the human frame, in a proper diet, and in the cause and prevention of disease."*
>
> Thomas A Edison (1847-1931)

THE FUTURE IS NOW !

A. Chapter I: Why Using Common Sense is the Only Way to Create More Effective Medicine

The largest crisis on our hands today is both the quality of our healthcare, and its enormous cost. We stand on the edge of an epiphany in medicine. First let's take a moment to look at where we are now. This understanding will serve as the springboard for positive change. In every instance I've attempted to use what I call the "Dalai Lama filter for communication": is it true, is it necessary, is it kind?

Though brilliantly effective in certain situations, like acute emergency medicine, the current underlying profit-centric approach does not do enough to prevent chronic disease or to promote health. A full 80% of our hugely increased current $3.8 trillion dollar healthcare expenditures are for complex chronic diseases. These are conditions like asthma, allergies, auto-immune disease, cancer, diabetes, depression, chronic pain syndromes, neuro-degenerative diseases, heart disease and obesity. According to the Human Genome Project, these conditions take place on dozens of genes. Therefore, getting a diagnosis, coupled with one, two or more medications, is not going to solve the problem.

The following information should make us think: "It's no coincidence that American obesity levels are rising side by side with environmental toxin levels. In 1990, less than 10% of the population in ten states was obese, and not a single state had an obesity rate higher than 14%, according to the Centers for Disease Control and Prevention. But in 2006 — just sixteen years later — only four states had obesity rates under 20%. Twenty-two states had topped 25%, and two (Mississippi and West Virginia) had ballooned past the 30% mark."[1] Imagine that, in 1990, ten states had obesity problems of less than 10% each and sixteen years later, forty-six states have obesity levels of greater than 20%, with 22 states greater than 25% and two greater than 30%! Talk about a quick supersizing of a country! We must ask, "What happened?"

Our healthcare system has been described as "broken." I disagree; I feel as though it is misdirected, and therefore, inappropriate. It does nothing to get at the true cause of disease, which is the impact of environmental toxins in our air, food and water coupled with multiple nutritional insufficiencies, and over-nutrition with high caloric, toxic, genetically modified foods. This, compounded by an environment of out-of-control microwave radiation, fear and lack of choices, which forces invasive medical approaches with potentially terrible side effects.

*"We live in the Age of Giants—In one day alone, we pump and burn
85 million barrels of oil.*

*In the same day we spew the waste of 27 billion pounds of coal into
the atmosphere."*

Paul Hawken, *Blessed Unrest*

*"The earth isn't something given to you from your parents but lent to
you by your children."*

K. R. Stridha

Dr. Sherry Rogers, internist and environmental specialist, is a prolific
writer and student of medical literature. In her book, *Detoxify or Die*, she states
that there is not a square centimeter on the planet that is not impregnated with
over one thousand carcinogens. The largest manufacturing sector in the United
States today is the chemical industry. According to Philip and Alice Shabecoff, in
their book, *Poisoned for Profit*, this industry has grown from $2 billion dollars in
1962 to $689 billion dollars in 2008. The United States "currently produces or
imports at least 27 trillion pounds of chemicals a year, which works out to 74 billion
pounds of chemicals per day. That's an 80 percent increase since three years ago."[2]

This approaches approximately one ton of chemicals for every man, woman
and child per year in the United States. A common statement when discussing
environmental medicine is that "genetics loads the gun, but the environment pulls
the trigger." Since the 1930s, the number of synthetic chemicals put into
commercial use has doubled every seven to eight years. According to Dr. Mark
Hyman, Chairman of the Institute for Functional Medicine, the average American
drinks one gallon of pesticides on their fruits and vegetables every year.

It is increasingly understood that as far as our children go, there is an
epidemic of serious chronic childhood illness to which these chemicals have been
found to cause or contribute.

"Increased exposure to atrazine (ATZ), used extensively in the US since the
early 60's corresponds to the beginning of the present obesity epidemic."[3]

Some of these problems include birth defects, cancers, asthma, heart disease
and a range of neurological illness including attention deficit disorder (ADHD) and
autism.

The rising incidence of obesity and diabetes, the epidemic of reproductive

2

problems, including infertility and miscarriages, are also understood to have environmental roots. One chemical at 1/25,000th the amount considered safe by the EPA is enough to cause an autoimmune disease.[4] There are over one hundred fifty autoimmune diseases and they are increasing in epidemic proportions. There are 24 million Americans suffering from autoimmune diseases. Because they are spreading to almost every industrialized nation, scientists the world over have dubbed it "the Western disease." Autoimmune disease in twin studies are shown to be 30% genetic and 70% environmental.[5]

The evidence of the effect of toxins on America's children is overwhelming and serves as an indictment of the chemical, nuclear and other polluting industries. "Disability, disease, and dysfunction among our nation's children have reached epidemic proportions. Of America's 73 million children, almost 21 million, nearly one out of three, suffer from one chronic disease or another. Cancer threatens the lives of 58,000 children. Those whose bodies and minds are poisoned with lead number 310,000. About 6 million or one in ten children suffer, and some of them die from asthma. Twelve million have some form of developmental mental disorder, from autism to ADHD, and serious learning disabilities that cloud their minds and torment their behavior."[6]

"In the 20th Century, a country's might was too often measured in what they could destroy. In the 21st Century strength should be measured by what we can build together."

Douglas Alexander, former UK Secretary of State for International Development

"Remember that your children are not your own, but are lent to you by the Creator."

Mohawk Indian

Women of childbearing age have toxic levels of mercury in their blood accounting for over 600,000 babies being brought into this world with a toxic load of mercury. Almost 2.5 million live with disfiguring, debilitating birth defects. A recent study suggests opioid use during pregnancy increases the risk of a wide variety of birth defects including the heart, spine and stomach areas.[7]

In this big picture, we have passively allowed ourselves to be poisoned. The fact that two thirds of the United States water is fluoridated with a carcinogenic, neuro-toxic waste product from the glass, aluminum and steel industries at a profit is criminal. Past senior scientists of the Environmental Protection Agency (EPA) have stated that the fluoridation of the American water supply is the greatest case of scientific fraud of the century, and that the EPA should act immediately to protect the public due to cancer, bone fractures, mutagenicity and arthritis. This assertion was made in 1992 and is only now starting to be acted upon. The only way out is for a critical mass of educated, concerned citizens to "abandon our lethal passivity in the face of the toxic juggernaut."[8] We need to creatively work to get the chemicals out of our water. The only known way to remove them is charcoal filtration, followed by reverse osmosis. This first step needs to be done immediately.

> *"In-utero exposure to medium/high magnetic fields was associated with 69% increased risk of being obese or overweight during childhood."*[9]

One thing is for sure, we are all better safe than sorry, especially when considering fundamentals such as air, soil and water. The precautionary principle, to be cautious right now about protecting our children from substances that may well prove harmful in the future, is not being acted upon. Dr. Harvey Kory, a pediatrician and author of the book/DVD *The Happiest Toddler on the Block* and Healthy Child Healthy World board member says this: "The government lets products be sold as long as they haven't been proven to cause harm. But unlike you and me, chemicals should never be considered innocent until proven guilty. In fact, we must consider them guilty until innocent. We must demand that the industry prove a substance safe before it is allowed to be sold to millions."

Dr. Candice Pert, former chief of brain biochemistry at National Institutes of Health is in complete agreement and states that, "we need to put the burden of proof on the chemical companies."

In his latest book, *World on the Edge: How to Prevent Environmental and Economic Collapse* Lester Brown says, "As the world economy expanded, some twenty-fold over the last century, it has revealed a flaw, a flaw so serious that if not corrected it will spell the end of civilization as we know it. The market, which sets prices, is not telling us the truth. It is omitting indirect costs that in some cases now dwarf direct costs." The collateral damage of industrial pollution fits the bill here. By rethinking the worldwide expenditure of 500 billion dollars per year to subsidize the production and use of fossil fuels, we can readily prevent the future expenditure of trillions of dollars for the treatment of future disease. This is ten times the 50 billion dollars spent to subsidize renewable energy including wind, solar and biofuels.

"Environmentally caused cancers are 'grossly underestimated' and 'needlessly devastate American lives ... proof of harm.'"
Dr. La Salle D. Leffall Jr., Chair of the President's Cancer Panel, May 2010

"Regulatory Agencies should reduce exposures even when absolute proof of harm was unavailable. Exposures happen in mixtures, not in isolation and children are most vulnerable."
Dr. Ted Schettler, Director of the Science and Environmental Health Network

"In 2009, fossil fuel consumption subsidies included 147 billion dollars for oil, 134 billion dollars for natural gas and 31 billion for coal. Governments are shelling out nearly 1.4 billion dollars per day to further destabilize the earth's climate."[10] How about deliberately pumping tons of deadly chemicals into the ground to destroy our water? The gas industry pumps a cocktail of 596 chemicals 8,000 feet underground to hydraulically fracture–(FRAC)–the earth to produce more gas. The water tables are at 1,000 feet. Because of the "Cheney/Halliburton Loophole" in the 2005 energy act, energy companies are exempt from the Safe Water Drinking Act and they don't have to disclose the 596 chemicals that may be contaminating our water. Imagine lighting your tap water on fire? Thankfully the Food and Water Watch Group started the concept of a global ban on fracking and has now been joined by 350 other organizations. Check out www.foodandwaterwatch.org.

"USA Today reported in September 2008 that hospitals and long term care facilities were dumping an estimated 250 million pounds of pharmaceutical drugs into public sewer systems every year."
KL Carlson, *Diary of a Legal Drug Dealer*

The citizens of this country must protect themselves from the polluting industries. The time for widespread installation of end point water filtration is now.

Municipal water systems are not only incapable of removing carcinogens and other deadly chemicals like hexavalent chromium, but also everyone else's pharmaceuticals are in the water as well. Tooling up America's preventive system will thus provide an abundance of much needed job opportunities in the water-cleaning arena alone. A "Persistent Polluters" industry-wide tax can be used to fund these efforts. Any industry that places ingredients that are harmful to human life in the environment would contribute. Instead of waiting around to prove that "this chemical causes that," either a popular vote or a simple clear-cut test showing epigenetic change to determine potential harm would satisfy the tax condition. This would remove the end run made by corporate attorneys to evade their responsibility. Every thinking citizen shares the same goal here—make those who pollute clean it up.

Lester Brown makes the salient point that, "since there is no other heavily armed superpower, the United States is essentially in an arms race with itself ... Given the enormity of the antiquated military budget, no one can argue that we do not have the resources to rescue civilization. The far flung, US military establishment, including hundreds of military bases scattered around the world, will not save civilization. It belongs to another era. We can most effectively achieve our security goals by helping to expand food production, by filling the family planning gap, by building wind farms and solar power plants and by building schools and clinics."

"We must all hang together, or assuredly we shall all hang separately."
Ben Franklin at the signing of the Declaration of Independence

"There are no secrets. There is no mystery. There is only common sense."
Onodaga Indian saying

Fortunately, Robert Gates' capabilities as a true eagle scout continue to be remarkable. The Pentagon quietly issued a report on April 8, 2011. The report is entitled "A National Strategic Narrative," and was issued under the pseudonym of "Mr. Y," which was actually two senior members of the Joint Chiefs of Staff: Captain Wayne Porter, USN and Colonel Mark "Puck" Mykleby, USMC. This report needs to be read by every American citizen.

The report creates a nonpartisan blueprint for understanding and responding appropriately to the changes of the 21st century world. "In one sentence, the strategic narrative of the United States in the 21st century is that we want to become the strongest competitor and most influential player in a deeply interconnected global system, which requires that we invest less in defense and more in sustainable prosperity and the tools of effective global engagement."[11] The report goes on to say that the move from control to credible influence, as a fundamental strategic goal, requires a shift from containment to sustainability. The focus must be first and foremost on investing our resources domestically in those natural resources that can be sustained, such as our youth and natural resources (ranging from crops, livestock and potable water, to sources of energy and materials for industry). Credible influence means we model the behavior we recommend for others, and that we pay close attention to the gap between our words and our deeds. It goes on to say that this begins at home, with quality healthcare and education, with a vital economy and low rates of unemployment, with thriving urban centers and carefully planned rural communities. We must seize the opportunity to be a model of stability, a model of the values we cherish, for the rest of the world to emulate. Swords into plough shares is now within our reach!

> *"Taking a patient-centered, whole person approach focused on long-term functional status will also help to address the current fragmentation of care and allow for the standardization of prevention strategies ... Centering our efforts on prevention is the only way to thwart the emerging pandemic of 'chronic disease.'"[12]*

People need more information, education and common sense medicine based on proven treatment regimens, predicated on the concept of least invasive first. They need choices, not more medication. Dennis Gottfried, MD, associate professor of medicine at the University of Connecticut Medical School, is author of *Too Much Medicine*. He notes that the respected nonprofit, nonpartisan policy analysis group, The Rand Corporation, recently released the shocking statistic that up to 30% of surgical procedures in the US are unnecessary. There is a time and a place for surgery. I have referred a half dozen patients for spine surgery over the years. I was one of them. I had a severely herniated disc at L5/SI that pierced my spinal cord like an arrow. A skilled neurosurgeon removed it, and I walked out of the hospital a few hours later. I am profoundly grateful for his expertise. But, as you go through this book, you will read about the safe resolution of a very significant number and type of cases, scheduled for a variety of surgeries, that were successfully treated without it. The skill sets described throughout this book can create the paradigm shift necessary to lift us into a new era of medicine that is more preventive, effective and appropriate, and less expensive.

"What people want is universal: security, the money to support their families, educational opportunities, nutritious and affordable foods, clean water, sanitation and access to healthcare. These are not entitlements, but rights according to the greater than 190 nations in the world."

Paul Hawken, Blessed Unrest.

'The ones that matter the most are the children. They are the true human beings."
Lakota Indian

Removing the conflict of interest that exists between industry and government can create a clean, sustainable environment and effective healthcare system. Separating the regulators from the manufacturers is a solid step in the right direction. According to our constitution, the core moral and legal responsibility of the President of the United States is to the people of the United States. Let's all make sure that he/she is both aware of this and is very successful at it.

"The Institute of Medicine, a prestigious group of physician experts and researchers, weighed in on this question ('evidence-based') and determined that any valid evidence supports 'well below half' of the practice of medicine."

Eric Topol, MD, The Creative Destruction of Medicine

Doctors were proven twelve years ago to be the third leading cause of death in the United States, published in the *Journal of the American Medical Association* (*JAMA*), July 6, 2000 by Dr. Barbara Starfield, MD. The landmark Starfield Study,

"Is U.S. Health Really the Best in the World?" concluded that every year in the U.S. there are 12,000 deaths from unnecessary surgeries, 7000 deaths from medication errors in hospitals, 20,000 deaths from other errors in hospitals, 80,000 deaths from infection acquired in hospitals, and 106,000 deaths from FDA-approved, correctly prescribed medicines. The total of medically-caused deaths in the U.S. every year is 225,000. This makes the medical system the third leading cause of death in the U.S., behind heart disease and cancer.

In recent interviews (12/09) with Dr. Starfield, which were posted on Dr. Gary Gordon's website (www.gordonresearch.com), several disturbing things became apparent. No systematic efforts have been instituted to remedy the main categories of medically-caused deaths. A lot of studies have been done; however, most of them indicate higher rates of death, so things are getting worse, not better! The main message from her study "has been obscured by those who don't want any change in the U.S. healthcare system." So even when an author has unassailable evidence within the medical-research establishment, the findings can, and often do, result in no changes to the system.

"Intellectual self-defense is just training yourself to ask the obvious questions. Sometimes the answers are immediately apparent and sometimes it takes a little longer to find them."

Noam Chomsky

Her papers on the benefit of primary healthcare have been widely disseminated, including through congressional testimony. She has done extensive research showing that family doctors who deliver primary care, as opposed to armies of specialists, produce better outcomes for patients. She notes that some of the most prestigious medical training institutions do not have family physician training programs or family medicine departments and "The Federal support for teaching institutions greatly favors specialist residencies, because it is calculated on the basis of hospital beds."

Dr. Starfield's findings are an explicit indictment of the U.S. healthcare industry, which includes insurance companies, specialty and disease-oriented medical academia, insurance networks, the pharmaceutical and device manufacturing industries—all of which contribute heavily to the re-election campaigns of members of Congress. Starfield says, "The problem is that we do not have a government that is free of vested interest. Alas, it is a general problem of our society—which clearly unbalances democracy."

> *"Another major deficiency of medicine is the use of experts to make recommendations or guidelines for a large proportion of decisions for which no or minimal data exists. Those guidelines, typically published in major specialty journals, have a pronounced impact, as they are believed to represent the standard of care, even though they are based on opinion with a paucity of facts. In fact, this should be considered 'eminence-based medicine.'"*
>
> Eric Topol, MD, *The Creative Destruction of Medicine*

The United States Food and Drug Administration (FDA) cannot divest itself from the vested interests. Although there is a large amount of literature on this, it is mostly unrecognized by the general population (the 99%) because the industry-supported media gives it no attention. The unfortunate fact is that the FDA is run by people who are not concerned with conflict of interest issues. Most of the decision-makers in the FDA have a vested interest in the drug industry or at the very least, allegiance based on prior and future employment with the industry. It is commonly referred to as a revolving door policy. The drug industry is a half-a-trillion-dollar-a-year industry which spends one billion dollars a month to fund 25% of all television ads.

The revolving door between government and industry is such that many people in the FDA effectively function as if their employer is big pharma and not the U.S. public. For example, the current head of the FDA has a history of working for the dental amalgam giant Howard Shein. You cannot find a more neurotoxic element than mercury, except plutonium, so why did this lead protector of our public health remove the information about harm of mercury from the FDA website?

New research shows mercury as one of the contributors to Alzheimer's disease even in low dose exposure, as from dental amalgam fillings. Research published in the November 15, 2010 issue of the *Alzheimer's Disease Journal* states: "Studies of low-dose human exposure, such as dentists and their staff, show that exposure to mercury is significantly correlated with neurological or psychological harm or both." If you go to the website www.factsontoxicity.com and search for the video titled "Mercury and Heart Disease," you can actually watch a growing neural bud stop growing and microtubules disintegrate in the presence of a small amount of mercury.

According to their own mission statement, "the FDA is responsible for protecting the public health by assuring the safety, efficacy and security of human and veterinary drugs, biological products, medical devices, our nation's food supply, cosmetics, and products that emit radiation. The FDA is also responsible for advancing the public health by helping to speed innovations that make medicines and foods more effective, safer and more affordable; and helping the public get the accurate, science-based information they need to use medicine and foods to improve their health."[13] Their basic mission and their actions are at odds with one another. The citizens of the United States have been systematically and intentionally failed, as is carefully documented, in Life Extension Foundation's books: *FDA:Failure, Deception and Abuse* and *Pharmocracy*.

Dr. Starfield's findings have been available for more than ten years and she says, "In these times, medical schools continue turning out a preponderance of specialists, who devote themselves to promoting the conflations of the complexities of human illness with massive drug treatments. Whatever the shortcomings of family doctors, their tradition speaks to less treatment, more common sense, and a proper reliance on the immune systems of their patients."

In Britain, 60% of National Health Services doctors are general practitioners (GPs). This is in stark contrast to the United States where 35% of doctors are GPs. Having agreed to "best practices," Britain's doctors are paid a bonus for carrying them out. According to T. R. Reid, in his book *The Healing of America*, the GPs in Britain generally make more money than the specialists—on average, about twice as much. The pay for performance has roughly doubled the GPs' annual income. The concept of paying for best practices and innovative breakthroughs has been voiced from the Institute of Medicine in their salient report, "Crossing the Quality Chasm, A New Health System for the 21st Century." Therefore, the application of the knowledge outlined in this book is key to relieving the national health deficits, which are undermining and weakening our economy and inexorably weakening our national security.

The pharmaceutical giants carve up the populace into "promising markets." For example, the targeting of little children by the psychiatry profession with drugs that have only been studied for four to eight weeks maximum is unsafe. The drugs being promoted cause the very disease they are supposed to treat. Watch the DVD on the "Marketing of Madness."[14] You will be shocked to learn that two thirds of self-help groups are funded by drug companies. This new campaign screening for mental health has school programs like Teen Screen for high school kids. The creator, Dr. David Sheffer, says that 84% of all kids are found to be depressed or suicidal by design. This is actually not a suicide prevention program, but a drug promotion one. Child suicide rates have skyrocketed 750%, from 1/100,000 to 750/100,000.

Legislators are incessantly lobbied (seven full time PHARMA lobbyists for each senator and congressman), and supported with pharmaceutical campaign monies ($280,373.83 annual monies per congressman).[15] The lobbyist industry has grown from zero dollars in 1970 to 25 billion per year today. With sixty lobbyists for each senator and congressman, corporations out-vote every citizen by sixty to one.

> *"According to the CDC one in ten kids are now diagnosed with ADHD. Ritalin has potential to cause sudden cardiac death. The cause is a functional disconnection; a lack of development or maturation— especially the right brain vs the left. The whole community—doctors, parents, teachers—needs to be aware of what's happening and what their choices are.*
> *Exercises help improve weaknesses*
> *and the problems are reversible."*
>
> Dr. Robert Melillo

With 4.9% of the world's population, the U.S. consumes 60% of the world's fast food and 60% of the world's prescription drugs. That is 1000 times more prescription drugs than any other country! A *New York Times* online article (July17, 2008) was titled "The United States Now Ranks Last in Preventable Mortality." In the 2010 update, the Commonwealth Fund's report "Mirror, Mirror on the Wall—How the Performance of the U.S. Health Care System Compares Internationally" noted that "the U.S. healthcare system ranks last or next to last on five dimensions of a high performance health system: quality, access, efficiency, equity and healthy lives." [16]

The Commonwealth Fund also noted that one area of concern in the United States is the infant mortality rate. Some experts are connecting the dots between the number of early childhood vaccines given in the U.S. (which number about 30) compared to the number given in other countries, like Japan with 13 vaccines. Vaccines have contents that overexcite the neuro-immune system leading to an out-of-control response that leads to nervous system damage and cellular death. The increased infant mortality rates correlate with the number of vaccines given.

The disconcerting truth is that we live amidst "paradigms of corruption."[17] The definition of insanity is to do the same thing over and over, and expect a different outcome. What we need are radical ("at the root") changes—keeping the best of what works and losing what doesn't. People's health has to come first. After all, that is collectively our greatest wealth.

What happened with respect to the treatment of chronic complex disease, and the function of medical schools, has been described as a failure of our leadership[18] to keep their eye on the ball. As the shift went from acute emergencies to chronic complex diseases as the major thrust of medicine, change in medical education has not kept up with the times. The application of medications that are successful in acute emergency situations, for the treatment of chronic complex disease, has not been successful. Dr. Jonathan Wright stated in his book, *Why Stomach Acid is Good for You*, "Symptom suppression is the standard treatment strategy for most diseases in conventional western medicine today. With the possible exception of antibiotics, very few drugs being marketed today can actually cure anything." [19]

Antibiotics can be miraculous when correctly used. However, an estimated 80% of the total amount manufactured annually is not used in medicine, but is applied in animal husbandry. This practice grows fatter chickens, turkeys, pigs and cows. But these drugs persist in the animals and are ingested by the consumer. These drugs persist in the consumer, where they destroy the good bacteria in the intestinal tract. This leverages an overgrowth of fungi and mold that creates a break in the intestinal integrity, fueling systemic inflammation and an overloaded, compromised immune system. This insidious reality lies like the iceberg in the path of the Titanic but its effects can be demonstrated and alleviated using PAK™ and Functional Medicine. Together, with the Union of Concerned Scientists (www.ucsusa.org), who have recognized this huge danger, we the people can bring back balance.

> "'We stand now where two roads diverge.' But unlike the roads in Robert Frost's familiar poem, they are not equally fair. The road we have been long traveling is deceptively easy, a smooth superhighway, on which we progress with great speed, but at its end lies disaster. The other fork of the road, the one less traveled, offers our last, our only chance to reach a destination that ensures the preservation of the earth."
>
> Rachel Carson, *Silent Spring*

If you take a look at how the U.S. healthcare dollar is spent (95% of all spending goes to treatment versus 5% for prevention) hospital care accounts for the largest share, at 31% of healthcare expenditures, physicians' services at 21%, and other providers at 10%. Prescription drugs, while accounting for only 10% of total expenditures, has been one of the fastest growing segments.[20]

A recent Institute of Medicine (IOM) report identified multiple challenges consumers face when using medications. Each year Americans spend more than $75 billion on prescription and non-prescription drugs. A study published in the Archives of Internal Medicine noted that improper medication use creates the expenditure of another $76 billion to fix the problems caused by the first $75 billion.[21] Insanity.

> *"The leading cause of death is fear*
> *and a lack of magnesium."*
>
> Dr. Norman Sheely

> *"In fact when you look at all the data, it looks like it should border*
> *on malpractice to fail to check a RBC magnesium in every disease,*
> *since it underlies not only arrhythmias, but is a major cause of sudden*
> *cardiac arrest, heart attacks, heart failure, high blood pressure,*
> *high cholesterol, cardiomyopathy, as well as diabetes, syndrome X,*
> *osteoporosis, depression, fatigue, muscle spasms,*
> *constipation and more."*
>
> Sherry Rogers, MD

The good news is that community pharmacists have teamed up with patients to educate them about the proper use of their drugs, resulting in a great reduction in adverse events. If we can teach the pharmacists, general and nurse practitioners to screen these people for potential adverse drug reactions looking for changes in Manual Muscle Tests (MMTs), while the potential medication is under the south pole of a 5,000 gauss magnet, their already good results could be exponentially multiplied.

Experts estimate that up to 30% of healthcare is unnecessary, emphasizing the need to streamline the system.[22] The U.S. Senate Committee on Finance, at their Health Reform Summit, discovered that 30% of the medical expenditures pay for tests, interventions and procedures for which there is no sound medical basis. *Time* published a special edition on Healthcare March 3, 2013. They cited a McKinsey and Associates analysis of our 2.8 trillion-dollar bill that noted .8 trillion was "unnecessary."

In 2005, 133 million (almost half) of all Americans lived with at least one chronic condition, and half of these people had more than one chronic disease. According to the CDC, after heart disease and stroke, at a cost of $448 billion dollars per year, the next largest silo, in terms of healthcare dollars, is for chronic pain at $333 billion dollars per year. This was eclipsed by the 2011 IOM study showing it to be closer to $700 billion dollars.

Let's digress for a moment and talk about heart disease and stroke. Scientific literature is loaded [23-31] with studies dating back twenty to thirty years showing two things: 1) the mineral magnesium is crucial for cardiovascular function, as it serves to both lower blood pressure by relaxing the arterial walls and normalize the rate of contraction of the heart, thus preventing deadly arrhythmias; 2) perhaps 95% of Americans are low in this mineral. The whole idea of people being calcium deficient is, in my opinion, somewhat outdated. The 2:1 calcium to magnesium ratio needs adjusting (read more in Appendix: Keeping a Positive Magnesium Status).

The average American diet only gives at best less than one-tenth of the magnesium people need. It is known as the "stress" mineral because stress depletes it. Additionally, the lack of magnesium creates an exaggerated response to stress. This is due to the simple fact that the key mineral for the full expression of the endocrine response to stress is the mineral magnesium. That is why, if this mineral is bio-unavailable, the body's response implodes one way or the other.

"Physicians are the slowest to realize what new information means, and slower still to apply that information to practicing medicine. The legal system often lays claim to being the slowest responding group, yet entrenched medical opinion changes glacially, if at all."
Richie Shoemaker, MD
Surviving Mold

Another study[32] showed that 85% of the public are deficient in getting the recommended dietary allowance (RDA) of magnesium, never mind the optimal amount need for living an active, stress-filled lifestyle. It is also depleted by alcohol, sugar, carbonated beverages, caffeinated drinks, pollution, prescription medications and most vitamin mineral and calcium supplements because of their 2:1 calcium to magnesium ratio. Mercury takes up and blocks magnesium receptors at the cellular level. Stress may be in the form of exercise, heat, cold, lack of sleep, lack of love; or lack of forgiveness, kindness, or understanding; or in the form of your self-talk, diet or pain.

I have discovered a functional diagnostic indicator for magnesium insufficiency called the Magnesium Stretch Test. Simply stated, in physiological terms, an intact muscle becomes inhibited after a quick stretch. When two or more random muscles show this, it correlates with a low normal or below normal RBC magnesium concentration. This is a much more accurate test for functional magnesium concentration than simply a serum level. In the last ten years only two new patients (out of thousands) have tested strong for the mineral. They were both very unusual, in that they both grew all their own food organically and never ate out at restaurants. In my opinion this test probably best represents the net effect of chronic stress at a biochemical level and once widely recognized and appropriately treated will create a health tsunami.

Finland held the first place award for the most heart disease in the world. So what did they do? They put magnesium, potassium, and lysine in their salt. This reduced heart disease and stroke by 70%! Dr. Jonathan Wright has copied this salt (Wright Salt) and made it available through his clinic website (www. tahomadispensary.com). Clearly, including these minerals and this amino acid in the protocols of the treatment of heart conditions are in the best interest of the American public.

In the official journal of the American Heart Association, *Circulation*, the "experts" publish the guidelines for all cardiologists on how to treat certain types of heart attacks. In their update (2007) they stated that vitamins played no role in treatment despite the huge evidence that doctors cut the death rate in the ICU in half with nutrients, or that they doubled the survival from heart attacks with nutrients.

Dr. Sherry Rogers recently wrote in her "Total Wellness" newsletter (March 2011), "After studying the official recommendations of the highest authorities in cardiology, it is clear they are clueless about the cause and cure of cardiovascular disease. In addition their focus on pharmaceuticals has produced some of the most unscientific papers I have seen in over 40 years of medicine." Less than 11% of cardiovascular recommendations are based on scientific evidence. The rest are based on pharmaceutical influence—87% of the "experts" have financial ties with the pharmaceutical industry.

According to the American Heart Association's website in a document updated August 2009, "The American Heart Association Pharmaceutical Round Table (PRT) is a strategic coalition of ten leading pharmaceutical companies and association volunteers and staff. It allows our association and members of the pharmaceutical industry to identify and pursue common objectives to improve cardiovascular health in the United States through research, patient education, and public and professional programs." (http://www.justice.gov/atr/public/busreview/1608.htm www. americanheart.org/ presenter.jhtml?identi ier 2366)

Alex Vasquez, DC, ND   Chiropractic Management of Chronic Hypertension

Heart disease ends the lives of 616,000 people annually in the United States. For half of these people their first symptom of heart disease is death from a massive cardiac arrest termed sudden cardiac death. People get stressed, causing their already low intracellular levels of magnesium to drop further which can trigger a spasm of their coronary arteries or a rupture of vulnerable plaque. Magnesium is not only responsible for the correct function of many key enzymes in the human body (400+), but is also the conductor of the body's mineral symphony. It helps stabilize cell membranes. It controls the body's use of potassium and has influence on calcium and sodium. It is a natural anti-inflammatory and blood thinner. It turns food into energy and powers the enzymes that create exact copies of our DNA, providing genomic stability. This means that a lack of magnesium creates an instability of your genes, arguably a huge potential factor in every single chronic disease. Not enough of it makes us tired, crave chocolate, lose bone, and causes higher blood pressure, tighter muscles, and pain.

The Karolinska Institute (where Nobel prizes originate) has found that, for every 100 milligrams of magnesium supplemented, there's a 15% reduction in type II diabetes. The cost of type II diabetes is enormous, with one out of every seven healthcare dollars spent on its treatment. In the last ten years, diabetes has increased 33% and is the fastest growing epidemic in the history of mankind. The collateral damage of blindness, kidney damage and limb amputation is horrific. It has been noted that from the time something is published in the literature, until it is practiced clinically, is currently forty to fifty years. It's clear that we can no longer wait to integrate and reorganize our clinical approaches. The lack of one mineral's (magnesium) mighty web clearly contributes to two thirds of the reasons people age faster than they should. It's critical necessity, scientifically proven, and widespread therapeutic application will save us trillions of dollars. You do the math. We can't afford not to.

"Every government degenerates when trusted to the rulers of the people alone. The people themselves are its only safe depositories. And to render them safe their minds must be improved to a certain degree."

Thomas Jefferson
Notes on the State of Virginia 1781

Pain affects more Americans than diabetes (20.8M), cancer (1.4M), and coronary heart disease and stroke (18.7M). The Institute of Medicine of the National Academies published a report in 2011 called "Relieving Pain in America" citing the fact that at least "116 million U.S. adults are burdened by chronic pain," costing our country billions of dollars. They also stated that the magnitude of pain suffered by individuals, and the associated costs, constituted a crisis for America, both human and economic. They stated that the need for a transformation in how Americans think and act individually and collectively regarding pain represents a moral and national imperative. According to the National Institute of Neurological Disorders and Stroke (NINDS), pain is the leading complaint among older Americans. "It's safe to say that 25 to 35% of the population is walking around with some type of chronic pain," says Michael R. Clark, MD, MPH, Director of the Pain Treatment Program at Johns Hopkins.[33]

"The most frequent cause of falling in elderly people was incorrect weight shifting."[34]

A recent study[35] found a strong association between chronic pain and fall risk. According to the National Safety Council's "Injury Facts" (2011 edition),

"The number of fall deaths among the 65 or older age group is four times as much as the number of fall deaths among all other age groups. From 1999 to 2007, the number of unintentional fall fatalities among the 65 and older age group increased 81%, while the fatality rate per 100,000 population increased 66% over this same period." Chronic pain measured according to number of locations, severity or pain interference with daily activities, was associated with greater risk of falls in older adults. Among people who reported severe or very severe pain, there was a 77% increased likelihood for a fall within one month compared with those who reported no pain. Even very mild pain increased the chance of a fall by 36%.

I took a look at the National Safety Council's 1995 "Accident Facts" to see what was going on then: "Falls were the leading cause of unintentional injury deaths of people 78 and over."

Fast forward to 2011: falls are the leading cause of unintentional injury death in the 65 and older age group. This means that there is a significant trend of accidental death by falling to an earlier age group with a 66% increase. This trend parallels the increasing lack of nutrient density in foods, increased stress, and increased pollution, all of which create stress MAPS in our bodies which destabilize our balance.

> *"Help publicly. Help privately. Help and you will abolish apathy—the void that is so quickly filled by ignorance and evil."*
>
> Tom Hanks

The first motor skill newborns develop is the ability to raise their head up and look around while they are on their belly. In an article by M. Schioppeto, et.al. published in *Neuroscience*, there are several relevant points regarding neck pain and balance: 1) Input is able to significantly alter posture control[36] as abnormal muscle spindle inflow can perturb and deteriorate postural control. Incoming (afferent) signals from the neck muscles may play a dominant role in calibrating all other sensory inputs. The density of the mechanoreceptors in the upper neck muscles (muscle spindle cells) is four to five times greater than more peripheral muscles like that of the thigh. There is an area of the brain that integrates what we are consciously thinking, seeing and saying (tongue movement), and coordinates this with input from the neck muscle spindles, our balance mechanism and all the functions of our autonomic nervous system (including heart rate, blood pressure, breathing and GI function). It is located on the lower part of the brain (medulla) in the upper neck. Thus, dysfunction here has possible implications throughout the entire body.

2) Physical therapy is more likely to succeed in reducing vertigo symptoms if patients present with an upper cervical spine dysfunction that is successfully resolved by manual medicine prior to physical therapy. [37] Chiropractic adjustments are five times more effective than Celebrex or Viox in treating chronic spinal pain. [38,39] These authors concluded, "In patients with chronic spinal pain syndromes, spinal manipulation may be the only treatment modality of the assessed regimens that provides broad and significant long-term benefit."

The use of low force respiratory adjustments to align the upper cervical spine significantly reduces the potential for harm as a consequence of chiropractic adjustment. The issue here is one of patient safety. The idea has been brought forth that a patient suffering from a dissecting aneurism of the vertebral artery has neck pain and will therefore seek treatment from a chiropractor or medical internist. This makes sense as to why these two professions see these types of pathologies. To what degree a high velocity cervical adjustment may add further risk of injury becomes instantly inconsequential with correctly performed respiratory adjusting. Widespread utilization of this technique will cause a diminution of naysayers, as the profession proactively pursues this course of action—especially in those patients at high risk (e.g., people with a genetic pre-disposing factor called fibro-muscular dysplasia).

"The time has come for a new paradigm of preventative medicine and a society-wide effort to educate our citizens about health and self care."

Andrew Weil, MD
Addressing the U S Senate Committee on Health, Education, Labor and Pensions

As far as the most recent evidence regarding the use of cervical manipulation in the treatment of patients with similar conditions, the comparative fatality rates are as follows: manipulation 7.5–10/10,000,000, medication 1/1,000, and surgery (anterior cervical fusions) 11.25/1,000. Spinal adjustments thus represent the safest approach from a treatment perspective.

In terms of web-like thinking, another aspect of pain that is interesting to note is that the chemistry of pain is similar to heart disease and cancer.[40] People with regional pain syndromes are significantly more likely to die from cancer.[41] Immune system function is an important factor in cancer control. Trauma, like whiplash injuries, alters the neuroendocrine axis, and thus alters the function of the immune system.[42, 43]

The neurendocrine axis, which controls our 24-hour or circadian clock, has profound effect on a variety of the body's systems. Recent studies have shown a relationship between disrupted circadian rhythm and vascular disease[44], metabolic syndrome[45], gut function[46], mood disturbances [47], cancer [48, 49] and chronic migraines [50].

When you take a hard look at where health dollars go, you realize that the $700B for chronic pain is just the tip of the iceberg. Closely related to this are the direct and indirect costs of arthritis at $81B and $128B respectively. Structural misalignment causes pain and leads to osteoarthritis, the most prevalent form of arthritis, and a major cause of disability in people aged 65 and older.[51] Protein metabolism, in the joint surface of a misaligned joint, stops after nine hours, and the cartilage around the joint de-mineralizes and degenerates within one week. One more magnesium caveat is that the cellular magnesium level controls protein synthesis. Stated another way, inadequate magnesium creates a cellular environment that is unable to manufacture protein. According to the researchers working on human proteins called the Proteonome, our bodies produce around 100,000 proteins with four million sequences.

Everybody needs physical medicine on a regular basis, otherwise you risk your body's own demise, as the destructive forces are incredible. The older you get the more positive action is important. As you will see, there are a wide range of co-morbidities linked to skeletal misalignment stemming from depression, balance, immune, digestive and blood pressure challenges.

You tune your car up, don't you? Why would you not do the same for your own body?

Every hour in the United States, there are 4,440 medically consulted injuries for people involved in either a motor vehicle accident or unintentional fall.[52] These are currently not treated appropriately. Fifteen years after a motor vehicle accident 70% of people have ongoing disability related to the accident.[53] Women and older people have a worse outcome. Sixty percent of symptomatic patients had not seen a doctor in the previous five years because the doctors were unable to help them.

"Never doubt that a small group of thoughtful committed citizens can change the world; indeed, it's the only thing that ever has."

Margaret Mead

Recent research (2009)[54] has revealed that up to 75% of human intervertebral disc cells die within the first 24 hours of trauma, mainly by necrosis (cellular death). The intervertebral disc tissue is very susceptible to disintegration if its glucose supply is interrupted. This is very important in all cases of spine traumas, especially whiplash cases. With immediate care and good blood supply, glucose metabolism can be re-established to save the disc. Degenerative changes in the spine start early. At 15 years of age, there is a 31% prevalence of disc degeneration. This rises linearly with age until by 70 years, 100% of lumbar spines show disc degeneration.[55] Osteoarthritis affects the facet (zygapophyseal) joints in 90% of individuals over 45 years of age.[56] Degenerated tissue has a greater effect on the nerve root than normal tissue. This appears to be caused by one or more chemicals released from cells in the degenerated disc (nucleus pulposis). One of these is tumor necrosis factor alpha, which is synthesized in the nerve root in response to signals from the disc.

Structure and function are hardwired together.[57] This means that when key (or nodal points) of alignment malfunction you need to be aware of these facts. Besides pain and arthritis, structural misalignment may be the prime component for other possible outcomes that may or may not be painful.

Two favorite web-related natural aphorisms are: "Where it is, it isn't" and, "Anything can cause anything." These include functional gastro-intestinal disturbances like gastro-esophageal reflux disease, irritable bowel syndrome, constipation and gall-bladder disease. This is a closely related $86 billion. Several other related annual health costs include: allergies at $11 billion,[58] asthma at $18 billion, depression at $83 billion,[59] drug-resistant infections at $50 billion, and sleep disorders at $5 billion. With the widespread integration of PAK™ and Functional Medicine, we have the likely capability of reducing the healthcare bill by $800 billion or more in the next five to ten years! When you add in the 200 billion for the costs of inactivity, we're up to 1 trillion or more with clean water, nutrient-dense foods, saunas and supplements. This will go a long way to lower the GNP spent on health from 18% to 10% or lower putting America back on track as a global model for a sustainable future.

According to the Occupational Safety and Health Administration (OSHA), more than a quarter of U.S. buildings are water damaged. Richie Shoemaker, MD (www.survivingmold.com) reveals that 24% of all children are genetically at risk for illness if exposed to a water-damaged building. The complex "stew" of biologically active chemicals initiates an immune system response that runs amuck that is called chronic inflammatory response syndrome or CIRS. There is a fungal DNA test called the Environmental Relative Mold Index (www.mycometrics.com) that he highly recommends.

> *"Unless we put Medical Freedom into the Constitution, the time will come when medicine will organize into an undercover dictatorship. To restrict the art of healing to one class of men, and deny equal privileges to others, will be to constitute the Bastille of Medical Science. All such laws are un-American and despotic and have no place in a Republic. The Constitution of this Republic should make special privilege for Medical Freedom as well as Religious Freedom."*
>
> Dr. Benjamin Rush, a signer of the Declaration of Independence

> *"Be not afraid of going slowly, but only afraid of standing still."*
> Chinese Proverb

Dr Shoemaker states that, "Mold illness will help in this emerging field of immunology, as the parallels to 'over-response' to antigens due to absence of protective antibody formation that are seen in mold illness apply to many other diseases, including auto-immunity and cancer."

Hippocrates, the Father of Modern Medicine, said, "Food first, medicine second, and surgery last." The Hippocratic Order of Treatment is, therefore, least invasive first. This is common sense. The point is, if we are going to trust something, we might as well not reinvent the wheel; and we'll do well to use the Nobel prize winners in Medicine and Physiology as our guideposts. Linus Pauling is the only person to ever singly be awarded two Nobel prizes: one in Chemistry and the other in Peace. He said, "Optimum nutrition is the medicine of tomorrow." When queried further about his vision for the future of medicine in 1982 he said, "The greatest breakthrough is the fact that nutritional therapy and nutritional supplements can be used more in the active prevention and treatment of disease with the result being an increased health span of 40 years, from 75 to 115."

An expert panel of eight top economists, including five Nobel Laureates, at the Cophenhagen Conference agreed that combating malnutrition is the top priority for child survival. They found that nutrition gave a 17:1 return on investment. "Each dollar spent on this program creates benefits (in the form of better health, fewer deaths, increased future earnings, etc.)" [http://www.copenhagenconsensus. com]. It is really a shame that fewer than 6% of graduate medical students get any training in nutrition. Think of the return on investment we could see if they did receive such training!

A recently published study (Jan 10, 2011) in the online journal "Pediatrics" revealed that children born less than one year after the last child have three times the incidences of autism. Dr. Gary Gordon believes that this suggests that maternal nutrition is compromised after one child and that all planned pregnancies need to be preceded by ideally one year of detoxification. It's scary to think that by doing nothing, the next trillion-dollar industry could be the caretakers of our autistic grandchildren.

According to a survey done by the Hast Research Associates (June 2009), "Ninety-six percent of primary care physicians believe the nation's healthcare system should place more emphasis on nutrition to treat and manage chronic disease." This challenges the United States National Library of Medicine, self-proclaimed as the largest medical library in the world, omission of most indexes for anything relating to natural medicine.

In March of 2012, the CDC reported that autism spectrum disorder (ASD) now affects 1 out of every 88 American children—a 23% increase from 2006 and a 78% increase from 2002. The increases are far too rapid to be of purely genetic origin. ADHD now affects 14% of American children. The Children's Environmental Health Center (CEHC) has published a list of 10 chemicals in *Environmental Health Perspectives,* an editorial by Dr. Philip J Landrigan (director of the CEHC), Dr. Linda Bimbaun (director of the National Institute for Environmental Health Sciences (NIEHS)), and Dr. Luca Lambetini (also of the CEHC). The top 10 chemicals are: lead, methylmercury, PCBs, organophospate pesticides, organochlorine, endocrine disruptors, automotive exhaust, polycyclic aromatic hydrocarbons, brominated flame retardants, and perfluorinated compounds.

The bulldozing of major scientific breakthroughs utilizing nutrition has been ongoing at our expense. Take for example polio. Dr. Frederick Klenner used intravenous vitamin C (6-20 grams in a 24 hour period) in a polio outbreak in North Carolina in 1948 and cured all 60 cases with no loss of muscle function within 72 hours of treatment. This was presented to the AMA at a meeting on June 10,1949 with a review of the presentation published in the *Journal of the American Medical Association* (JAMA) soon thereafter published by Galloway and Seifert. In spite of this, the twenty-first edition of the *Cecil Textbook of Medicine* (WB Sanders Co, 2000) clearly states that, "no specific treatment is available for polio," adding that "supportive care" is essential for dealing with pain and increasing the chances of survival.

Half of all diseases can be considered untreatable and for the other half the drugs only work half the time with major side effects. Imagine a car that starts only half the time, and whose brakes don't often work.

Severin Schwan, CEO Roche
Economist 12.10.2009

The textbook goes on to say, "The American Public appears to have been hoodwinked into believing that more interventions lead to better health; and most people that I meet are completely unaware that the U.S. does not have the best health in the world. The U.S. public does not recognize that not only are some drugs dangerous, but that many drugs are overused or inappropriately used. The U.S. public does not seem to recognize that inappropriate care is dangerous; more does not mean better." These sentiments are voiced by a growing number of medical educators including Jonathan Wright, Julian Whitaker, Gary Gordon, Marc Micozzi and Sidney Wolfe.

If prescription drugs taken as prescribed are killing more than one million Americans per decade, the studies on which those drugs are based must be fraudulent, or at the very least, massively incompetent. This makes the whole literature suspect. Marcia Angell, past editor of the famous *New England Journal of Medicine*, has written extensively about the need for change in her book *The Truth About the Drug Companies: How They Deceive Us and What To Do About It*. She believes that drug companies should, "... no longer be permitted to control the clinical testing of their own drugs. There is too much evidence that the practice biases the research in favor of the sponsor's drug." She goes on to propose that an Institute for Prescription Drug Trials be established within the National Institutes of Health (NIH) to administer clinical trials of prescription drugs.

" We must be good to one another. ... We're a nation of community. A government that remembers that the people are its master, is a good and needed thing. And I respect old fashioned common sense. I am going to stop ocean dumping. And we must clean the air. There is

In 2009, the Nobel Prize in Medicine was won by three Americans: Elizabeth Blackburn, UCSF, Carol Greider of Johns Hopkins, and Jack Szostak of Harvard Medical School. In the 1970s they discovered the telomere, or tail of each chromosome. Previously thought to be junk (or non-functional) DNA, they discovered that these segments are critical for healthy cell division and function. With each cell division the telomere shortens, lessening the level of gene activity.

"The dynamic interface between mechanics and biology influence the effectiveness of the healing response."

Ken Hildebrand, MD, et al. The Basics of Soft Tissue Healing and General Factors that Influence Such Healing; Sports Medicine Arthroscopic Review: Sept 2005; vol 13; no 3; pp136-144

Most cells have a preset number of divisions that numbers around 60. Telomere length is emerging as a marker of biological age that independently predicts morbidity and mortality.

Current research has shown that the enzyme telomerase, a cellular enzyme, adds to the length of the telomeres. People with the highest levels of vitamin D have telomeres five years longer than those with the lowest levels of vitamin D. Green tea supports longer telomeres. Omega 3 fatty acids have been shown to increase telomeres.[60] Multivitamins,[61] vitamins C, E and folic acid have also been shown to increase telomeres, as have stress reduction[62] and exercise.

By exiting what some have called the dark ages of medicine, with its failed pain treatment model and lack of common sense, a truly remarkable future is approachable that is at the same time fiscally responsible, kind, and environmentally sustainable. Once it's clear that the pain driving a person to the emergency room is not due to broken bones, cancer metastasis or infection, then the patient can be referred from the hospital to a Soft Tissue Injury Clinic.

"We continuously swat at flies and swallow camels."

Dr. George Goodheart, Founder of PAK™ Commenting on traditional healthcare

"You are, by accident of fate, alive at an absolutely critical moment in the history of our planet.
Anything else you're interested in is not going to happen if you can't breathe the air and drink the water.

Don't sit this one out, do something."

Carl Sagan

A team approach can start to immediately resolve their stress MAPs, which the recent scientific literature strongly supports. The team can utilize multiple disciplines, such as chiropractic medicine, professional applied kinesiology, functional medicine, deep muscle therapy, acupuncture, new forms of electrical stimulation (i.e., Frequency Specific MicroCurrent, lasers and interferential) and lifestyle counseling (First Line Therapy).

In their article, "From Sick Care to Health Care–Re-engineering Prevention in the US System," Farghoil Fani Marvosti, MD, MPH and Randal S. Stafford, MD, PhD say, "All healthcare professionals will need to embrace a coordinated multidisciplinary team approach," (New England Journal of Medicine 2012;367:889-891). The patient may then follow up at a community-based healthcare center. As reported in Dan Buettner's book; *The Blue Zones*, there are areas where people live to old age with no disease, more precisely, in these "Blue Zones," ten times more people reach the age of 100 compared with people in the United States. Part of the secret of the "Blue Zones" is the spirit of community. The time has come for Community Based Health Teams (CBHTs): places where a person can go to get educated, adjusted, muscle balanced, massaged, checked for other aspects of primary care, detoxify in a Far InfraRed Sauna (to outgas toxins), de-stress, eat and get clean food from the local CSA (community-sponsored agriculture) in an environment of neighbors, friends and healers. It is only through a lifetime of ongoing, integrated preventative medical care, coupled with an educated self-responsible populace, that we can actually stop the heart disease, cancer, auto immune, neuro-degenerative and diabesity epidemics that stand ready to crush the life out of us: physically, mentally, financially and above all spiritually.

Years ago I received a call for help from a gentleman who said that he couldn't move due to severe back pain. He was stuck, bent over a bathtub on his hands and knees, unable to move. He had been giving his infant daughter a bath when his back "went out," severe pain freezing him in the kneeling-over-the-tub position. He weighed 450 pounds. The emergency room at the nearby University of

Massachusetts Medical School said they would have to get a crane, chainsaw a hole into the side of his house, and lower him by crane into a dump truck, since he was on the top floor of a three-floor house.

I went over and got him standing in just a few minutes. The point of this story is to show that by doing the right thing morally and applying the right tools physically, with a sense of urgency and awareness, a disaster can be avoided. This is analogous to our current healthcare crisis.

Quick use of the right tools can really make a big difference. Logic proclaims least invasive first.

Sixty years ago 90% of our food came from within 50 miles, not the 1,500 miles of today. The average plant, from seed to table, is treated with or exposed to 1,500 chemicals. Getting people back to the land will precipitate positive change.

"Scientists reporting in the Proceedings of the National Academy of Sciences have recently concluded that running has a positive impact on the hippocampus, which is the section of the brain responsible for learning and memory. Exercise triggers significant physiological and structural changes in the brain that can improve cognitive function and help prevent mental decline."
Proceedings of the National Academy of Sciences
USA, January 10, 2010

Redirecting the 40 billion dollars used to fund corn and soy annually by the USDA, and expanding it to 200 billion, and using it instead to leverage the creation of one million small local farms could put us on the right track for soil repletion and the creation of jobs. Pushing the already ripe interests in local growing, with an eye on regional best crop studies and nutrient density, has the potential to create a very bright innovative food future.

Let's give people the incentive to move with a motion tax credit. Creating a safe environment with "green roads" (dedicated to walking, running, biking or rollerblading only) will instantly reduce the majority of the 200 billion dollars currently associated with the costs of inactivity. People will be smarter, fitter, less stressed and have direct access to personal community networks. This will have a huge positive ripple effect to lower overall health costs.

Smart electronic medical records to cut redundancy will provide huge savings. Health Savings Accounts (HSAs) have been found to increase the use of preventive care. They have grown from 660,000 in 2004 to 18 million in 2009.

According to Dr. Dave Janda, 40% [63] of the people who signed up for HSAs were previously uninsured and 56% of the purchasers had incomes of less than $15,000 per year! Research at the Mackinac Center for Public Policy in Michigan concluded that anywhere from 200 to 800 billion dollars per year would by saved with HSAs.[64]

Dr. James Forleo's book title says it all: *Health is Simple—Disease is Complicated.*

We must take care of our bodies, exercise them, hydrate them with clean water, fuel them with nutrient-dense organic foods, all while living and learning about a lifetime of detoxification through nutraceuticals, saunas, and right thinking to prevent disease. At the same time we will be both getting to know, love and educate each other and help one another build the sustainable model society. Making the entire country a "Blue Zone" is one worthwhile goal.

"Medical education should prepare students well for the clinical problems they will face. However, that is not happening for 'chronic disease.'"

Journal of the American Medical Association 2004; 292: 1057-105

Chapter II   Functional Medicine (FM): A Systems-Based Approach Utilizing the Web of Wellness

If you think about what is right in medicine today, you most likely think of acute emergency medicine: the removal of a diseased appendix, the setting of a broken bone, or the suturing of a laceration. This takes up about 20% of our healthcare dollar. The other 80% is spent on complex chronic diseases.

Dr. Jeffrey Bland, biochemist, legendary teacher, writer, and innovator founded the concept of Functional Medicine. Dr. Bland has sought to understand the cellular mechanisms of diseases as they relate to nutritional biochemistry and their effect on genetics. He has authored a monthly audiotape to professionals for 30 years and over 20 annual Functional Medicine Symposiums. This is new model of medicine will completely replace the current one since it is evidence and not economic or eminence based. His resource websites are the Personalized Lifestyle Medicine Institute (www.plminstitute.org) and the Institute for Functional Medicine (www.functionalmedicine.org).

Through continuous improvement to healthcare practices, it is the vision of the Institute for Functional Medicine to improve the health of individuals worldwide. "Functional Medicine is a dynamic approach to assessing, preventing and treating complex chronic disease."[1] The need for an evidence-guided, systems-based approach for chronic complex diseases has never been greater. By changing the way healthcare is practiced, Functional Medicine represents the paradigm shift, from pharmaco-centric, to personalized medicine. This paradigm shift is about thinking in terms of networks instead of pathways.

Perhaps the best way to simply understand what this new approach has to offer is by using the analogy of the tree of medicine (see figure 1). Here the uppermost branches and leaves of the tree represent the various medical specialists. Typically, these doctors will render a diagnosis, and offer one, two, or more medications to symptomatically treat the condition. When the mapping of the human genome was finished just over a decade ago, it revealed that chronic complex diseases take place on dozens of genes. Thus, changing the signaling of just one or two of these genes would not appreciably change the disease process.

The top of the trunk of this tree represents a group of fundamental biological processes, organizing systems and core clinical imbalances, which compose the total integrated functional process of the body. These can be studied clinically to determine their state of balance. Increased understanding of the human body has irrevocably demonstrated that it functions as an orchestrated network of interconnected systems, rather than distinct systems working in isolation from one another. Perhaps the easiest way to appreciate this is by considering how these organizing systems form a web (see figure 2). A web implies that each component is connected to, and therefore affects, every other component. The more you are aware of and address these interrelationships, the more quickly healing takes place.

> *"Each new discovery is another indication of how important consciousness is for healing. We are learning to see our cells and our bodies as malleable, influenced by every thought and feeling that flows through us. We can claim responsibility for the quality of thought and feelings we host, selecting those that radiate benevolence, good will, love and kindness. Doing this, we are doing more than conscious epigenetic engineering on our bodies, we are loving the whole world into health."*
>
> Dawson Church, PhD—*The Genie in Your Genes*

As you drop lower on this tree trunk, you come to the causes of the core clinical imbalances known as the antecedents, triggers and mediators. Our genetic predispositions interplay not only with our mental, emotional and spiritual influences but also our experiences, attitudes and beliefs. All of this takes its roots from our personalized lifestyle and environmental factors.

A person's body-mind is their overall spiritual and psychological attitude. Recent research has shown that people with a positive mental attitude have 50% less all cause mortality. Ninety percent of peoples' self-talk is negative. Over 100 genes have been found to be directly under our conscious control. Turn your camera lens inwards several times a day and see what you are saying to yourself. You might be surprised!

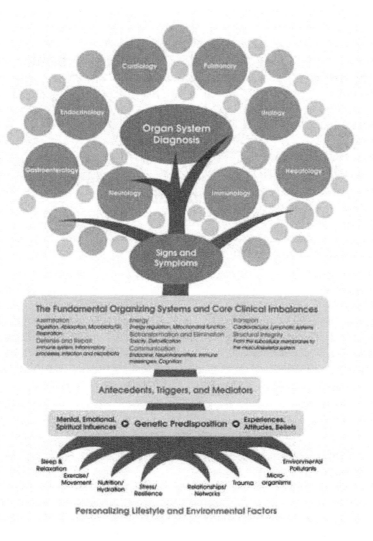

(c) 2005 The Institute for Functional Medicine

FUNCTIONAL MEDICINE
Web of Wellness

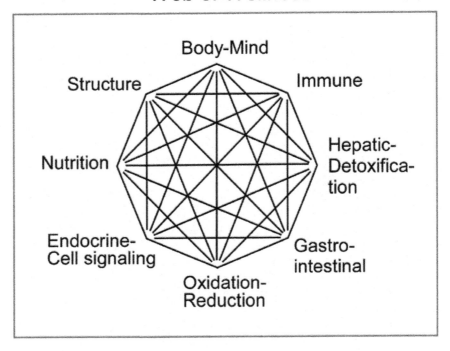

Artwork courtesy of Institute for Functional Medicine[48]

*"Each time a man stands up for an ideal, or acts to improve the lot of
others or strikes out against injustice, he sends forth a tiny ripple
of hope, and crossing each other from a million different centers of
energy and daring, those ripples build a current which can sweep
down the mightiest walls of oppression and resistance."*

Robert F. Kennedy

*"Just for fun, another reason to avoid the whites: chlorine dioxide, one
of the chemicals used to bleach flour (even if made brown again, a
common trick), combines with residual proteins in most of these foods
to form alloxan. Researchers use alloxan in lab rats to induce
diabetes. That's right—it's used to produce diabetes. This is bad news
if you eat anything white or 'enriched'. Don't eat white stuff unless you
want to get fatter."*

Timothy Ferris, *The 4-Hour Body*

Immune and inflammatory balance play another key role in systems biology. Consuming a food plan that has a net anti-inflammatory effect is key here, but it requires both education and effort. The Paleolithic and Mediterranean plans provide a good backbone. Consuming carbohydrates that turn to sugar slowly and don't stress the pancreas, known as low glycemic load, is important. The avoidance of "white" as in flour and sweeteners is important. The avoidance of all refined grains is another component. Whole grains like brown rice, steel cut oats, buckwheat groats, and quinoa provide some positive choices. Eating lots of fruits and vegetables of a wide variety of colors (preferably organic) is a good idea. At least make an effort to eat the Environmental Working Group's "clean 15" and avoid the "dirty dozen," which are the fruits and vegetables with the least and most pesticides respectively. You will find the list at www.ewg.org.

Eating free-range poultry and grass-fed beef, or wild game like elk and venison, provides a better choice for two extremely important reasons. The fat in grass-fed beef has more conjugated linolenic acids, which tend to burn fat and strengthen the immune system. Wild game as well as grass-fed beef and chicken is typically devoid of both potentially carcinogenic hormones and pesticides built into genetically modified corn.

Fatty fish should include sardines and wild salmon or halibut. Care must be taken with choices when it comes to farm-raised fish. You need to do some research here. One website worth knowing about is the Technology Entertainment Design network (TED). Google TED video and watch chef Dan Barber tell of his love affair with a particular kind of farm-raised fish. The whole idea of TED is to expose people to life-changing, world-improving ideas. A person is given 16 minutes to communicate a positive thought process. With two meetings a year since the early 80s, one in California and the other in Scotland, they have posted over 800 of these presentations on their website (www.ted.com).

The use of eggs made by free range chickens and fortified to increase omega 3 fatty acids is a way to increase your omega 3 intake. In general, striving to eat organic dairy products will overcome the tendency for dairy products to contain concentrated chlorinated pesticides. The abundant use of nuts and seeds, and their butters, is a lifestyle change worth the effort, with a great return on investment.

Since half of your immune system, responsible for 77% of our antibody production, is wrapped around your small intestine, it's important to take steps to preserve the health of this digestive and detox organ. Your intestines contain three to five pounds of bacteria, molds and viruses, made up of 1,800 different genuses with between 15 to 35,000 species. Known as your gut biome, this important intestinal biomass is estimated to manufacture greater than one million compounds for the body.

An estimated 80% of the antibiotics made in this country are not used in medicine but in animal husbandry to grow fatter chickens, turkeys, pigs and cows. Eating these drug-laden foods destroys our good bacteria and make us prone to mold overgrowth, which leads to inflammation of the small intestine, and ultimately, a breakdown of its barrier function, known as a "leaky gut," occurs. This creates a cascade of inflammation and immune dysregulation. Recent research shows this to be an underlying cause of autoimmune disease.[2,3] The downstream effect is more stress on the hepato-biliary tree (liver-gallbladder), a net loss of energy, a source of food and chemical sensitivities, and poor nutrient absorption. One of the areas giving us new information is the relationship of the gut micro-flora to the overall function of the immune system, especially with respect to chronic fatigue syndrome and metabolic disorders like obesity.[4,5]

The uptake of toxins from the gut (endotoxemia) is dramatically increased with the typical diet[1] and initiates obesity.[2]

1) Penyala S et al. Gastroenterol 2012; 142: pp1100-1101
2) Carni PP et al. Diabetes 2007;56; pp1761-72

A person's structural integrity is important at all levels—from a single cell all the way through the entire neuro-musculoskeletal system. Our cell membranes are double layered, having phospholipids on the inside and outside and essential fatty acids in the middle. These cellular skins are very thin. Ten thousand of them fit into the thickness of this piece of paper. You would have to run a marathon—26.2 miles—to get around the fat in your 400 trillion cell membranes if they were spread out in a one cell thick layer. Every cell membrane has two to three million receptors which are protein-rich docking sites. These proteins extend through the cell membrane. The receptor end on the outside senses the environment and signals the other end—the effector—to direct the creation of proteins by our DNA. Thus, the cellular membranes are actually the brains of the cell.

> *"Biochemist Barbara Corkey, dubbed 'the queen of metabolism' by Ron Kaln (past president of the Joslin Diabetes Center) suspects food additives and other environmental factors play a role in the biochemical changes that lead to type II diabetes. Her research suggests that monoglycerides—like mono-oleoyl glycerol, an emulsifier added to foods like cupcakes and artificial sweeteners like saccharin—stimulate the beta cells to secrete insulin, but not in a normal way. 'Usually,' says Corkey, 'calcium is involved in stimulating beta cells to produce insulin, and when stimulated they increase their oxygen consumption. Instead, the beta cells underwent some unexpected chemical changes and released molecules called reactive oxygen species, which have been implicated in cell damage, inflammation and obesity.'*
>
> *Her work pointing to the fact that a person can't get type II diabetes without mal-functioning beta cells, now widely accepted by scientists, was a paradigm shift largely precipitated by her work. 'Metabolic disease has always interested me,' she says. 'It's a system where pathways all interconnect and talk to each other. And so if you push on one button over here, it has consequences everywhere else.'"*
>
> *"Why We Are Fat"*
> Barbara Moran - Bostonia, Winter-Spring 2012

You have to eat, digest and absorb the right foods to get all the right fats for healthy cell membranes. Avoiding bad fats, such as those in fried and processed foods, is important. Examination of arterial plaque was found to predominantly contain adulterated omega 6 polyunsaturated oils.[6] "Those that start out containing good essential fatty acids (EFAs), but they are ruined in commercial processing and sold at the supermarket in thousands of products."[7] The use of cold processed, refrigerated oils, stored in a dark container to prevent breakdown by ultraviolet light is necessary for healthy cell membranes.

Eating foods that contain living essential fatty acids, and far less, if any, processed fats, is critical to any body-balancing regimen. The right fats help to create the right cellular signals so that cellular communication flows freely.

"All of the diseases of aging are accelerated by micro-nutrient deficiency and the majority of Americans are aging faster than they should. I do not believe that politicians are going to be helping very much."

Dr. Bruce Ames, Chair, Dept of Biochemistry UCLA

"The one who tells the stories rules the world."

Hopi Indian

Your hormones' sensitivity, and neurotransmitters' production and delivery are affected by a variety of factors. Many environmental pollutants look—on the molecular level in the body— like estrogens (xenoestrogens or environmental endocrine disrupters—EEDs) and these may block the related hormone function. Xenohormetic changes mean that small amounts of a foreign substance (xeno-) can create big changes (hormesis). Frederick von Soal is a professor at the University of Missouri where he studies endocrine disruptors. Bisphenol A (BPA) is a synthetic estrogen made from petroleum. Von Soal fed BPA to mice in dosages 25,000 times lower than what the plastics industry has published as a "no effect" or safe level and found that it, "wrecked the male reproductive system."

In most autoimmune diseases, a pattern of hormone disturbance exists, with elevated estrogen and prolactin, accompanied by lowered cortisol, DHEA and testosterone.[8] Certain nutrients like fish oil, 5-hydroxytryptophan, and vitamin D3 have been shown to modulate the neurotransmitter serotonin. This neurotransmitter is considered key for balanced brain function.

Other nutrients build organ reserve, and thus, promote balanced hormone production. Environmental chemicals create imbalance in the brain.

In addition to the use of betaine hydrochloride as a digestive enzyme replacement for the stomach enzymes, there is another component you need to know about. That component is salt (sodium chloride). The chloride in the salt is essential for the production of adequate amounts of hydrochloric acid. I don't recommend regular table salt, which is 99% sodium chloride and .01% chemicals, for free flow. What I do recommend, to the people who eat plenty of fruit and vegetables, is a type of sea salt mined off the Normandy Coast of France for the last several hundred years, called Celtic Salt. This is 84% sodium chloride and 16%

trace minerals. This will greatly enhance the quality of the taste of your food, while providing valuable minerals at the same time. If you don't eat enough fruits and vegetables, No Salt (brand name for potassium chloride) or Dr. Wright's salt is a better choice, as potassium is a vascular protector.

Digestion, absorption and microbiological (gut biome) function is important because a full 50% of your immune system—your mucous associated lymphatic tissue (MALT) and gut-associated lymphatic tissue (GALT)—sits in the lining of your small intestine. Seventy percent of the body's circulating antibodies are made here. The small intestine is also responsible for half of the body's detoxification, while the other half is detoxified by the liver. The absorptive surface of the small intestine is the size of a tennis court. Adequate parasympathetic nervous system (feel, rest, and relax) activation at meal time is crucial since this system is what signals your digestive glands to produce their juice. It's a good idea to drink one to two glasses of purified water five to ten minutes before a meal. This hydrates the gastro-intestinal tract so that it may function at optimal efficiency.

> *"The area most susceptible to damage and difficult to repair is your intestinal flora."*
> Dr. Sid Baker - *Detoxification is a Lifetime Strategy*

Slowing down, taking several long deep breaths, and enjoying someone else's company are good ways to further improve your digestion.

The intelligent process of taking proactive steps to amplify the function of your gastro-intestinal tract is known as the Four-R program, and is a cornerstone of Functional Medicine. The first "R" in this restoration program is Remove: removing any pathogens, antigens or toxins. The second "R" is Replace: replacement of stomach acid or pancreatic enzymes if necessary. Third is Re-inoculation: with prebiotics (bacterial fertilizer) and probiotics (bacteria themselves). The fourth "R" stands for Repair: repairing of the mucosal membrane.

One excellent product, called Endefen, developed by Metagenics, actually produces multi-dimensional support for the upper GI tract. This product supports the growth of gastric mucosal cells, thickens the protective gastric mucin layer, enhances GI immune function and selectively promotes Bifido bacteria and Lactobacillus growth to promote healthy flora. The choice of a probiotic that possesses characteristics that allows it to survive in the presence of bile or stomach acid is key. One such strain is the Lactobacillus HCFM strain, which has been the subject of over 50 research studies.

I tell patients that their stomach is an oven that cooks their food with hydrochloric acid. There's a huge misunderstanding in medicine today with respect to what creates gastroesphogeal reflux (GERD), which has been hammered with strong medications to stop acid production. The production of hydrochloric acid takes six times more energy to produce than any other molecule in the human body so its overproduction is indeed rare. The body has to concentrate both hydrogen and chloride a hundred thousandfold to drop the pH of blood at 7.4 to 2, the pH which cooks the food. Only one person in a million has the rare Zollinger-Ellison syndrome with too much acid from a gastric tumor (gastroma). The real cause of reflux is not enough acid, so the undigested food sits longer in the stomach due to the fact that the pyloric sphincter valve, at the emptying end of the stomach, is pH sensitive. This means that unless enough acid is made to lower the pH to 2 (very acidic) this valve stays closed and the undigested food with its small amount of acid can reflux. This is true especially if the person's body is structurally misaligned with a stress maladaptation pattern that causes them to have a diaphragm strain or hiatal hernia. This causes the lower esophageal sphincter to be above the diaphragm so that it is not reinforcing its closure. This represents the structural dysfunction driving this common condition, as I describe in a paper called "The Structural Diathesis of GERD: Safe, Cost Effective Therapy Using PAK™" (International College of Applied Kinesiology, Proceedings of the Annual Meeting, 2008-2009, p.241-243).

The liver and gallbladder, along with the small and large intestine, make up a good part of the body's detoxification/biotransformation and elimination systems. The liver may be likened to the engine that cleans your blood, and the gallbladder its oil filter. With the passage of a meal from your stomach into the small intestine, the gallbladder empties its bile (90% cholesterol, 10% bile salts, phosphatidyl choline and taurine) into the small intestine where it is reabsorbed back to the liver, into the gallbladder and back out again. This occurs in a healthy body two times per meal. This removes toxins the liver has trapped, emulsifies fats, and acts as an intestinal lubricant. The healthy transit time (from mouth to rectum) is 18 hours, and the average American's transit time is 52 hours! Teaching people how to "change their oil" is key.

"Functional Medicine (FM) is both comprehensive and patient-centered. It offers a new model of cutting edge systems, biology, synthesized with whole person medicine, by evaluating a matrix of root causes. FM can look further 'upstream' to understand the physiology and patho-physiology, and not simply treat the end stage."

"It is important to keep in mind that the essence of functional medicine is contained in the very simple questions: What harms us? What makes us thrive?"

Dr. Jeffrey Bland

Dr. Sid Baker notes that, "detoxification is the biggest item in each individual's biochemical budget."[9] The majority of our energy (80% for an adult) is spent daily on manufacturing the molecules needed to detoxify us. The "total load" is the term applied to the sum of both exotoxins (i.e., those delivered through food, water, air and the environment, and lifestyle) and endotoxins (i.e., those produced by the body and enteric bacterial metabolism). The detox molecules are in high demand and short supply in this toxic world. In fact, 25% to 35% of Americans have elevated liver enzymes.

The gamma–glutamyl transferase (GGT) is an extracellular enzyme that is anchored to the plasma membrane of cells. "It hydrolyzes and transfers gamma—glutamylmoleties from glutathione to other receptors. As such it is critical for the function and metabolism and recycling of glutathione."[10] Increase of the GGT enzyme to upper levels of normal is the area of the web where chemicals from our environment, (i.e., obesogens like pesticides, heavy metals, and persistent organic pollutants), talk to our genetic software (epigenome) and direct it to create the diseases of today. Dr. Jeffrey Bland recently stated, "The drugs of today treat the conditions that arise from the alteration of our genes from our environment."

Functional Medicine utilizes a vast array of foods and nutrients to allow the eliminative organs to function at optimal levels. A few examples may serve to illustrate this point. Foods like beet greens, or supplements made out of them, are very helpful to thin out the bile in the gallbladder which has a tendency to thicken. This causes a slowing of fat digestion and elimination in general, since bile lubricates the gut tube. Vitamin C is important for the production and excretion of bile acids, which are the toxins' actual transport out of the liver. Herbs like milk thistle (silymarin) and anti-oxidants like alpha-lipoic acid have been shown to protect the liver.

Because of the huge exposure everyone now has to environmental chemicals and heavy metals, the nutrients necessary for the liver to trap and remove them are in high demand, but short supply. Due to the brilliant work of Dr. Jeffrey Bland and his dedicated staff at the Metagenics Functional Medicine Research Center and the MetProteomics Nutrigenomics Center in Gig Harbor, Washington, several major breakthroughs have been achieved. At the top of the list of their breakthroughs is the development of personalized support programs for people whose metabolisms have been distorted by their unique gene-environment connections.

Starting back in 1991, Dr. Bland published his first paper on the disease-toxicity connection describing the results of a detoxification nutrition and diet program on liver detoxification enzyme activities. What followed was a paper in 1995 relating these enzymes to the clinical symptoms of chronic fatigue syndrome and fibromyalgia.[11] Their initial research led to the development of **medical foods**. These are powdered products, which when mixed with water become a meal with a known physiological action (see Appendix: Medical Foods).

"From the perspective of 'health' as organized structure and meaningful function; and 'disease' as the reversion to chaos, destruction of structure and the loss of function: the task of healthcare providers is essentially to restore order, and to acutely reduce and proactively prevent/eliminate clinical-biochemical-biomechanical-emotional chaos; in so far as it adversely affects the patient's life experience as an individual, and our collective experience as an interdependent society."

Alex Vasquez, D.C., N.D.

In the last few years, Bland's team performed some very interesting ethno-botanical research. They identified native people in the African Congo that had no heart disease, diabetes, cancer, blood pressure problems or obesity. They carefully observed their diet and identified components of the acacia nilotica plant as having active phytonutrients contributing to their good health. They tested their specific phytochemical supplement against a modified Mediterranean style, low glycemic load dietary program on variables associated with metabolic syndrome and cardiovascular disease. The found that these increased the effectiveness of the diet.[12] The study was then repeated in a university setting which concluded that the "Supplemented lifestyle program that used a soy/phytosterol-containing medical food and the rho iso-alpha acids and acacia pro-anthocyanidins led to significantly greater improvement in multiple risk factors. It represents a potentially powerful nutritional approach to the cardiovascular disease risk management of individuals with both metabolic syndrome and elevated LDL-C."[13]

Having a quick meal replacement with such profound benefits is really a gift.

41

As Aristotle commented, "Health is a matter of choice, not a mystery of chance." The range of choices of the medical foods falls into the following general areas: weight loss/gain, lowering inflammation/pain, improving glycemic control, and improving energy through improved liver detoxification. Every so often, female patients arrive with a history of debilitating menstrual challenges. Utilizing the Ultra Clear Plus medical food for one to two meals a day for a couple of weeks premenstrually, along with increasing magnesium levels, and a full body tune-up, is a recipe for success.

By this point everyone should be aware of the term insulin resistance, with its related metabolic syndrome. Metabolic syndrome is implicated in cardiovascular diseases, type II diabetes and cardiovascular disease. The control of insulin and blood lipids is not only accomplished with the phytonutrients in the aforementioned medical foods, but also in a stand alone product developed by Metagenics called Insinase.[14]

The development and execution of a product that naturally increases the production of the enzymes in the human body made to excrete heavy metals is another major breakthrough for this research team.

"More than 70% of Americans will die prematurely from disease caused by or compounded by deficiencies of the antioxidant network. Thanks to the antioxidant advantage, these conditions can be prevented, controlled and in some cases even cured."

Lester Packer, PhD
Past Director of the Packer Lab, University of California At Berkeley

"Dedicated, committed effort can bring about significant changes of consciousness and understanding. Unless you develop an ongoing, living, democratic culture that can compel the candidates, they're not going to do the things you voted for."

Noam Chomsky

The intense pollution in our environment has left the average person today with 1,000 times more lead in them than a skeleton of 300 years ago.[15] Since bone turns over at a rate of once every 16 years, and heavy metals like mercury, lead, arsenic and cadmium are exponential in their harmful effects, it behooves all of us to have a plan in place to help eliminate these to minimize their damage to our bodies. Studies at Harvard have shown that a higher bone lead contributes to cataract formation and six times more heart attacks.[16] Recent studies have implicated mercury as a cause of high blood pressure[17] (it blocks the magnesium receptors) and systemic inflammation.[18]

The enzyme metallothionein is one enzyme that has been identified whose specific function is to remove heavy metals. The product Metalloclear, manufactured and distributed by Metagenics, was shown to increase the body's production of metallothionein messenger RNA levels by 37 fold. There was increased urinary excretion of cobalt, cadmium, lead, barium, mercury and arsenic. This product, used in conjunction with other chelating agents, creates a powerful, yet safe detoxification program.

The health of our cellular signaling network is directly related to our cellular membranes, both outside and inside our cells. Research done by Dr. Lester Packer at Packer Labs at the University of California at Berkeley over a period of fifty years revealed that exercise depleted the body of vitamin E and other antioxidants and that they had to be replaced for exercise to produce its desired effects.

As molecular biologists, Dr Packer and his team discovered that out of the 500-plus known anti-oxidants, five of them have a dynamic interplay that allows them to recharge one another. Thus, they act like a shield to bolster or strengthen the entire human defense system. These five key antioxidants are Vitamins C and E, CoQ10, lipoic acid and glutathione. What makes network antioxidants special is that they can "recycle" or regenerate one another after they have quenched a free radical, vastly extending their antioxidant power. Dr. Packer wrote *The Antioxidant Miracle* in 1999. Everyone should read this book as this information is critical to know.

The *Maine Fishing Law Book* contains the warning that children under eight, and pregnant and nursing women should not eat any freshwater fish; adults and children over eight can eat two fish meals per month. This is due to the high levels of mercury in the fish.

It is clear that the mercury in the fish is man-made and comes from the atmosphere. Researchers in Canada investigated levels of mercury in loons in pristine Nova Scotia lakes and found levels twice as high as anywhere else in North America. Most evidence points to coal-fired power plants in the Midwest not equipped with scrubbers; so far, environmental regulators have been unsuccessful in requiring scrubbers.

This charismatic bird (the loon), whose ancestors roamed the earth 65 million years ago, can fly at speeds up to 80 miles per hour and can dive to depths of 200 feet or more. It would be a tragedy if they were wiped out by our country's inability to control airborne mercury pollution.

John Lund, The Maine Sportsman, Sept 2011

Besides free radical quenching, another one of the networks FM concerns itself with is that of estrogen metabolism. The diseases of estrogen metabolism are known to include cancers of the head, neck, throat, breast, prostate and uterus. The study of estrogen does not involve one chemical, but actually three: estrone, estradial and estriol. The way these leave the body is varied as well. They may leave the body through a 2-, 4-, or 16-hydroxylated pathway in the urine. The mechanisms and influences of these metabolites are sophisticated to study because of their short life and low level of concentration. Due to the pioneering work of Dr. Eleanor Rogan of the Eppley Institute at the University of Nebraska Medical Center, this network is starting to be understood.

The 2-OH pathway has been found to be safe. The 4-OH pathway, though, is not a good pathway for your body to be excreting estrogens through. This pathway creates damage to the DNA that seems to be a source of cancer initiation. These urinary quotients may be measured in a urinalysis by your FM provider. Cardiovascular exercise, fish oil and the increased intake of the cruciferous family of vegetables creates the desired result of greater 2-OH estrogen excretion. The component indole-3-carbinol (I3C) of the crucifers has been the most researched crucifer.

In addition to taking a global history and really listening to the patient's story, the practice of letting them communicate their symptoms on the Medical Symptoms Questionnaire (MSQ) (sample in Appendix), lays the groundwork for an in-depth analysis. The use of specific lab tests for biochemical baseline analysis is usually followed at some point with the use of a Bio Impedance Analysis (BIA) test. Developed to study the effects of space travel on the human body by NASA, the BIA non-invasively measures body compartments. It measures your total body water, as well as intracellular and extracellular water. This helps determine hydration and toxicity, as an elevated extracellular water is a sign of toxicity. It measures your total body fat and lean muscle mass, so if you lose weight, you can tell if it's from losing muscle mass (negative) or from burning fat (positive). The reading known as the "phase angle" is an instantaneous snapshot of your overall cell membrane health. The range runs approximately from 2 to 10 and is age and sex adjusted. It's quick, noninvasive and gives you personal numbers needed to improve and maintain your health.

"The marketing to keep people imprisoned in poor lifestyle habits is very effective."

"Life style medicine is about finding a personalized way of applying the science of nutrition, the science of exercise and movement, the science of sleep and restorative activities, the importance of relationships and resiliency in stress.

The underlying knowledge is deep and robust—its application is in the domain of primary healthcare and not public health. All of the studies show that lifestyle medicine has better outcomes than any single medication or groups of them. Lifestyle medicine is recognized in every national guideline—heart disease, cancer, diabetes, etc., however it is not taught!

Not to use lifestyle medicine is a black mark on medicine. Professor Halsted Holman, MD, when speaking to a recent graduating class at Stanford Medical School actually apologized for only preparing them for the 20% acute care patients and not for the 80% chronic complex disease majority which they will see."

David Jones, MD - President of the Institute for Functional Medicine

C. Chapter III: Professional Applied Kinesiology (PAK™): Browser for the Functional Medicine Web of Wellness

Professional Applied Kinesiology (or PAK™) provides an, "integrated, interdisciplinary approach to healthcare."[1] Dr. George Goodheart Jr., a second generation Detroit, Michigan chiropractor, originated PAK in 1964. It enables the functional evaluation of several of the components of Functional Medicine's Web of Wellness. By utilizing the manual muscle test (MMT) as a diagnostic indicator, a healthcare provider can determine the potential involvement of a person's emotional integrity, structural alignment, gastrointestinal function, liver detoxification, immune and endocrine balance with respect to both acute and chronic health conditions. This is well documented in the scientific literature with over 100 peer-reviewed journal articles on the methods and outcomes of PAK™.[2]

Necessity is truly the mother of invention. It all began in the early 1960s when a frazzled patient with a shoulder problem pressured Dr. Goodheart into a situation that created something which he described as, "Giving me the answer to a question I was not familiar with." One day while passing by his front desk, a patient sitting in his crowded waiting room brazenly yelled out and asked when his shoulder problem was going to get fixed. Once in the exam room, Dr. Goodheart noticed the patient's shoulder blade was sticking out (i.e., a winged scapula). Along the front side of this patient's chest, on the same side of the winged scapula, was a chain of palpable soft tissue nodules, which disappeared as he continued to rub them. At the same time, the winged scapula assumed its normal position. The patient could now move his shoulder without pain.

"Mind body techniques, diet, exercise, and group support are not complimentary, alternative medicine and they're not conventional; they are basic healthcare and they should be available to everybody."

James Gordon, MD
Director of the Center for Mind Body Medicine

This sent Dr. Goodheart to the anatomy texts to see what had happened. It didn't take him long to figure out that the anterior serratus muscle had inserted into the top 10 ribs in a semi-circular fashion across the lateral chest wall. By rubbing these insertion fibers in a back and forth manner, he had reset the muscle's function.

By studying the work of Kendall and Kendall,[3] Dr. Goodheart was quick to develop the art and science of not just muscle testing, but also muscle therapeutics. This led him to discover that a muscle's function could be inhibited by any one of a number of potential circuit breakers. At the level of the muscle itself, he found that either the beginning or end of the muscle's attachments—known as the origin and insertion respectively—could be partially torn from the bones. The tendons at the ends of a muscle insert into the outer shell or periosteum of a bone with small, root like structures known as **Sharpey's fibers**.

Overuse of a muscle can avulse or tear these fibers from the bone. These avulsion tears can effectively inhibit a muscle's function. Transverse frictional massage at the origin and insertion of a muscle is a basic technique of muscle therapeutics today.

Subsequently, muscle tissue came to be recognized in functional terms, as an organ unto itself; an understanding which formed the early basis for the emerging technology of PAK™. The belly or middle of a muscle is wired into the nervous system by the presence of several specialized nerve endings, one of which is known as spindle cells, due to their shape as seen under a microscope. They detect the change of length and the rate of change of length of the muscle. When they were manually tractioned apart from the middle, the spindle organs were stimulated to "fire" and this up-regulated or facilitated the muscle's contractile power.

Conversely, compression of the spindles inhibited or weakened a strong muscle. This is primary care medicine, as muscle spindles are the primary input into the brain. Posture is an indicator of brain function.

"There is an approach to healthcare that helps the doctor understand functional health disorders (the early stages of disease processes) and that provide direction toward optimal treatment of these dysfunctions when they are still in the reparable stage."

Dr. George Goodheart, Jr.

It is interesting to note that the density of these spindle cells increases as you go up the spine, with the highest concentration in the muscles at the suboccipital area (the muscles that attach our upper neck to the base of our skull). "Muscles responsible for fine and precise movement have a significantly higher concentration of spindles than those that must accomplish gross movement."[4] The small suboccipital muscles have 150-200 muscle spindles per gram of muscle tissue and the intertransverse muscle in the cervical spine have 200-500 muscle spindles per gram versus the rectus femorus (thigh muscle) which has 50 muscle spindles per gram of muscle tissue. Suboccipital muscles are quite specialized, having only spindle receptors. The high density of spindles in these muscles is necessary because they have direct feedback to the area of the brain (the intermedius nucleus of the medulla) that coordinates autonomic responses like balance, digestion, blood pressure and heart rate, with postural changes. Two of the suboccipital muscles, called the rectus capitus posterior minor and obliqus capitis inferior, directly attach to the posterolateral cervical dura mater so that when we look up they pull this tubing away from our delicate spinal cord. This tissue is called the myodural bridge.

At the ends of a muscle, where the muscle belly tapers into tendons, are other specialized mechanoreceptors known as golgi tendon receptors. These have the special job of protecting the muscle spindle cells in the muscle belly from harm. For example, if you were bending your elbow to lift a heavy shopping bag, and the bicep muscle was going to rip or tear because of the excessive weight, the golgi tendon receptors would fire, causing the tendons to stretch, protecting your bicep muscle from injury. The golgi tendons can be up- or down-regulated with manual therapy just like the neuromuscular spindle cells. Activating golgi tendons and muscle spindles in a variety of ways (e.g., adjustments, massage, exercise, yoga) is good for brain health.

Over the course of several years, Dr. Goodheart studied and incorporated various neurological, vascular, lymphatic, skin, fascial and electro-magnetic (acupuncture meridian) circuits into the growing body of muscle-testing knowledge, known as Applied Kinesiology (AK). He taught and studied with a core group of chiropractors in the United States, known lovingly as "the dirty dozen."[12] In 1976, The International College of Applied Kinesiology (ICAK) was founded to promote the teaching and research of AK.

In the mid-1990s, two facts became abundantly apparent. First, a large number of organizations around the world were using techniques from AK for a wide range of therapeutic approaches to health and healing. Some were professional and some were not. Second, as the need to distance the professional organization from the rest of the groups using AK was recognized, the ICAK leadership found that the term AK could not be copyrighted, because it had been in the common vernacular too long. Thus, the term, Professional Applied Kinesiology (PAK™) was proposed and accepted by the membership majority.

> *"The evidence now shows, with greater consistency and clarity than ever before, that inflammation or injury produces specifically identifiable inhibited muscles. Controlled clinical studies have shown that dysfunction and pain, specifically in the ankle, knee, lumbar spine, temporal mandibular joint, and cervical spine, will produce inhibited muscles."*
>
> Scott Cuthbert, DC
> *The Muscle Weakness Revolution Is Here*

This was done so that the standards of professional excellence, and reproducible results, based on the original tenets of Dr. Goodheart and provided by healthcare professionals, could be differentiated from those that were not.

As the intricacies of the PAK™ organization and its wide range of muscle therapeutics grew, so did another key area of understanding. This was the development of a particularly powerful diagnostic tool known as the "challenge." At any given moment one can't simultaneously read while someone else is talking to you. This is due to the fact that we have only about 10% of our nervous system (cortical volitional output) to consciously work with. The other 90% carries out a multitude of functions in what is called the autonomic, automatic or subconscious nervous system. The majority of cortical output goes to parasympathetic areas in the brain stem to control and regulate sympathetics. The fact is that we live in a receptor-based nervous system. Specialized nerve endings called mechanoreceptors (like the neuromuscular spindle cells and the golgi tendon receptors) are both position and pressure sensitive. These special receptors are wrapped around all of our joints, muscles and organs. Specialized mechanoreceptors called integrins spot weld areas of the cell's membrane called focal adhesions to the extra-cellular matrix.

It is through this receptor network that the brain carries out the vast amount of tasks that it does at any given moment.

The fact that an intact muscle became inhibited when a joint that was misaligned was slightly more misaligned was understood to be a key component of the new field of functional neurology or articular neurology. This technique, utilizing the body's functional neurological response, could be used to quickly and precisely determine not only which specific joints were misaligned, but also if the correction given was adequate to restore function. The challenge, in my opinion, stands out as the most powerful non-invasive diagnostic tool available today, and it represents the unique diagnostic contribution of PAK.™

Let's take a moment to appreciate PAK™ for the powerful breakthrough that it is. At the core of our body the normal vertebral complex (Appendix page 414) consists of a single motor unit, two vertebrae connected by an intervertebral disc. The vertebral bodies interconnect at the back via interlocking joints called facets. These sliding, gliding joints are richly innervated with both position (mechano) and pain (noci) receptors. This complex, as the basic unit of spinal function, or spinal biomechanics must allow for flexion, extension, rotation and lateral bending. At the same time, it also has to allow the spinal cord nerve roots (the dura-arachnoid sleeve) to come out through the intervertebral foramina without getting compressed or stretched. There is a small, instantaneous axis of rotation with motion here that facilitates neurological (propulsion of cerebrospinal fluid with its molecules of emotion and nutrients to the distant organs) and intervertebral disc health (glucose and other nutrients from the vertebral end plates into the disc). This inherent motion self-lubricates the intervertebral disc and facets with nutrients and natural painkillers for your pain-free existence. To bring clarity to a functional understanding of the brain and nervous system, let's talk about the dural membranes. The brain sits in a hammock of ligaments called "the tough mother" or dura mater. These form a tent that divides the brain into three major compartments: the cerebellum, right and left hemispheres. They line the inside of our cranial bones, and form an outer tube that surrounds the spinal cord that extends down its entire length. Inside this tube are two more layers of tubing that surround the spinal cord allowing freedom of motion. When we inhale and the three curves of our spine straighten out, this shortens the spinal cord which contracts the brain at its base, but lifts and widens it from the top and sides. This creates a slightly lateral expansion of the four hollow ventricles that both promotes cerebrospinal fluid production and flow into them. When we exhale the curves of our spine relax, allowing the brain to expand, pushing the cerebrospinal fluid out of the ventricles and down the spinal cord. From here it exits the spine along the nerve roots as it flows to the various muscles and organs. The cerebrospinal fluid carries oxygen, glucose and the body's informational substances right into the structures to which the nerves go. The richest blood supply to the spinal cord is from C1 to T4. This is also the fastest area of cerebrospinal fluid flow. It's the back part of the spinal column (the dorsal horn), where the spinal nerve roots originate, that is richly endowed with the body's natural pain relievers (opiates). Normal functional motion really does create a naturally pain-free state and an enormous flow of informational substances from the brain to the body at every moment.

> *"The body heals itself in a sure, sensible, practical, reasonable, and observable manner.*
> *The 'healer within' can be approached from without. The opportunity to use the body as an*
> *instrument of laboratory analysis is unparalleled in modern therapy;*
> *if one approaches the problem correctly, making the proper and adequate diagnosis and treatment, the response is satisfactory to both the doctor and the patient."*
> Dr. George Goodheart, Founder of PAK™

This is important to understand because normal function here prevents disease. Research dating back to 1921 showed a 100% correlation between diseased organs (visceral diseases) and spinal segmental levels of sympathetic involvement.[5] A dissection of 50 cadavers from the University of Pennsylvania found, "In general, the ordinary diseases of adult life." The author's theory was that the sympathetic nerves going to the organs were irritated by spinal curves that increased sympathetic tone, increased vaso-motor spasm (arterial spasm) and reduced blood flow. "The spine becomes stiff first and old age follows." The author described the process of spondylosis (vertebral malfunction) as the interdependent misalignment of the sacroiliac joint combined with lateral curves of the lumbar spine. The stages of this process of subluxation degeneration were described in the 1970s by doctors Felesia and Riekman in their Renaissance Seminars, (see Appendix: "Spinal Decay").

> *"It is known that a primary segmental dysfunction of the locomotive apparatus can cause referred pain in the inner organs (Schwartz, 1974). The reverse is also observed, that is, diseases of inner organs can reflexo-genically induce tendomyotic changes (somato-visceral, viscerosomatic reflexes)."*
>
> Korr 1975, Beal 1984

A healthy intervertebral disc is key not only for optimal spinal complex motion, but also for the length of your life. According to a recent 20-year study, there is a strong correlation between losing height and mortality.[6] The disc is made up of two distinct parts. A central ball bearing called the nucleus pulposis allows for all the necessary vertebral complex motions (i.e., flexion, extension, lateral bending and rotation). This places the nuclear material under a tremendous amount of pressure so that it is held in place by 15 to 20 rings of ligaments called the annulus fibrosis. These rings run at alternating thirty-degree angles to provide support and motion. There is a direct blood supply to the discs up until about age 20 at which time the arteries disappear. From that point on the discs get their nutrition by passive inhibition of fluid from the end plates of the vertebral body above and below the disc. So you truly are only as young as your spine is flexible. During the day there is a gradual loss of fluid from the spinal discs to the extent that a person loses an inch of height from the time they get up in the morning until they go to bed at night. That's why a firm mattress is key. Your discs imbibe water as you sleep and your spine lengthens one inch–if you are on a good mattress (see Appendix: "Mattress Matters" p.274).

The strength of the disc is related to its fluid and proteoglycan content. Proteoglycans are molecules composed of a protein attached to a sugar. Proteoglycans are hydrophilic and therefore bind water. These are also known as glycosaminoglycans and include such structures as chondroitin and collagen. These tend to decrease with age and therefore so does the disc water content. Trauma dehydrates the disc leading to degenerative changes by creating a disruption of the disc's glucose supply. Because the disc receives most of its nutrition by diffusion, it is facilitated by spinal motion.[7] Degenerative changes follow fixation with their inflammatory chemicals. Spinal manipulation decreases those inflammatory intermediates, reversing the manifestation of inflammation. Motion is life.

"More than 85% of patients who present to their primary care provider have low back pain that cannot reliably be attributed to a specific disease or spinal abnormality."
Roger Chou, MD, et al., Annals of Internal Medicine, Oct 2007

As illustrated, the challenge technique may quickly and accurately detect intervertebral discs that are in trouble. This technology may also be used to monitor the recovery—or lack thereof—as both a clinical guidepost and patient motivator. (see: Appendix illustration, p.264).

Collagen is the most widely distributed proteoglycan throughout the human body. Vitamin C is necessary for its production in human beings, who along with a few other species (bats, guinea pigs, gorillas) lost their ability to make vitamin C. Oxidative stress depletes vitamin C, which increases degenerative diseases of all types. The free radical cause of disease is scientifically proven for all degenerative diseases. Spine diseases are no different. As a matter of fact, disease in either the facet joints or the disc is not reliably correlated with age. These two areas are richly innervated with pain nerve endings and once injured are the source of chronic pain.[8] It is interesting to note that neurologists look for problems with the trunk flexors with the deep tendon reflex (which tests the anterior primary rami out of the spinal cord). The posterior primary rami is what innervates the facets and the muscles that control the spine. This is a good example of looking for pathology (severely compressed motor nerve roots) versus segmented dysfunction (a functionally abnormal position). The ability to identify and remove disc compression and facet imbrication with the "challenge" is a godsend.

These tools enabled an in-depth understanding of the body's adaptation or lack thereof from stress and trauma to ensue. The combination of postural analysis, challenge, adjustment, muscle isolation, testing and correction proved to be incredible assets to the tool kit of the PAK™ providers. The idea of the web-like nature of the body's inter-connectedness permeated the developments in PAK™, creating a truly layered and unique approach to health and function. A couple soft tissue examples readily come to mind. The first is the skin and its receptors. The skin is one of our largest organs, forming a protective barrier that also serves to maintain our fluid matrix and body temperature. It also serves as the conductor of our movement symphony.

For example, if you are sitting and your right ankle itches you simply reach down with your right arm and scratch the area. In order for this to happen, the skin on your right shoulder stretches and communicates to the underlying muscles (via a local spinal cord pathway), "Hey team, we are moving so you need to relax." The shoulder muscles relax in concert as you bend and reach your ankle. A robust symphony has just occurred and all is well, as all the concert players performed as they should. An abrasive injury, like the repetitive carrying of a heavy bag with a shoulder strap on your right, could set you up for a right shoulder problem. As the shoulder strap rubs the skin it activates the stretch reflex causing it to get stuck in a feed-forward pattern. This is probably due to a crushing of the local cellular cytoskeletons into a pattern from which they can't spring back. This results in a constant inhibition of the underlying muscles, which, until found and corrected, may be major contributors to areas of chronic body dysfunction. Once identified, aberrant skin receptors are readily corrected with motion in an up-down, left-right sequence to reset them.

A second example is the internal skin or fascial connection that exists to connect the body as a whole. Everyone has a layer of contiguous fascia that helps form our extra-cellular matrix and another whole system of communication. This closed system has been found to create circuit breakers—termed stress receptors—in areas separate from and at a distance from the area that is complaining. When a muscle suffers from overuse or trauma, a related area of fascia on the head or hands may develop a wrinkle or lump. These wrinkles, or stress receptors, act like a circuit breaker and represent a twist in the fascia (think local extra-cellular matrix adhesion or strain) that literally turns off the related muscles. These need to be accurately and firmly massaged to reset the aberrant muscle-fascia circuitry to an uncompensated and fully functional state. These receptors act as deep balancing centers to promote full function at all costs and are one reason that deep muscle therapy on a regular basis is so important.

> *"When educational intelligence can communicate with innate intelligence, a point at which the not-too-distant future may hold, then a correct diagnosis and treatment will be made and rendered."*
> DD Palmer
> Son of the founder of Chiropractic Medicine, B. J. Palmer

The current footprint of the International College of Applied Kinesiology (ICAK) is global. The original ICAK chapter founded in the US now has chapters in Australia, Austria, Benelux, Brazil, Canada, France, Germany, Italy, Korea, Russia, Sweden, Switzerland and the United Kingdom. PAK™ today is practiced mostly by medical doctors outside the US. It is recognized as a medical specialty in Austria. Due to its reliability and cost effectiveness, PAK™ is poised to revolutionize healthcare, along with FM, as the fastest growing integrative medical specialties today.

Acupuncture became integrated into PAK™; the relationship between the internal glands and organs of the body to the external muscle groups opened up whole new vistas. Attitude or body-mind balance was one of the key branches of the web that became partially unglued with the solidification of the relationship between specific emotions and acupuncture meridians. The body has 12 paired flows of electromagnetic energy called acupuncture meridians or meridians for short. Every two hours the energy or "chi" shifts from one meridian to another so that in a 24-hour period the energy flows throughout the entire system. The function of this system is to nourish the organ and glandular systems with electromagnetic energy. Recent research[9] has shown that this cellular signaling system runs along specific deep tissue planes, helping us to understand another reason that proper body alignment impacts both the coherence and flow of information.

Dr. John Diamond, an Australian psychiatrist, discovered and developed the specific emotional correlates to the specific meridians. Understanding and treating the specific emotional components associated with disease causation and promulgation with easy, non-invasive methods was born. The implications of this were not lost to Dr. Goodheart, who felt Dr. Diamond's work was one of the biggest breakthroughs ever in PAK™. His work provided a fertile basis for the use of PAK™ in evaluating and treating the emotional correlates of disease (outlined in *Meridians and Their Emotions;* see Appendix: "Meridians and Their Emotions"). The Neuro-emotional Techniques (NET) was further developed and is taught through the work of Dr. Scott Walker.

Dr. Roger Callahan carried this work into the field of psychotherapy, where it has virtually exploded. Dawson Church, PhD, elegantly describes the recent research in epigenetic medicine and the new biology of intention in his book *The Genie in Your Genes: Epigenetic Medicine and the New Biology of Intention.*

> *"Above all else, it seems to me that it is our role as human beings always to join learning to loving-kindness. Learning to learn, learning to love, and to be kind are so closely connected and so profoundly interwoven, especially with the sense of touch, it would greatly help our rehumanization if we could pay close attention to the need we all have for tactual experience."*
> Ashley Montague

At the same time as this work was unfolding, Dr. Candace Pert, chief of brain biochemistry at the National Institutes of Health was busy mapping out the new human physiology—the Body Mind Field—that served to provide a molecular basis that both reinforced and further expanded these PAK™ findings. She discovered the cellular receptor for the body's own morphine called endorphin. This is the cause of the well known "runner's high." The substances made by our bodies that alter our moods are known as neuropeptides. Each has a specific receptor on the cell membrane to deliver its specific message. These receptors are capable of changing shape, thus affecting the ion channels they are associated with as well as changing their location.

All of our cells are intelligent entities that have two to three million receptor docking sites on their cell membranes for the two to three hundred informational substances found in our bodies. Mind can now be understood as the constantly changing flow of molecular information at the level of cell membranes. "Emotions are the link between the spiritual realm and the physical realm," says Dr. Pert in her audio book, *"Your Body is Your Subconscious Mind."* [10] She encourages bodywork to keep your Body Mind—which she likens to a field—unstuck and flowing for greater well being. The concept of getting and keeping your body tuned-up is one key to vibrant health. Dr. Pert says, "When you mind the body, you mend the mind."

One concrete example of the "unstuck" aspect with respect to overall health that we should all be aware of is our heart rate variability. A healthy heart rate is chaotic, representing a dynamic range, with lots of neurotransmitters and neuropeptides being simultaneously expressed. Increases in heart rate variability are associated with "in sync" autonomic nervous system branches. So when the sympathetic and parasympathetic divisions are not fighting one another, this state is called entrainment. Recent research has shown that chiropractic adjustments increase heart rate variability,[11] which is a really good thing since low heart rate variability is predictive of mortality from all causes.[12]

The fact that organs and glands shared the same stem cell origin as muscles added another important layer of diagnostic information to PAK™. Although separated by distance and function, external muscle groups and internal organs and glands still share the same coaxial cable. This means that they share the same nerve supply, blood supply, lymphatic or waste matter drainage and the same electromagnetic circuits or acupuncture meridians. A provider may evaluate a patient's digestive, endocrine, immune, and hepato-bilary (liver-gallbladder) systems by isolating and testing external muscle groups to find potential red flags in their Web of Wellness (AM J Path;2008 Nov;173(5) 1243-52).

"We are our own Genetic Engineers"
Rob Rakowsky, DC

In essence, PAK™ provides a quick non-invasive way to fine tune the individual's predisposition to incipient problems in key areas of the Web of Wellness so that they may be quickly resolved. The Four R program for gastro-intestinal health may be delivered in a manner that is both accurate and cost effective. For example, in practice, the restoration of balance usually results in significant improvements in short order, bypassing the need for more expensive treatments. This is not to say that comprehensive stool, digestive and parasite testing is never done, but that it may be used more judiciously. You can think of the PAK™ approach as a layered one, where the areas of greatest need in the patient's story are addressed first. In this way low cost treatment (e.g., a digestive enzyme) may be administered first, with its larger return on investment prior to the use of more expensive approaches with their inherent collateral damage. Allowing time for "the smoke to clear" gives the more difficult to approach problems time to surface. It's a kind of "active watchful waiting," says Dr. Goodheart and "Treatment helps define the diagnosis."

STRUCTURE/ FUNCTION TAKE AWAY:

One of the most common downstream effects of a cranial stress MAP—regardless of whether the cause is trauma, infection, poor nutrition or electro-magnetic—is a functional compression of the vagus nerve at its exit from the skull just behind the jaw joints at the occipito-mastoid sutures. Reduction of the cranial stress MAP provides instant up-regulation of the functional deficits created by the vagus nerve dysfunction. It is part of the reset button from allostatic load to allostasis.

In my clinical experience, the typical stressed individual will show a reproducible pattern of imbalance. The majority will have an inhibition of the stomach related muscles (the pectoralis major-clavicular division). This coincides with a diminished production of hydrochloric acid, the chief digestive enzyme of the stomach. This is usually abolished with insalivation of betaine-hydrochloride and/or zinc. The reason for this is the high energy requirement for the production of this enzyme, along with prolonged stress and poor eating lifestyle habits depleting both of these and slowing the parasympathetics necessary for its formation. Zinc is needed for the production of this enzyme (and about 300 others including superoxide dismutase (SOD) used to neutralize free radicals from environmental chemicals). It is in high demand and short supply for two reasons: It is not appreciably stored in the body for more than a day or two, so a very nutrient dense diet or regular supplementation is required; and second, the carcinogen most present by molecular weight (10,000 times greater than all others) are pthlates or plasticizers, which use up the body's zinc stores. A less common consequence of low zinc levels is inhibition of the muscles associated with the pancreas (the latisimus dorsi). Research has shown that induced zinc deficiency took four generations to replete in test animals! Sometimes this weakness will be negated with insalivation of the stomach's digestive enzyme, betaine hydrochloride.

"In 1969 the United States Department of Agriculture found that only 17 out of 50 states had adequate amounts of zinc in their agricultural soil. Until zinc and other essential nutrients are restored to optimal levels in all agricultural soils throughout these United States, there will be an increasing requirement for supplemental zinc to ensure better health."

Dr. Jonathan Wright, *Nutrition and Healing*, June 2007

The stomach and pancreas are paired digestive organs, so supporting one often enhances the other. On occasion, the individual will need pancreatic enzymes to boost function. I have seen patients diagnosed with chronic pancreatitis respond beautifully to up-regulation of the stomach with the use of betaine hydrochloride. The guesswork to determine when to replace stomach acid or pancreatic enzymes is replaced with a straightforward answer from the Manual Muscle Test (MMT).

Further down the digestive tract, the next organ system we encounter is the small intestine with its tennis court size of absorptive area. This 23-foot tube is lined with millions of micro-villae, at the base of which is a pore that lets digested foods into our portal venous system to be carried to our liver to be utilized for body functions. The related muscles are the abdominals and the quadriceps. Inhibition of these muscle groups is associated with diminished function of the small intestine as well as your low back and knees.

"In my studies from looking at what we know about Round-up, it's a potentially powerful inducer of lymphomas and leukemias. This is being ignored because of the massive money made by Monsanto, the maker and leader in the industry of GMO foods."

Russell Blaylock, MD, *Bombshell*, S. Somers page 189

Impaired hydrochloric acid production by the stomach leads to undigested food passing into the lining of the small intestine and this over time sets a person up for food sensitivities. The undigested food acts to congest the lymphatic drainage of this huge system resulting in a reduction of some of its key functions—namely nutrient absorption and detoxification. Bacterial overgrowth may lead to intestinal biofilms that may constrict or partially block the emptying of the common bile duct (gallbladder/pancreas). Small intestine congestion may create inflammation and congestion in the sinuses as they share common embryological origin. There is also an intricate world of bacterial species necessary for both normal intestinal and sinus function which science is really just beginning to appreciate.

In addition to congestion with undigested foods fueling sensitivity to these foods, a small intestine with an unbalanced biome (collection of bacteria, molds and viruses) creates the environment for bacterial and mold overgrowth. Mold overgrowth is fueled by its presence in grains, the overuse of antibiotics in the animal husbandry field, and the fact that 25% of all buildings in this country are water damaged[13] and contain mold. The integrity of the small intestine's barrier is reduced, allowing large macro-molecules to pass through the pores which fuels systemic or body-wide inflammation. Genetically modified foods, present now in 90% of our processed foods, rip open the gut lining due to the presence of insecticides. It is the loss of this barrier's integrity that fuels auto-immune disease and cardiovascular disease. Cardiologist Dr. Marc Houston states that if you don't heal your gut, you'll never heal your arteries. Inflammation in the gut leads to inflammation in the brain, promoting neurodegenerative changes as well.

Four significant reflex points have proven over the years to be effective with respect to answering the remove and repair aspects of the Four R program. One point, halfway between the lower sternum (Xiphoid) and the right nipple, signifies liver overload problems secondary to ongoing food and/or mold sensitivities. Inhibition of an intact muscle while touching this point (a positive therapy localization) indicates a need to look at the integrity of the small intestine to determine whether antigen-antibody complexes or endotoxins are stressing the liver. A positive therapy localization to the umbilicus is indictative of a small intestine mold overgrowth. Potential anti-fungals may be tested here for efficacy. Point number three lies one inch medial to the upper part of the left hip bone (the anterior superior iliac spine) and when positive may indicate a parasitic infection. Once again, potential anti-parasitic compounds may be evaluated here.

The next reflex point lies approximately three inches from the umbilicus on a line towards the liver (at 10 o'clock). This is indicative of a leaky gut and a need to repair the integrity of the small intestine lining. The more current term "metabolic endotoxemia" is now replacing leaky gut as it better describes the panoply of systemic effects.

> "We now know that most autoimmune diseases are caused by and/or perpetuated by chronic infections, food allergies, a pro-inflammatory lifestyle, hormonal imbalances, and exposure to chemicals and metals that cause immune dysfunction. When the cause(s) of the disease is treated, the disease is cured. When the disease is cured, lifelong medicalization becomes unnecessary, the patient is free to fully resume his/her life, and doctors are liberated from their roles as drug representatives and can resume their proper positions as healers."
>
> Alex Vasquez, DC, ND, *Chiropractic Management of Chronic Hypertension*, page 84

To my knowledge, this has yet to be clinically correlated with a positive lactulose-mannitol test, which is the "gold standard" diagnostic test for a leaky gut. This is high on our "to do" list (see Appendix: "Key Gastroinestinal and Immune Function Areas" p.281). Familiarize yourself with these areas, get them treated and keep them monitored for your own health and well being.

The pectoralis major–sternal division is the liver-related muscle. Abnormal inhibition here signals a lack of optimal liver function. The reflex point for ongoing food and mold sensitivities lies over the anterior liver, halfway between the lower sternum (xiphoid) and the sternum. This frequently coexists with a leaky gut and is usually indicative of a need for more of the key nutrients necessary for detoxification. Specific products designed to up-regulate these pathways are indicated and with the toxic world we live in, should be used on a regular basis (see Appendix: "Key Gastrointestinal and Immune Function Areas" p.281). Your ongoing health and high levels of energy depend on optimal function here.

STRUCTURE/ FUNCTION TAKE AWAY:

The diaphragm works as a commutator pump which activates the electromagnetic flow of energy in the extra-cellular matrix. Pelvic spinal MAPs create functional hiatal hernias that grossly down-regulate the flow of energy in your acupuncture meridians. This may result in reflux symptoms, and reduces the flow of chi and with it the intelligence of your energy field.

The gallbladder-related muscle is the popliteus, a small muscle at the posterior aspect of the knee. A bilateral weakness of this muscle together with pain on palpation to the gallbladder (a positive Murphy's test) suggests gallbladder dysfunction. The use of lipotrophic (fat mobilizing) agents in foods, like beets and their greens or concentrated beets (betaine), Vitamin C, taurine and phosphatidyl choline are other lipotrophic agents. Metagenics Lipogen or Standard Process AF Betafood work wonders here.

There are three areas of diagnostic challenges relating to the gross structural function of the gastrointestinal tract you really need to know about so that they can be diagnosed and treated promptly and correctly. One involves the stomach and the other two the large intestine. The term hiatal hernia refers to a strain of the stomach up through the opening for the esophagus. Like anything else in the body that goes wrong this may create zero to catastrophic symptoms. At the low end of the spectrum a person may experience low energy and at the high end life-altering heart burn and upper abdominal pain. It has been my clinical experience that the majority of functional hiatal hernias may be successfully corrected with a full body tune-up. This basically balances the feet and pelvis, removes spasm of the psoas muscles that contract secondary to the sacroiliac sprain, which created the situation to begin with by pulling the diaphragm downwards. This must be accompanied with proper patient education and lifestyle change when necessary (e.g., not eating a meal less than two or three hours before going to bed).

> *"I am convinced we can seriously lower the incidence of adverse food sensitivity related health problems with the combined use of optimal prebiotic with probiotic, but I do not believe that there is a probiotic product that will implant so efficiently that we can stop taking it. The chemicals in our water, food and air are in our intestine and they will continue to alter the flora."*
>
> Dr. Gary Gordon, President, Gordon Research Institute

The ileocecal valve (ICV) is a true sphincter valve that separates the end of the small intestine (ileum) from the beginning of the large intestine (cecum). Located in the right lower abdominal quadrant, this valve opens to allow the gastrointestinal contents to pass from the end of the small intestine into the colon. I use the analogy of going from the dining room into the pantry for processing before removal, as one of the functions of the large intestine is to remove water to make solid waste. The ileo-cecal valve (as the pantry door) should open and close on a regular basis as needed. Problems crop up when the valve malfunctions and gets stuck closed (a closed or spastic ICV) or open (an open ICV). Constipation and auto-toxicity are the respective problems. Abdominal pain is often not consciously present. You must be tested by a skilled provider. Correction of the spinal-related segments (L3) leads to a quick and lasting fix.

At the end of the large intestine in the lower left quadrant is a thickening of the muscular wall (taenia-coli) in the sigmoid section (think plumbing under your sink) as the descending colon ends at the rectum. This ileo-colic area may spasm and create pain or intestinal malfunction as well. Once again, correct identification leads to quick and lasting elimination of symptoms. This is usually created by dysfunction at L4 (anterior) and may reflect a need for more iron.

The use of the MMT to test for food, mold and chemical sensitivities has been successfully utilized. Research has substantiated a clinically significant correlation to foods that tested positive upon salivation with those found in IGG blood tests.[14] The official teaching of this methodology involves the actual insalivation of the substance to be tested. Innovations such as the work of Dr. Michael Lebowitz have utilized a ceramic magnet, by passing the gustatory receptors in the mouth and directly challenging substances against the body's electro-magnetic field. Based on the work of Dr. William Philpott, the south pole of a magnet pushes the vibratory field of the substance being tested into the energy field of the patient. The net result is that any substance creating an immune system stress results in the tested muscle becoming inhibited. I have utilized this method for many years and have seen great clinical results.

The usefulness of drug sensitivity testing under a magnet provides a safe method to screen for adverse drug reactions or ADRs. It is my belief that accelerated research validation in this area will provide enormous returns on investment. Your chance of an ADR is too great to be treated in any other way. The teaching of this skill set to all those who prescribe should be priority one.

MMT, when correctly integrated, has the potential to create the greatest return on investment of anything ever seen in modern medicine. This is true especially if you consider that by their own admission, drug manufacturers know their drugs are hit or miss, working only half the time. Until genomic profiling is in full gear, don't play pharma roulette. Bring your medications to a PAK™ provider near you and request that they test them for potential sensitivity. This one step may save your life or the life of someone you love.

> Vaccines "have little or no effect. We've got an exaggerated expectation of what vaccines can actually do. I'm hoping American and European taxpayers will be alerted and start asking questions."
> Dr. Tom Jefferson is coordinator of the Cochrane Vaccines Field, Rome, Italy.

> "Improved nutrition, stress management techniques, walking and psychosocial support actually changed the expression of over 500 genes."
> Dean Ornish, MD

Using the thymus-related muscle, the infraspinatus, is helpful in establishing an accurate differential diagnosis for the answer to the question of bacterial versus viral as it relates to the cause of infection. We know that antibiotics are overused and this is in no small way due to the fact that no quick test has been developed to test for viral versus bacterial infections. The return to optimal function for an inhibited infraspinatous with insalivation of an antiviral like olive leaf extract, lauric acid or virex (a Nutriwest product) has created a very reproducible, favorable outcome for many of my patients. Once again research in this area is desperately needed, as are providers skilled in this art to apply this new science.

Viral infections are a big problem that are not adequately dealt with in our current medical mainstream. Several examples quickly come to mind. The common cold is a viral-induced illness that has an enormous amount of antibiotics inappropriately thrown at it. The Epstein-Barr virus (EBV), causative agent of both mononucleosis and some cases of high blood pressure, quickly succumbs to the naturally occurring antiviral lauric acid. Although in the literature for decades, this information remains hidden. Alzheimer's Disease has been recently found to be directly associated with a herpes 1 viral infection, which 90% of the population carries (think cold sore or fever blister). The fact that the brain has levels of vitamin C that are almost fifteen times higher than they are outside the brain is good to know.[15] Vitamin C contributes to the manufacture of several neurotransmitters including acetylcholine, dopamine and norepinephrine. It is a potent anti-viral and most kids and adults are chronically low in it. As mentioned earlier, it is also necessary for the formation of bile in the liver to emulsify fats and remove wastes. Linus Pauling tried to show heart disease was no more than a chronic depletion of vitamin C from the arterial walls. Dr. Tom Levy's books, *Curing the Incurable* and *Stop America's Number One Killer*, cover this and do an excellent job of elucidating other aspects of vitamin C.

> "Depression is considered the leading cause of disability in the US, according to the National Institutes of Health, but only a relatively small percentage of Americans receive adequate treatment for the condition. In a recent survey of 16,000 households in the US, half of these with clinical depression received no treatment at all, and only 21% of Americans receive care consistent with the American Psychiatric Association Guidelines."
>
> Andrew Cusco, PhD
> Duke Health News, March 2010

The human pappiloma virus (HPV) is another common viral infection causing genital warts and cervical cancer. It's estimated to infect 15 to 40% of the adult population in the United States with one million new cases per year. The successful use of Indole 3-carbinol, [16,17,18] folic acid,[19-24] epigallatocatechingallate,[25] and vitamin A[26-29] are well documented. The CDC's website reveals significant side effects from the HPV vaccine. The center received a total of 18,727 reports of adverse events following Gardisil HPV vaccination, with 1,498 of them (8%) considered "serious," such as the neurological disorder Guillain-Barre Syndrome, blood clots and 84 reports of death. Diane Harper, MD, professor and vice-chair of research at the University of Missouri-Kansas City

School of Medicine, was the principal investigator for clinical trials for both Merck (maker of Gardisil) and GlaxoSmithKline (maker of Cervorix). Research by her team found that the incidence of cervical cancer in the United States (3.0 per 100,000 women) is actually lower than the incidence of adverse effects from the vaccine that's supposed to protect against it (4.3 per 100,000). This is an unacceptable risk-to-benefit ratio.

> *"Probiotics and prebiotics, by balancing the intestinal microbial population, have powerful immune-stimulating properties. Zinc supplementation fights immune senescence by enhancing the appropriate cytokine signaling to mobilize response to infection. Sulfur-containing anti-oxidants such as N-acetylcysteins help replenish the body's stores of natural anti-oxidants."*
>
> *Lisa Antone*

> *Vaccination is Not Immunization by Dr. Tim O'Shea is a thought-provoking book on the vaccine controversy (www.thedoctorwithin.com).*

There are a few basic nutrients whose need may be revealed by the MMT. If every muscle tested appears inhibited, the patient may be grossly dehydrated. Of course just having the person open their mouth, putting a finger to the tongue and looking at the finger to see if it glistens, is a quick and easy way to check hydration status. A good thing to know is what to do if a person drinks a good amount of water yet still indicates a need for more. This may show as inhibited muscles (especially GI tract related) or as a low hydration on a BIA measurement. This may occur if the person is not consuming enough salt. Sodium chloride is essential for proper fluid balance. A good sea salt like Celtic Salt may be all that is needed.

Multiple muscle fatigue after two or three contractions has been correlated with a lack of essential fatty acids. This stems from one of several causes: either the person is not taking them in or fails to digest and absorb them or both. Current knowledge is that we have to have both essential fatty acids—omega 6 and omega 3s — daily in a four to one ratio to have good health, which directly stems from optimal cell membrane function.[30,31]

> *"One of the first duties of the physician is to educate the masses not to take medicine."*
>
> *Sir William Osler, aphorisms from his bedside*

Since the mid 1990s when this ratio was conclusively proven, organic sunflower oil and organic flax oil at the preferred 4:1 ratio has been distributed by Body Bio (www.bodybio.com). You have to be able to digest and absorb these fats to utilize them as well. The repetitive muscle test showing positive here is a window into this system. Appropriate steps to evaluate your dietary habits, intestinal inhabitants and gallbladder function are in order.

Muscle inhibition after the tapping of a joint—the shock absorber test—signifies a lack of trace minerals (e.g., like zinc, copper, chromium and manganese) necessary for ligament stability. The use of a good multi–vitamin mineral to replete the body's mineral need is indicated.

The inhibition of muscles after being stretched has been shown to correlate with either a low normal or slightly below normal level of Red Blood Cell Magnesium (see Appendix: "Tricks to Keep a Positive Magnesium Status" p.285).

The supra spinatous muscle is the only muscle that has shown on electromyography to fire 24/7. It is the brain-related muscle and is commonly inhibited in those experiencing sleep disorders, mild depression, cognitive dysfunction or other brain-based illnesses. Nutrients to improve brain function may be screened in this way. Recent research at Harvard Medical School and Massachusetts General Hospital[32] was funded by the National Institute of Mental Health. This double-blind, placebo-controlled trial evaluated SAMe (s-adenosylmethionine) as an adjunctive therapy in those suffering major depression who were resistant to FDA-approved drugs. Those receiving SAMe had double the response rate and remission when compared to placebo.

The teres minor, muscles located in the rotator cuffs of our shoulders, relate to the thyroid gland and may be found to be inhibited bilaterally. Often an iodine-containing supplement will be helpful here. Care must be taken to rule out an auto-immune thyroid problem (with blood tests for the key thyroid antibodies, thyroid peroxidase and anti–thyroglobulin), because giving more iodine to those patients will worsen their problems. According to Datis Kharrazian, DC, in his book *Why Do I Still Have Thyroid Symptoms? When My Lab Tests Are Normal: A revolutionary breakthrough in understanding Hashimoto's disease and hypothyroidism,* a remarkable 27 million Americans suffer from thyroid gland dysfunction. More than half of these are caused by to an auto-immune disorder called Hashimotos disease. Dr. Kharrazian's well written and researched text clearly delineates the thyroid's web-like relationship to gastrointestinal (bacteria), adrenal function, hydrochloric acid production, brain chemistry and liver detoxification.

The gastrocnemius and sartorius are two adrenal-related muscles that may reveal imbalances to this key stress-handling endocrine gland. The state of the function of the adrenal glands may be further ascertained with the Ragland blood pressure test. A person's blood pressure is taken with them lying down and then again standing after a one-minute equilibration period. A healthy response from lying to standing is an increased systolic (1st number) blood pressure of 8-10 mm Hg pressure. A flat line or dropping systolic number indicates a weakened or exhausted state. When the adrenal related muscles are inhibited, various adaptogens or vitamins and minerals may be found to improve or facilitate the related muscles, signifying up regulation of these endocrine glands.

> *"Basically, when intuition and the heart are united, even for a short period of time, miracles occur. At a deep, subconscious level, the greatest suppressed fear inside conventional medicine is that there might be something safe and simple that works! Suppose, just suppose, that all of these alternatives work as well as or better than drugs or surgery and without potential side effects?"*
>
> C. Norman Shealy, MD, PhD, *Medical Intuition*, page 60

Salivary testing for the adrenal glands may also be performed with a test called the adrenal-stress index panel. This is a four-point salivary cortisol measurement (8AM, 12PM, 6PM,11PM), along with dihydroepiandosterane (dhea). Your doctor can get this test through Diagnos Techs (www.diagnostechs. com). It is called the adrenal stress index test (ASI). This test may accurately indicate the adaptive status of the adrenal gland whether healthy, alarm, resistive or exhausted and thus guide treatment.

There is another very important way that PAK™ may help to identify a malfunctioning adrenal system. Dr. Goodheart made the observation that both the adrenal glands and the ligaments at either end of the spine (occiput-C1 and sacro-iliac) had similar responses to staining with a specific chemical. This indicated a shared embryological relationship to their development, which clinically has stood the test of time. One clue to malfunctioning adrenals that otherwise may not be found is instability in the spine at the upper neck or low back areas. The body sometimes is very good about hiding the actual cause of a problem, but with an increased awareness of the body's intricate interrelationships these may be uncovered.

I recently had a very fit patient who had acutely injured his low back after having lifted weights in a gym, and then going home and bending forward to pick up a piece of paper. Careful checking of the digestive, nutritional and endocrine reflexes revealed no particular cause. All the adrenal related reflexes and muscles were facilitated. It was not until the patient touched his adrenal lymphatic reflex point and I simultaneously touched his upper neck ligaments that this weakness was found, which subsequently allowed him to adequately heal his low back problem. Our bodies certainly are intricately simple and simply intricate!

Equally potent as chemical cues, mechanical forces serve as important regulators at the cell and molecular levels. Every cell has its own filamentous cytoskeleton as well as its surface membrane, intracellular organelles and nucleus. "Recent insights into cellular mechanotransduction—the molecular mechanism by which cells sense and respond to mechanical stress—reveals that a wide range of diseases included within virtually all fields of medicine and surgery share a common feature: their etiology or clinical presentation results from abnormal mechanotransduction."[33] Recent understanding from the field of cellular structural physiology reveals one intensely interconnected field of cellular membranes. "Tissues are composed of groups of living cells held together by an extracellular matrix (ECM) comprised of a network of collagens, glycoproteins, and proteoglycans."[34] Cells adhere to ECM through the binding of cell surface receptors known as "integrins." These appear to function as cell surface "mechanoreceptors" in that they are among the first molecules to sense a mechanical stress applied at the cell surface.

"Blood vessels of the cranial dura mater are the most pain sensitive intracranial structures. The biochemical origin of pain 'the origin of all pain is inflammation and the inflammatory response.'"

Soto Omoigui
Medical Hypothesis 2007

Mechanical forces are translated into chemical signals. They transmit this signal across the plasma membrane to the cell's cytoskeleton. These, in turn, are transmitted to the cellular organelles and chromosomes to manufacture proteins. A healthy cell membrane, when appropriately stimulated, orchestrates protein synthesis for matrix metalloproteinases and all other regulatory proteins. These create and maintain structural integrity, maintaining the body's blood brain, periodontal and gastrointestinal barriers.

Cell-generated tensional forces appear to play a central role in the development of virtually all living tissues, even in neural tissues such as retina and brain. Mechanical stress to integrins may eventually lead to changes in gene transcription and govern other cellular behavior regardless of the presence of hormones or other regulatory factors. The correct amount of motion stimulates ground substance (extracellular matrix), organizes collagen and increases collagen. Abnormal mechanotransduction may act as a common denominator for many ostensibly unrelated diseases. Physical medicine in the form of chiropractic adjustments, muscle balancing, postural correction, acupuncture and massage therapy have well known therapeutic value because they alter mechanotransduction and cell signaling. They flood the cerebellum with signals that amplify the healing response of the parasympathetic nervous system.

Expanding out from the cellular level to that of the whole body, we can now begin to appreciate how alignment or lack thereof creates such a basic component of health or disease. Only by understanding the normal function of the human body can we appreciate what goes wrong and become more aware of the best ways to proactively care for ourselves.

As complex as the human body is, by looking at the four key areas that are the pillars of body tensegrity/geometry, we can readily understand and care for our body. The four key nodal areas are the cranial complex, the pelvic-spinal complex, and upper and lower extremities. Each of these complexes has core functions that are intimately interrelated. Let's answer three key questions: What are these complexes? What are their job descriptions? How does stress/trauma effect them? Knowledge builds confidence and confidence enhances self-responsibility.

"I was taught in osteopathic medical school that by the time we reach puberty (at the very latest), all the bones of the skull are fused solidly together. It is as though we have one solid bone on top of our necks, except for our lower jaws (which continue to move) and the tiny bones in our middle ear cavities (which vibrate and move in response to various sounds). In other words, at my present age, my head should essentially be solid like a coconut shell with my brain inside of it. This is simply not so. Our research at Michigan State University (1975-1982) did indeed prove beyond any doubt that skull bones continue to move throughout normal life."

John E Upledger, DO

There are 22 bones that make up the skull or cranial complex. This complex may be divided into two catagories: the vault bones, which have a direct association with the brain (or the dural meningeal tissue that surrounds it) and the face, which includes those indirectly associated with the duramater. The cranial bones are separated from one another by articular seams known as sutures.

"For years anatomists believed that sutures functioned as primary growth regions of the skull and only served to hold the skull together. However recent studies suggest another important function for sutures: they permit independent cranial motion throughout the skull."[35] When the sutures are viewed under an electron microscope, the observant eye can see that they are clearly built for motion with an intricate network of nerves and arteries. One example of the functional aspect of the cranial sutures is that of the bull elk. When bull elk fight, their heads are down so that they can battle to become the dominant or alpha bull. However, when they run through the thick aspen trees they tilt their heads back and the moveable suture at the top of their skulls allows their rack to fold in to clear their way through dense trees.

Due to the attachments of the dural membranes and the functional shape of the sutures between the cranial bones, they move in a predictable sequence that allows for not only production and distribution of cerebrospinal fluid, but also optimal function of the neuroendocrine axis, which is where the brain folds in upon itself and becomes the endocrine system. This area is located in the middle of your brain just a few inches behind your eyes. The pituitary, hypothalamus and pineal make up the neuroendocrine axis which is also referred to as the hypothalamic pituitary adrenal (HPA) axis. There are four hollow areas in your brain called ventricles—two lateral ones, a third and fourth one. This is where cerebrospinal fluid (CSF) is made by the ultrafiltration of blood. These ventricles are tucked away, up inside the middle of our brains, alongside and in the middle of our neuroendocrine axis. This intimate structural relationship ensures easy access for the informational substances made by the neuroendocrine glands to the CSF for instantaneous delivery throughout the body.

"There is universal agreement that 50-75% of patients with major depression exhibit hyperactivity of the HPA axis."

J Clin Psychiatry; 1989 May 50 Supp 13-20

In at least 40% of depression cases in older people, an underlying physical disorder can be causing or exacerbating the depression.

How to Use Herbs, Nutrients and Yoga in Mental Healthcare
Richard Brown, MD, Patricia Gerberg, MD

The dural membranes tighten when we inhale due to their attachments around the brain with extension throughout in the entire spinal column. This has the effect of lifting the brain and filling the ventricles with CSF. As we exhale the spinal curves reform, relaxing the dural membranes, propulsing the CSF out of the brain, down the spinal cord and out along the nerve roots of the spine. From here it travels along spaces in our nerves to the organs and tissues that the nerves supply.

The central gear train mechanism in the cranial complex is known as the spheno-basilar mechanism. The occipital bone at the base of the our skull has a hole in it (the foramen magnum or the grand opening) for the brain and spinal cord to extend down through.

"The semiconductor properties of the connective tissue acting in resonance have a speed and power that far transcends other signaling mechanisms."

Dawson Church, PhD, *The Genie in Your Genes*

The occipital bone is what actually sits on the top of our spine. The first cervical vertebrae it rests on is the atlas, named for its action of supporting the globe of our skull. The part of the occiput in front of the foramen magnum is called the basilar portion, and this is the part that attaches to the sphenoid bone (at the spheno-basilar symphysis).

The sphenoid bone is a butterfly-shaped bone that sits behind our eyes. The butterfly's outer wings make up the very touch sensitive areas we know as our temples. There is a saddle that sits on the butterfly's back that is called the turkish saddle or the sella turcica. In this saddle sits the pituitary gland. The gear train mechanism—the sphenobasilar symphysis—rocks up and down with breathing. This creates a forward and backward rocking of the turkish saddle which physically massages the pituitary gland. By its connection to the hypothalamus, pineal and surrounding ventricular system, it helps express the contents of the neurendocrine axis. This motion creates a continuous flow of neuropeptides and neurotransmitters from these master endocrine glands to provide the basis for crucial bodily functions. Our sleep wakefulness, anti-tumor surveillance, reproductive system, stress handling (thyroid/adrenal), mood and structural integrity (collagen strength/ligament tone) are a few examples. It is estimated that the baseline for over 100 physiological parameters emits from this area. Although the motion is only a few hundredths of a millimeter, the downstream effects are profound.

> *"Low back pain (LBP), can be seen as a marker for a change in the health status of an individual with often wide ranging consequences. Recent studies that have evidenced the negatively reinforcing consequences of co-morbid conditions for healthcare costs lead to appreciation of comprehensive management approaches geared to work across chronic illnesses. Nonetheless, the association of LBP with psychiatric medications here supports prior studies that have found an association between mental health and LBP."*
>
> Ashole Nimgade, MD
> "Increased Expenditures for Other Health Conditions After an Incident of Low Back Pain" Spine, (35) 7, pp 769-777, 2010

Stress and trauma may impair the elaborate function of the cranial stress complex, which I refer to as cranial stress maladaptation patterns or MAPs. There are at least seven specific causes of cranial stress MAPs. The first three causes of stress MAPs involve trauma: the first is slipping and falling, hitting your head, or walking into a pole or tree. The second is having an invasive dental procedure, such as a tooth extraction, multiple fillings, a root canal or reconstructive dentistry with crowns, bridgework or implants (an unbalanced bite or malocclusion and missing teeth may also be added to this list. A heavy handed hygienist may adversely stress the cranium, but this is at the low end of causation).

A motor vehicle accident (MVA) is the third trauma that leads to cranial stress MAPs. Even in a low-speed 3 to 5 miles per hour collision where there is little or no vehicle damage, the momentum of the vehicles is exponentially multiplied into the soft tissues of the occupant's head, neck and spine. These accidents lead to dysregulations of the hypothalamic-pituitary-adrenal (HPA) axis with the physiological substrate of chronic pain and fatigue.[36] Currently 1 out of 8 people seeks emergency room (ER) care for falls and MVAs annually. Having up-to-date information and knowing the best way to proactively correct stress MAPs is important for good health.

The other four causes are less direct as you will see. A systemic infection like the flu, urinary tract or sinus infection, is the fourth cause of cranial stress MAPs. Immunological warfare takes precedence over optimal neuromuscular function. A severe cold that settles in the chest with lots of coughing is another potential candidate for a cranial stress MAP in this catagory.

The fifth cause, exposing your head or body to close range electro magnetic fields, will definitely create a cranial stress MAP if given enough time. One of your three neurendocrine glands—your pineal gland—is your global positioning system (GPS). Known by the ancients as the seat of your soul, this gland allows us to differentiate north from south, east and west. This master endocrine gland is very electro-magnetically (EMF) sensitive. Car seat heaters, electric blankets and water bed heaters all work to quietly stress this gland. Cell phones, cordless phones and WIFI in your home or school create radio frequency that may create cranial stress MAPS. The cell phone industry's chief scientist and researcher, Dr. George Carlo, proved that micro-nuclei, the proven precurser to cancer, was beyond a shadow of a doubt, caused by cell phone use. He published his findings in the book *Cell Phones, Invisible Hazards in the Wireless Age in 2001*. Several more studies[37,38,39] have also weighed in reviewing damage done to the brain.

> *"Taken together, the long term epidemiologic data suggest an increased risk of being diagnosed with an ipsilateral brain tumor related to cell phone usage of 10 years or more." There is also "significantly elevated odds for the development of ipsilateral parotid gland tumors among heavy cell phone users."*
>
> Vini G Khuranh, et al. "Cell Phones and brain tumors: A review including the long-term epidemiologic data" *Surgical Neurology*, Sept 2009; 72; pp205-215

In her book *Disconnected*, Devra Davis says, "Mobile phones can take as little as ten minutes to trigger changes in the brain associated with cancer."[40] Recent research shows how cell phone microwaves prevent DNA self-repair.

The sixth and probably most common cause of cranial stress MAPs is chewing food when in need of magnesium since calcium contracts a muscle and magnesium relaxes them. This is in light of the fact of the massive magnesium needs of the population at large. I tell patients chewing food when low in magnesium causes their jaw muscles to act like a winch jamming their cranial sutures together when they chew food. The seventh cause is not producing enough stomach acid even though adequate magnesium is being ingested. Adequate hydrochloric acid is needed to not only digest proteins, but also to cleave the ionic bonds of minerals so that they may be absorbed in the small intestine. Prolonged stress, hot humid weather, eating too fast and not relaxing while eating are guaranteed to create this situation given enough time.

> *"Whether it's called 'energy medicine', electromedicine or something else all together. I believe this is the future of healing. I predict that the growing body of research exploring the relationships between our bodies and various energy sources—both nutritional and environmental—will eventually force the medical establishment to become more holistic in how it treats disease."*
>
> Dr. Stephen Sinatra, *Heart Health & Nutrition*, March 2010

About 20 years ago, a woman came to the office for the treatment of acute sciatia neuralgia and was profusely weeping throughout the entire visit. She had ongoing deep melancholy that she described as "Empty Nest Syndrome." Evidently she had been like this for over a year since her youngest child had left the house to go off to college.

After careful examination and treatment, I advised her to use a flexible ice pack with a moist towel wrapped around it (to decrease pain and improve blood flow to the injured ligaments) at home and return the next day for a follow-up treatment as she had a severe pelvic-spinal stress MAP. To our mutual surprise, the constant weeping had ended. The cranial corrections done the previous day had the effect of bolstering the strength of her adrenal glands, which I knew were intimately associated with the sacroiliac ligaments. The disappearance of the "Empty Nest Syndrome" led to the realization that it was the normal functioning of the neurendocrine axis that gives normal tone to the entire ligamentous system or tree, if you will, of the body.

> *"It's only by focusing on promoting human health that we'll get the kind of healthcare system we really need."*
> Michael Lerner, PhD

I am in the process of organizing the specific research parameters to understand the mechanisms involved in this clinical breakthrough. The highly functional neuroendocrine axis results in delivering the message of tone that results in systemic strong ligaments that allows physical medicine to work wonders at reducing acute and chronic pain without recidivism. Previous research has shown an increased collagen synthesis in rabbits by 200% in an *in vitro* rabbit model.[41] New technological research breakthroughs [42,43] are shedding light on the autonomic nervous system, neuroendocrine axis and immune system.

I tell patients that when their cranial bones are not functioning properly, their ligaments become like rubber instead of stainless steel packing bands. At this point they are either an accident waiting to happen or multiple accidents that have already happened. For ease of understanding I have divided the cranial area into three divisions, or floors, from the bottom up.

> *"The spine of all human beings, composed of muscles, ligaments and bones are pre-stressed tensegrity cantilevers."*
>
> Donald Ingber, MD, PhD, "The Architecture of Life"
>
> Scientific American:
> Jan 1998, page 56

Due to the multifactorial inputs that stress and trauma have, nine common stress MAPs have emerged. A cranial stress MAP must be recognized and corrected as it may cause local structural problems such as Bell's Palsy, temporomandibular joint (TMJ) dysfunction or contribute to local problems like vertigo or otitis media. Additionally, the systemic effects of interruption of the smooth function of the neuroendocrine axis may lead to not only gross structural instability and pain, but a vast array of related problems (e.g., temperature control, mood, reproductive, digestive, balance control, cardiovascular and immunologic).

The next complex includes that of the pelvis and spine, which I designate as the pelvic-spinal complex. The foundation of the spine is the pelvis, consisting of the triangular wedge-shaped sacrum (a fusion of five vertebrae) with the coccyx (a four-bone fusion) hanging from it. This sits wedged between two innominate bones or ilia. The strong sacroiliac ligaments—from both the front and back—allow for stability of the spine's foundation. They only allow a very slight (two degrees) range of motion and move like a gyroscopic figure eight when we walk or run. As our cranial-sacral system moves to pump cerebral spinal fluid (CSF), the sacrum moves into flexion and extension. The literature (top of the page) depicts the huge amount of impact of these stress MAPs. For example, bone spurs or osteophytes at the sacroiliac joint have been observed in 85% of men and 50% of women in their 50s.[44] Back pain is the number one cause of disability worldwide.

"Musculoskeletal conditions are an enormous and emerging problem in all parts of the world and need to be given the same priority and resources as other major conditions like cancer, mental health and cardiovascular disease."

Scott Haldeman; DC, MD, PhD
Chair 2000-2010 Bone and Joint Decade Task Force on Neck Pain and
Its Associated Disorders

The spine, which sits on the pelvis, is made up of 24 vertebrae (5 lumbar, 12 thoracic, 7 cervical) that make up three curves. These three curves give the spine, as an organ, 20 times more strength in terms of flexibility and resilience.

Two of the curves are forward facing (lordotic) and these are in the lumbar and cervical areas. The backward facing (kyphotic) curve is sandwiched in the middle in the thoracic spine. Each of the 12 thoracic vertebrae except for the last one (T12) articulates with two ribs that forms the rib cage.

The presence of the three spinal curves and the shape of the articulation between the vertebrae make the spine truly, intricately simple and simply intricate. Recall the normal vertebral complex with its two vertebrae connected by an intervertebral disc.

"In order for healthcare professionals to help manage chronic diseases, the impact of stress on physiological systems and understanding of the neurendocrine-immune system must be appreciated."

Dr. Datis Kharrazian
Neurotransmitters p.131

Each disc is composed of two parts. There is a central ball bearing called the nucleus pulposis which allows for flexion, extension, lateral bending and rotation. Because it is under a tremendous amount of pressure, it is held in place by 15-20 rings of ligamentous tissue that alternate opposing 30-degree angles to provide increased strength and flexibility. These are called the annulus fibrosus.

There are pain sensitive (nociceptive) mechanoreceptors in the outer layers of the annulus. Up until we are 20 years old there is a direct blood supply to these tissues. Around this age the vascular supply disappears and the disc must rely on passive inbibition of fluid through the end plates of the vertebrae above and below it to obtain its nutrients. In the course of a day the force of gravity compresses about one inch of fluid out of the discs. A good night's sleep on a firm mattress resets the fluid loss. Thus, we are one inch taller in the morning than we are when we go to bed at night. Spinal stretching needs to be performed on a daily basis. Loss of the spine's physiological function results in disease. Structure governs function and vice versa. Spinal exercises prevent degradation of the spinal joints, improve vascular and nerve supply to the glands and organs and lessen the burden of chronic disease; they should be taught and performed in all schools on a daily basis (see Appendices:16-18).

There is a reciprocal relationship in the vertebral column that sounds spiritual in nature—as above, so below. This has been termed the Lovett Brothers relationship. When the bottom vertebrae, or L5, rotates the body right so does the top vertebrae or atlas. This coordination occurs to allow our eyes to stay level with the horizon at all times to provide balance. Stress/trauma challenges and changes the body's inherent structural stability throughout the spine in a predictable pattern. Simply stated, once the sacroiliac ligaments are injured, the physical base of the spine—the sacrum—becomes unlevel and creates asymmetry and biomechanical compensations throughout the entire spine. The normal predictable pattern of motion with walking that allows the multiple functions of the human physiology to simultaneously take place is thus interrupted.

The third complex involves the feet or the tarsal tunnel complex. Each foot has 26 bones that make up three primary arches. Much like the carpal bones in the hands and wrists with their carpal tunnels, the feet have tarsal bones with their tarsal tunnels. The feet provide shock absorption, balance and strength for the rest of the skeleton.

Stress in its many forms causes the heel bone (calcaneus) to go backwards. This causes the arches to become compromised. The"Plantar vault" that they form together is "sprung." The third and fourth metatarsal bones drop, along with bones on the inner and outer arches. These biomechanical lesions cause the inhibition of large pelvic muscles which, contributes to stress MAPs in the pelvic spine organ. The bone just above the calcaneus—the talus—migrates either inward or outward creating unleveling and subsequent rotation of the tibia/knee above it.

Dr. Goodheart discovered that the six acupuncture meridians, which began or ended on each foot, cause specific paired muscles to fire, thereby contributing to body balance while in motion. Piezo-electrical sparks stimulate acupuncture meridian-related muscles at distant locations, providing improved neuromusculoskeletal system function. These may also be negatively affected and add one further layer of musculoskeletal instability. The discovery of these gaits was exciting, as this represented a new addition by Dr. Goodheart to the 5,000-year-old body of knowledge of acupuncture.

> *"Screening for specific, common clusters of risk factors and linked interventions, on the basis of skills that can be readily developed in the current clinical workforce, has the potential to improve the efficiency and effectiveness of care and associated outcomes. As noted earlier, there was a consensus that LBP care is often ineffective, sometimes even injurious, and patients should be better informed about choices and long-term consequences. There may be significant advantages for patients who view LBP as simply a condition, and not as a disease that requires medical diagnosis and treatments. However, this shift in perspective is unlikely to change unless providers develop new skills to provide reassurance and reshape patients' cognitions, develop better therapeutic alliances, and the ability to work with patients' expectations."*
>
> Glenn Pransky, MD, et al. "Are We Making Progress?"
> The Tenth International Forum for Primary Care Research on Low Back Pain, Spine 2011;36:1608-1614

It is by the overall understanding of integrated body biomechanics that we can prevent and minimize the need for invasive medical procedures. The web-like structure of the body is revealed with PAK™ and its secrets have slowly unfolded. A bright future awaits the health of mankind as its clinical application flourishes. The cure to our "national and moral imperative" is in our hands. Immediate and intense application is now the key to success.

> *"What the caterpillar calls the end, the rest of the world calls a butterfly."*
> Lao Tzu

1. Failure to Thrive

A five-month-old baby girl was brought in for treatment by her parents. Her father, a medical doctor, noted that she was a normal vaginal delivery. Her mother was "a little bit small" throughout the pregnancy. After birth, the baby screamed incessantly for the first two months. They "figured out" that it was "somewhat related to acid reflux," and she would make dystonic reactions from the reflux. They put her on Zantac and she "had some good results with that." She had a couple of "breakthroughs," so they switched her to Prevacid, with an "eight percent better mood response." Her father noted that she had kind of a "floppy head," and was unable to hold her head straight. Her head would always tilt to the left. He also noted that her left leg seemed "different than her right." She was borderline underweight for her age, and thus, was exhibiting a failure to thrive.

Our physical examination revealed an extremely distraught five-month-old girl. She screamed incessantly throughout her entire first visit. We utilized surrogate testing to evaluate her neuro-musculoskeletal integrity as well as her digestive reflexes. Energy field transfer, or surrogate testing, is professionally taught to be used as an "avenue of last resort" (i.e., newborns, paralyzed individuals or otherwise severely incapacitated individuals). The technique consisted of placing the child over the mother's shoulder while the mother was seated on the treatment table. The mother's arm was used to evaluate the response of the challenges to the child. Since they were in close approximation, their energy fields blended and the net result of the challenge on the child could be tested using the mother's nervous system: the surrogate.

Challenge revealed a right-left-right cranial stress complex MAP, a category two left pelvic-spinal complex MAP, and a bilateral tarsal tunnel complex MAP. Extra pelvic-spinal complex lesions included T1 through T7 right with ribs right, and C5, 6, 7 right left right (RLR). All of her right cervical facets were imbricated.

Gastrointestinal reflexes suggested the presence of a leaky gut with the resultant metabolic endotoxemia. This means that her small intestine (where food is absorbed to go to the liver) was no longer working efficiently. Normally, only digested food is selectively absorbed through special pores that open and close at the base of the microvillae that line the small intestine. Various factors, especially including mold overgrowth, can cause the lining of the small intestine to get irritated, changing the pore's function from that of a turn-style to that of a swinging door, allowing undigested food and bacterial endotoxins to leak into our immune system. This leads to a cascade of increased low-grade inflammation (metflammation). The food that leaks through the pores is engulfed by white blood cells. The white blood cells, carrying the partially-digested foods, are called circulating immune complexes (CICs). Two things now happen: 1) We become sensitive to these particular foods because they are treated as foreign invaders. 2) These circulating immune complexes cause inflammation wherever they settle (e.g., the brain/nervous system in erratic behavior, such as ADD or ADHD; or the GI tract in failure to adequately absorb nutrients or irritable bowel syndrome; or the vascular tree and its diseases). These substances are key promoters of total body inflammation and their burdens' symptoms may range from fatigue, arthritis, weight gain, allergies, asthma and skin problems to sinusitis, neurodegenerative disease, immune dysfunction (autoimmune diseases) and cardiovascular disease.

"The upper cervical spine contains most of the proprioceptive afferent (incoming) signals to the central nervous system. The brain requires appropriate afferent proprioceptive input from the upper cervical spine to organize itself during early development. Birth injury to the upper spine robs the brain of the required proprioceptive afferent input it requires to organize itself, including visuomotor function.

Typical early signs displayed by babies with upper cervical injury include asymmetric posture, tilted head, torticollis, using only one posture for sleeping, asymmetrics of movement patterns, asymmetrics or swelling of the face/head, asymmetrics of the gluteal muscles, asymmetric development and range of motion of the hips, fever of unknown origin and deformities of the feet.

Later symptoms displayed by these children at age five or six include restlessness, concentration difficulties, a reduced capacity to absorb stress, headaches, postural problems and diffuse symptoms like sleep disorders."

H. Biedermann, MD
Surgery Department, University of Witten, Herdecke, Germany

On the first visit, her cranial, pelvic-spinal and tarsal stress MAPs were gently reduced with respiratory adjusting. The mother was to return on her second visit so that we could evaluate and clear her gut of food and mold sensitivities (major contributors of leaky gut) so that her milk would not have circulating immune complexes that could aggravate her baby.

The mother noted that soon after her first visit, maybe a day or two later, the alarm reaction of constant screaming stopped. She had now become quite a peaceful baby.

Two weeks later, on her second visit, her mother informed us that the baby had just spent a couple of days in the hospital. She was diagnosed with failure to thrive. Her weight was at 12 pounds. She was supposed to be gaining approximately a half ounce per day. The bottom of her range was 12.5 pounds, so she was just under by a little bit.

Testing the mother revealed sensitivities to several molds and foods, including peanuts, bananas and oats. The baby was given a complete second set of respiratory adjustments that included the further reduction of the pelvic-spinal MAPs. Muscle work was also performed to strengthen and balance her neck flexors and extensors.

On her third visit, two-and-a-half weeks later, her parents noted that not only was her attitude 100% better, but she was holding her head up straight. Her range of motion with regard to her neck was much better. Mom was retested for allergens and they were all negative. The baby received some fine-tuning to her upper neck and lower spinal areas.

On her fourth visit, two weeks later, her parents noted that she had been doing relatively well until earlier in the week when she received a set of vaccines, followed by a massage. At that point, her colic seemed to really have kicked up, and for the previous two days she had been miserable. We found that her diaphragm was strained, most likely due to misalignment of her lower thoracic and upper lumbar spinal areas, which we realigned.

She was next seen seven months later. As a healthy, happy one-year-old she was thrusting her left hip laterally when walking. This had been ongoing for a few weeks. We found and corrected a left tarsal tunnel complex MAP and a category two left pelvic-spinal complex MAP. Her failure to thrive was now history.

Discussion:

The concept of a grouping of the signs and symptoms associated with fundamental disorders of the cervical spine into a framework through a model has been published by Heiner Biedermann, MD,[1] a surgeon in private practice at the European Workgroup for Manual Medicine, Koln, Germany. Workgroup has treated more than 35,000 children over the past 15 years. The Kinematic Imbalances (KISS) due to suboccipital strain is the name given to this entity to facilitate easy recognition. "By using this concept as a term in communication with other caregivers (physiotherapists, speech therapists and others) of infants and children," Biederman states, "we may be able to improve the contact between pediatricians and specialists of Manual Therapy in Children (MTC) ... to widen their scope of available therapeutic options and to include the 'functional approach' in their therapeutic consideration."

All of this work takes on even greater significance when one considers the area of the brain created by input from the upper three cervical vertebrae and the cranial nerve five (the trigeminal nerve). With input from the first three cervical joints and muscles of the upper neck combined with those of the orofacial muscles, the trigemino-cervical nucleus in the brain takes its shape. According to Raphael Poritsky, PhD, "Our first conscious muscular act is nursing at the breast. The neuronal pathways mediated and stimulated by nursing form the beginnings of our awareness of 'self' as well as the neuronal substratum upon which all future emotional and mental experience is interpreted and reported. The tactile and oral sensations that accompany this important act, namely pleasure, warmth, and security, are conveyed centrally primarily by the trigeminal nerve ... and its myriad connections. Conceivably whether a person is basically happy and content in life, whether he or she is trusting of other human beings, and whether he or she is capable of loving another human being may all depend upon the sufficient stimulation, activation and persistence of these neurons, their connections and their neurotransmitters."[2]

In an effort to promote a better understanding of the KISS score contributors—for parents and caregivers—what follows are the relevant questions regarding newborns that the European Workgroup uses to improve their accuracy of the diagnosis:

Posture: Leading symptom is a fixed posture in the newborn,
KISS I is a fixed lateral flexion (baby on back, head tilt to one side with shoulder elevated to ear on side of tilt).
KISS II is a fixed retro-flexion (baby on back with head in hyperextension with arms over head while sleeping).

Heiner Biedermann, MD, says that during delivery, "A majority of newborns suffer from microtrauma of brain stem tissues in the periventriculer areas. Only when we are able to look for specific signs in the case history will it be possible to advance our understanding of the impact of birth trauma on the clinical pattern of complaints of our patients." During the first year the most important direct signs of functional problems of the occipitocervical junction is asymmetry and fixed posture.

Delivery: Was the duration less than one hour, one to three hours, or three to six hours?
Was the presentation oblique? Was the child a twin?
Was it a forceps or a vacuum delivery? Was it a Caesarian?

First Months:	Bad sleeper during first months (6 to 12 months) or later? Child wakes up at night?
	Crying at night—how often?
	Problems with breastfeeding on one side?
	Signs of colic?
	Lack of tone of facial muscles?
	Neck region hypersensitivity?

General Health:	Headaches?
	Mouth open often?

Sensorimotor Development:	Slower than normal? This includes postural movement, language, concentration and social integration.
Asymmetry:	Visible after birth or later, looks only to one side; moves only one arm or leg?
	Back of head smaller on one side, face smaller on one side? Bald spot on back of head?

Important Predisposing Facts:

When an infant is born, his/her brain is one-fourth its final, mature size, while the body is only one-twentieth its final size.
Joseph Chilton Pearce, *Magical Child*

KISS Indicators in 4- to 6-year-old children:
Symptoms at this age may include learning disabilities, children that are reported as being clumsy or slow; difficulties in learning to bike or rollerskate.

Dr. Biedermann makes the point that the newborn is special due to the fact that after birth, most of their activities are governed by spinal or cerebellar reflexes. One of the few accessible areas to therapy is "the spinal engine," specifically at the upper cervical area. Biedermann notes, "A cesarian delivery is no guarantee that the cervical spine was not mechanically strained." He goes on to say that manual therapy is much more effective before verticalization (or upright posture is achieved). He makes the point that the balance between function and form is tilted in the newborn towards function. Incessant crying or headache may be relieved in one session (as in the case aforementioned). The ability of MTC to reduce these problems in newborns is far greater than is appreciated by the average pediatrician or general practitioner.

It is Biedermann's hope that, "KISS and KISS-induced dyspraxy (coordination/movement) and dysgnosy (learning/development issues) tools may facilitate the interprofessional dialogue between pediatricians, neurologists and manual therapists in the best interest of our young patients."

The pathogenic importance of asymmetric posture and motion in small children is often played down, if recognized at all.[3] Nature selects for bilateral symmetry. Bilateral symmetry means developmental stability, which means fitness and health. Asymmetry is inefficient for energy maintenance and is selected against in nature. The immense pathogenic potential of the proprioceptive afferents (incoming signals) of the suboccipital region, until now, has been "widely underestimated."[4]

The 20th century mathematical genius, Amalie Noether, called the most "significant" and "creative" female mathematician of all time by Albert Einstein, invented a theorem that united two conceptual pillars of physics: symmetry in nature and the universal laws of conservation. In 1915, Einstein published his General Theory of Relativity. Noether worked with some of the complexities of the theory to formulate her revolutionary theorem. It basically says that wherever you find some sort of symmetry in nature, some predictability or homogeneity of parts, you'll find lurking in the background a corresponding conservation of momentum, electric charge, energy or the like. According to Lisa Randall, a professor of theoretical particle physics and cosmology at Harvard, the connections that Noether forged are "critical" to modern physics. They are also critical to good health and form the matrix of modern chiropractic theory.

In experimental studies of the biomechanics of delivery, injury of the intracranial and subcranial structure is the rule, not the exception. The ability of most newborns to overcome and repair these lesions shows the enormous capacity of the not yet fully developed brain to cope with trauma at this stage .

A Wislchnik, et al.

This area has been studied from another perspective as well. Iatrogenic illness means injury or illness that is physician-induced. Abraham Towbin, a Harvard researcher who studied children who died from Sudden Infant Death Syndrome (SIDS), published his findings in 1969.[5] Upon autopsy of 133 children, he found evidence of either broken blood vessels in the upper neck or complete severance of the spinal cord in 132 of the children. All newborns should be checked after birth for stress MAPs. The process of labor and delivery is stressful for a baby as well as the mother.

At any rate, Towbin went back to the ob-gyn physicians who did the deliveries and queried them as to how much force was needed "to extract" the child from the mother's womb. He found that 100% of them said that 90 pounds was not enough, and the majority said 100 pounds was not enough. Towbin knew that 90 pounds was enough to rupture the arteries surrounding the upper spinal cord and 100 pounds was enough to sever it.

> Once you realize that helping others is also helping yourself, the size of the overall problems become irrelevant. You're not a one-man or one-woman army out to save the whole world. You help simply because it does good and it feels good.
> David Edwards, from Interviews, www.thesunmagazine.org

The bottom line is that labor and delivery are stressful for both the mother and the child. Well-adjusted mothers have fewer complications in labor and delivery. Estimates are that 48-56% of woman develop pelvic or low back pain during pregnancy. Clinical outcomes of patients with pregnancy-related lumbopelvic pain (PRLP) treated according to a diagnosis-based clinical decision rule (DBCDR) demonstrated that.

Eighty-two percent experienced clinically significant improvement in pain and 73% experienced clinically significant improvement in disability.[6] I was amazed to find that more woman than men—45% for women to 35% for men—suffer from lumbar radiculapathy (radiating leg pain), secondary to a herniated disc.[7] Well-adjusted newborns and mothers thrive robustly. Professional Applied Kinesiology (PAK™) treatment visits at these key points as well as throughout people's lives will reap profound benefits.

> "Integrity does not consist of loyalty to one's subjective whims, but of loyalty to rational principles."
>
> Ayn Rand

2. Neonatal Bloody Stools

A newborn of one month was brought in for treatment of severe gastrointestinal dysfunction. Since birth his stools were full of mucus and blood.

Physical examination revealed an alert one-month-old boy. Palpation of his abdomen revealed marked sensitivity and ropiness throughout the entire area of the large intestine. The mother was quite concerned over the situation for two reasons: 1) the proposed medical examinations were very invasive for a newborn. 2) the timing could not have been worse as the family was poised to move from Boston to Hawaii.

Surrogate testing revealed several abnormal digestive reflexes including a leaky gut, and ongoing food and mold sensitivities in the child. Since the child was being exclusively breastfed, this meant that her mother had to be tested and treated for intestinal dysbiosis. The subsequent downstream production of circulating immune complexes were getting into her milk, affecting the baby's gastrointestinal tract. Upon testing, the mother was found to have an overgrowth of mold. She was instructed to use a natural antifungal derived from olive leaves. Additionally, she was instructed to avoid sugar-containing foods (not only white sugar but also honey, molasses, corn syrup, maple syrup and dried fruits). She was sensitive to wheat, corn, oats, cow's milk and chocolate. Because it takes three weeks for antigen-antibody complexes to clear from the bloodstream, she was advised to avoid those foods for that length of time.

Challenge revealed a category two right pelvic spinal MAP with extra pelvic-spinal lesions as follows: C5, 6, 7 RLR and T1-5 R with ribs right. These were corrected with gentle respiratory adjustments.

The family subsequently moved to Hawaii, and the baby's problems completely resolved with this one intervention.

Discussion: The positive outcomes of this intervention prevented the use of massive amounts of radiation to this newborn. At this age, radiation from "routine" diagnostic studies, especially CT scans (computerized axial tomography), pose a substantial and largely unrecognized threat to one's health. One CT scan exposes patients to the equivalent amount of radiation received by atomic bomb survivors in the low dose range, equal to 300 chest X-rays.

Published studies document that these excessive amounts of radiation will result in catastrophic new numbers of cancer (as many as 29,000 new cases of cancer per year according to an article on this subject by the Life Extension Foundation). About 70 million of these diagnostic procedures are now done annually, up from 3 million in 1980.

"After the verb to Love ...
To Help is the most beautiful verb in the world."
Berth von Suttner

Should you or your loved ones be facing a radiographic procedure, there are several classes of nutrients that have been studied for their radio-protective capabilities. The soy isoflavone, genistein can protect mice from ionizing radiation after a single dose.[1] A radio-protective enzyme inhibiter known as the Bowman-Birk Inhibitor (BBI)[2] activates genes involved in DNA repair. This survives processing in commercial soybean products (e.g. soymilk, soybean concentrate, and soy protein isolates), making it a highly accessible radio-protectant.

Circumin from turmeric has powerful radio-protective effects. It has a dual effect: its antioxidant effects protect normal tissue from radiation, and it up-regulates genes responsible for cell death in tumors.[3] Garlic and ginger also offer radio-protection. Garlic supports the glutathione antioxidant system and down-regulates X-ray-mediated increases in the NF Kappa B system.[4] Ginger extracts boost glutathione activity and reduce lipid peroxidation. Ginkgo Biloba reduces "clastogenic" factors—DNA damage artifacts in the blood of people exposed to radiation.[5] Ginseng extracts protect against radiation-induced DNA damage.[6] A North American ginseng extract was recently found to protect human white blood cells from DNA damage even up to 90 minutes following radiation exposure.[7] Silymarin, a milk thistle extract, is well known to protect both liver and prostate cells from carcinogens. It has also been found to protect liver tissue from radiation damage as well.[8] As a precursor to glutathione, N-acetyl cysteine (NAC) powerfully supports natural intracellular antioxidant systems, making it an effective radio-protective agent.[9]

Some versatile molecules found in plants are called polyphenols. The best-studied and most potent radio-protective agents in this class are EGCG, resveratrol and quercetin.

(a) *Epigallocatechin gallate (EGCG),* derived from green tea, protects animals from whole-body radiation blocking lipid oxidation and prolonging life span.[10]

(b) *Reservatrol* protects mouse chromosomes from radiation-induced damage. Its antioxidant properties prevent radiation toxicity to the liver and small intestines, two tissues most immediately sensitive to radiation's ill effects.[11]

(c) *Quercetin* is probably the most potent anti-inflammatory of all the known 500 plus bioflavinoids. It protects proteins and lipids from otherwise lethal doses of gamma radiation.[12] It provides both chromosomal and mitochondrial DNA radio-protection.

Key vitamins and minerals offer proven antioxidant protection. Fifty years of research on the effect of exercise on cell membranes done at the Packer Institute at UCLA resulted in the following understanding: Out of 500-plus known anti-oxidants, five recharged each other and thus were identified as the anti-oxidant "network." They are vitamins E, C, alpha-lipoic acid, coenzyme Q10 and glutathione. Vitamins A, C and E have been shown to protect airline pilots from radiation-induced chromosomal damage (an occupational hazard).

(a) Controlled animal studies have shown that vitamin A can reverse radiation-induced gene expression abnormalities that could lead to cancer.[13] Other studies have show that vitamin A can actually prevent radiation-induced death of healthy cells.[14]

A paradigm shift in medicine has to occur now; the environmental degradation may pose too big of a threat to our survival as a species. All the following contribute to leaky gut:

- Genetically modified foods create multi-organ system damage/failure and are present in the majority of our processed foods

- Toxic heavy metals and industrial chemicals in our air and water and seafood

- Pesticides and insecticides on our fruits and vegetables

- Antibiotics, hormones and more pesticides in our dairy

(b) Vitamin C, as a member of the antioxidant network, helps protect DNA and chromosomes from oxidative damage. Radiation-induced death of human blood cells is inhibited by vitamin C,[15] which has also been shown to counteract radiation-induced "long-lived radicals" that destabilize chromosomes and induce cancerous mutations.

(c) Vitamin E, like vitamin C, stabilizes free radicals, reducing their toxicity. It also enhances the growth-inhibiting effect of radiation on cancer cell tissue, while simultaneously protecting normal cells.[16]

The minerals zinc, selenium, manganese and magnesium are essential cofactors for the cellular antioxidant systems, such as, glutathione peroxidase, superoxide dismutase and catalase. Zinc supplementation has been shown to protect bone marrow, but not tumor cells, from radiation-induced damage.[17]

A study presented at the 2002 Essential Fatty Acid and Human Nutrition and Health International Conference in Shanghai, China showed you can avoid the ill effects of radiation (usually for cancer cell treatment), which create more cancer cells: "The results showed that EPA and DHA (both EFA derivatives) inhibited radiation-caused cancer tumors, when given two weeks prior to and after radiation treatments, by 80-100%."[18]

> *"Inspiration is not garnered from the recitation of what is flawed; it resides, rather in humanity's willingness to restore, redress, reform, rebuild, recover, re-imagine and reconsider. 'Consider' (con sidere) means 'with the stars.' Reconsider means 'to rejoin the movement and cycle of heaven and life.'"*
>
> Paul Hawken, *Blessed Unrest*

3. Un-Descended Testicle (Cryptorchidism)

A three-month-old boy was brought to our office for care. One of his testicles had failed to come out of the body's cavity and descend into the scrotum. The family wanted a less invasive approach than the surgery recommended.

Physical examination revealed a healthy three-month-old boy. His left testicle was found to be undescended. Surrogate testing revealed a category two right pelvic-spinal MAP.

Resolution of this, and the abnormal spinal aspects accompanying this (i.e., sacral, lumbar, thoracic and cervical), completed the initial treatment approach. A subsequent visit two weeks later revealed that the previously un-descended testicle had descended into the scrotum. A second set of respiratory adjustments to the sacrum, and relevant spinal areas of compensation, was given to finalize the gross skeletal realignment. Surgery had been avoided, and the family was ecstatic.

From a clinician's point of view, this is a beautiful example of structure's intimate relation to function. It's said, the two are inextricably linked. I can only theorize that the stretch in the inguinal ligaments caused by the pelvic distortion, closed or pinched off the opening for the testicle to descend. Once this restriction was removed, it allowed nature to unfold as planned.

This is another reason that all newborns should be checked after delivery. Active prevention is a prime facet of a healthy lifestyle that needs to begin immediately after birth.

"Intelligent discontent is the mainspring of civilization. Progress is born of agitation. It is agitation or stagnation."

Eugene V. Debs

4. Autism

A three-year-old boy was brought in for the treatment of autism. His mother noted that he was diagnosed with the condition one year previously. The diagnosis was based on the following behaviors: repetitive play behaviors, no tolerance for change, and loud screams elicited while in the presence of strangers or other children. She noted that she had been working with a phone coaching program called "Relationship Developmental Intervention" for fifteen months to try to improve his behaviors. Other issues included crying frequently, fatigue and gut-related issues with food sensitivities and poor digestion.

His mother had a history of allergies, and was milk intolerant until age 12 and she was, "probably autistic, no friends." The father also had a history of allergies. The extended family history revealed slight autism in the paternal grandmother. The child's medical history revealed that he was a full-term baby weighing 7 lbs. 8 oz., delivered vaginally with no complications. He had "a lot of vaccines" as an infant. Thimerosal, a mercury-containing preservative, was in his DPT vaccine. He had no trauma or surgeries. His mother had stopped breastfeeding him five weeks previously. At that time, he "went downhill" and fatigued easily even after nine hours of sleep. He cried a lot and had diminished language and pronunciation skills. He was fragile and irritable.

"My caveat is that heavy metals always have an adverse effect on ALL children."

Dr. Gary F. Gordon, MD, DO, MD(H)

His diet was sugar, gluten, soy and casein-free. He could only tolerate peas, cauliflower and pears. Reactions to any other food included headaches, "stimming" (repetitive motions), blank stares, loss of interactive capabilities, and a rash on his buttocks, with a red ring at the anus.

His homeopathic pediatrician ran a hair and stool analysis. The hair analysis was negative for heavy metals, and showed a number of low minerals, suggestive of mal-absorption. Stool analysis showed normal digestion/absorption and gut immunology markers. The metabolic markers involving short chain fats and bile acids were normal. The ratio of the two major bile acids was elevated, probably due to an imbalance in the intestinal bacteria. Beneficial bacteria were lacking, and one potential pathogenic bacteria was found in abundance. Small amounts of normal fungi were present and he had an abnormal imbalance of gut bacteria, known as dysbiosis.

His mother tried a food elimination diet based on the work of Nambudripad (NAET) without any helpful changes. She also used probiotics and a multivitamin, based on the aforementioned test results. His bowel movements were once every two to three days.

Physical examination revealed a quiet, withdrawn, underweight three-year-old. Posturally, his head was level and both his right shoulder and left hip were elevated by one inch. Both feet were moderate to severely pronated. His spine was straight. Structurally, surrogate testing revealed a pure right cranial stress MAP, a category two right, pelvic-spinal MAP and a bilateral tarsal tunnel complex MAP.

"Evidence that increased acetaminophen use in genetically vulnerable children appears to be a major cause of the epidemics of Autism, Attention Deficit with Hyperactivity and Asthma."
William Shaw, PhD, Journal of Restorative Medicine, 2013

Positive reflexes were found in his endocrine system relating to his neuro-endocrine axis, thyroid and adrenals. This is a typical compensation pattern for a cranial stress MAP. His digestive reflexes indicated a lack of stomach hydrochloric acid, a leaky gut with a subsequent weakened liver, and reflexes suggestive of food and mold sensitivities. He scored 51 on the Medical System's Questionnaire (results greater than 50 are significant).

We adjusted the patient from head to toe, correcting his cranial, pelvic-spinal, and tarsal tunnel stress MAPs. We then tested him for food and mold sensitivities. This was performed using the technique of Michael Lebowitz, DC, with a small vial of either molds, powdered foods or liquids as placed under the south pole of a diagnostic magnet. This magnetic field drives the frequency of the vibration of the substance into the energy field of the patient. If the patient's immune system reacts negatively, it inhibits a strong muscle.

We identified five molds, which the antifungal Citricidal (a liquid grapefruit seed extract) neutralized. Six grains, six dairy products, three vegetables and three proteins tested positive for sensitivity. We had the patient avoid the offending foods for three weeks using two drops of Citricidal in water, twice a day, increasing to three times per day after a few days.

"Antidepressants (selective serotonin reuptake inhibitors - SSRIs) taken by a mother within one year of pregnancy results in two times the chance of an autistic child and four times the chance if taken in the first trimester of pregnancy."

The Center for Disease Control and Prevention,
National Center for Health Statistics, Sept 2011

We also recommended the use of apple cider vinegar, two to three teaspoons in four ounces of water, to improve stomach function, specifically to aid digestion of proteins. The small and large intestines were re-inoculated with a probiotic containing sixteen friendly species of bacteria, along with fertilizer for these (artichoke flower, a prebiotic).

The patient was adjusted once a week for two weeks, to clear the remainder of his structural MAPs, and then retested for foods and molds three weeks later. No molds showed positive at this point, and just two foods, one grain and one protein.

At this point, we ordered a provoked urinalysis to check for heavy metals. This is considered the gold standard for finding heavy metals, because the heavy metals like fat and immediately get tucked away in the fat of our organs. He did, in fact, have slight elevation of lead, mercury and arsenic, as well as a number of rare earth elements. A slight elevation is significant in the presence of other heavy metals, since they synergize one another's effect to become exponentially more dangerous. We recommended the intermittent use of dimercaptosuccinic acid (DMSA) to chelate these; three days on, two weeks off, for six repetitions.

91

"DMSA chelation increased the urinary output of toxic and neurotoxic metals. Our data supports evidence that detoxification treatment with oral DMSA has beneficial effect on ASD (Autistic Spectrum Disorder) patients."

Eleanor Blancok, Busch, et al.
"Efficacy of DMSA Therapy in a sample of Arab Children with Autistic Spectrum Disorder" Media - *A Journal of Clinical Medicine*, Vol 7, no 3, 2012, pp214-221.

The patient was seen three weeks later with no molds positive, ten foods showed sensitivity, and he had a positive leaky gut reflex. Due to this, we used a glutamine-containing powder, as the amino acid is the basic food of the cells lining the GI tract.

Working with detoxification, elimination and re-inoculation programs, one month later, two molds showed up and eight foods. His behavior and intestinal function were steadily improving. After approximately six weeks of care, the mother was elated to, "have [her] son back." He was pretty much back to normal, without exhibiting any of the previously abundant repetitious play behaviors. Tolerance for change was normalized, and there were no longer any loud screams elicited in the presence of other children or strangers. Her loving child was back!

At the end of July, the patient was markedly improved, and only had two "bad days." His mom noted that he was 185 on childbrain.com and now he was 45 (less than 50 is "no autism"), which is on the verge of mild to none in terms of autism. The patient was seen monthly from August to November, at which time they moved to California.

Epigenetic side-effects caused by a drug may persist after the drug is discontinued.

Medical Hypothesis, 2009 Nov:73(5):770-80

As a clinician, the ultimate moment with this child was when just before leaving the office on one of his final visits, he looked up at me and said, "I love you, Dr. Maykel."

From continued contact with his mother, I found out that this little boy has turned out to be a mathematical genius, and he continues to enjoy good health. His mother is a warrior for her son's health, doing absolutely everything she can to facilitate his well being. She has told me that the intervention at my office was the process that "absolutely turned him around."

Discussion:

Michael Ganz, Assistant Professor of Society, Human Development, and Health at Harvard School of Public Health, authored the first study to comprehensively survey and document the costs of autism to U.S. society. The study, which appears in a chapter titled, "The Costs of Autism," in the newly published book, *Understanding Autism: From Basic Neuroscience to Treatment* (CRC Press, 2006) estimates a $3.2 million dollar cost to take care of an autistic person over his or her lifetime. Caring for all people with autism over their lifetimes costs an estimated $35B in the U.S. per year. The federal autism research budget has been historically less than $100M per year. Ganz hopes his research can help focus attention on directing more resources toward finding the prevention and treatment options for autism.

> "Acetominophen is suggested for pain management following vaccinations. In 1983 the average U.S. child received 8 immunizations before age two. In 2011, the average was 25, a 313% increase."
>
> Ann Z Bauer, et al; *Environmental Health*; May 9, 2013

He notes for comparison, estimated annual costs of other conditions, including Alzheimer's disease ($91B), mental retardation ($51B), anxiety ($47B), and schizophrenia ($33B).

Autism is the most prevalent and pervasive developmental disorder, and the most common of all childhood disorders. During the last two decades, the chance of a child being diagnosed with autism has skyrocketed from one in 10,000 to one in 91[1] (2009), and now is one in 61[2] (2010). It affects an estimated 1.5 million Americans, and is increasing at a rate of 10-17% each year. It is four times more common in boys than girls. Ganz states that the exact cause of autism is not known, and there is currently "no cure for the disorder."

In a 2005 paper[3], Mark Geier showed that exposure to mercury from Thimerosal-containing vaccines (TCV's) administered in the United States was a consistent significant risk factor for the development of neuro-developmental disorders (NDs). The United States is in the midst of an epidemic of neuro-developmental disorders, with one in six children affected. Thimerosal is an ethyl mercury-containing preservative that has been added to many vaccines that are still being given to U.S. children and pregnant women (e.g., influenza, tetanus-diphtheria, meningitis, and monovalent tetanus).

> *"For both the young and the old, excessive vaccination is now, in my opinion, a major contributor to neurological disease. American youth, followed closely by British youth, are the most vaccinated people on the planet, and there is compelling evidence that we are paying a heavy price for this policy. There is a direct connection between childhood mortality for children under the age of five and the number of vaccinations they receive."*
>
> Russell Blaylock, MD
> The Blaylock Wellness Report, Nov 2011

Standard vaccine practices in the United States have exposed many children to levels of mercury that have exceeded Federal Safety Guidelines, and the U.S. Environmental Protection Agency's (EPA) permissible mercury limit. This study showed a significant association between "Thimerosal-containing DTP vaccines and neuro-developmental disorders, in comparison to Thimerosal-free DTP vaccines, for each of the following neuro-developmental disorders, including: autism (80% increased risk), speech disorders (160% increased risk), mental retardation (220% increased risk), personality disorders (130% increased risk), and thinking abnormalities (370% increased risk)."

This study showed that there were, "significant associations between cumulative Thimerosal exposure and outcomes." As the Centers for Disease Control and Prevention have expanded childhood immunizations, there has been an increase in neuro-developmental disorders in the U.S. Five other U.S. epidemiological studies have, "found a significant association between Thimerosal-containing childhood vaccines and neuro-developmental disorders." Research on Thimerosal by a major congressional committee has shown that the preservative is directly associated with the autism epidemic.

> *U. S. children receive 17 aluminum-adjuvanted pediatric vaccines containing a total of 5 mg of aluminum by two years of age. Brain aluminum kills microglia and astrocytes, releasing their glutamate causing excitotoxic damage and death of neurons. The official incidence of autism in U. S. children now stands at 1 in 50.*
>
> Russell Blaylock, M.D. "Aluminum Induced Immunoexcitotoxicity in Neurodevelopmental and Neurodegenerative Disorders," Current Inorganic Chemistry, 2012,Vol 2, no 1.

Published in May, 2003, the House Committee on Government Reform, the chairman, representative Dan Burton (R-Indiana) concluded that the CDC's research on Thimerosal was "fatally flawed" and charged that the CDC and FDA "failed in their duty to be vigilant." Federal health officials were complicit in covering up scientifically-validated associations between vaccines and neurological damage. The Committee's final report summarized their findings:

> Thimerosal used as a preservative in vaccines is likely related to the autism epidemic. This epidemic, in all probability, may have been prevented or curtailed, had the FDA not been asleep at the switch regarding the lack of safety data regarding injected Thimerosal and the sharp rise of infant exposure to this known neurotoxin. Our public health agencies failure to act is indicative of institutional malfeasance for self-protection, and misplaced protectionism of the pharmaceutical industry. [4]

A deeper look into this problem goes upstream into the mother's body and into the environment she creates for her growing baby. According to Doris Rapp, M.D., the average child "marinates" in over 300 neurotoxins in the mother's amniotic fluids.

According to the CDC, Autism spectrum disorder (ASD) now effects one of every 88 American Children—a 23% increase from 2066 and a 78% increase from 2002. These increases are too rapid to be a purely genetic origin. Five recent papers have listed the possible environmental causes. April 25, 2012

Recently, the environmental working group (ewg.org) got together 90,000 signatures to stop the "pre-polluted baby syndrome." The environmental contribution including exposure in early pregnancy to the organophosphate insecticide-chlorpyrifos, thalidomides, misoprostol, valproic acid and maternal rubella infection have powerful proof of concept evidence.[5]

The overall toxicity of the environment needs to be addressed especially with respect to mercury. We need to clean up "Dirty Coal" plants along with food sources, such as high fructose corn syrup. The average daily consumption of high fructose corn syrup in the US is 50g/person and a recent study shows that 45% of the samples contained significant amounts of mercury.[6] Another implication co-contributor is a lack of vitamin D.[7]

Our cell membranes are roughly analogous to an Oreo cookie. The outer and inner layers (the chocolate) are made of phosphatidyl choline (PC). In fact a 10-year-old child's cell membrane is 90% PC. Lying sideways in the cell membrane (the white of the cookie) are our essential fatty acids: Omega 6 and Omega 3 fatty acids. These fats are 18 to 20 carbons long. The optimal ratio of Omega 6 to Omega 3 fats is 4 to 1. Our cell membranes are very thin: 10,000 of them fit into the thickness of this piece of paper. They scintillate at 100 billion times per second. When exposed to environmental toxins, "renegade" fatty acids are formed, having lengths of carbons much longer (28 to 30) than normal. These create a buckling of the cell membrane (known as a ceramide bridge). Cumulative cell membrane damage leads to cellular dysfunction, and eventually cellular death. [8,9,10,11,12]

> By reframing the vaccine debate and offering, for the first time, the opportunity to have a rational and scientific discussion on how to create a safer and more effective vaccination program in America today, a movie called The Greater Good challenges viewers to think again. Peer reviewed research by Dr. Shaw shows that aluminum in vaccines causes motor neuron death.
>
> The FDA's response? "No interest" in following it up according to Dr. Shaw.

The use of phosphatidyl choline, butyrate, and folinic acid (a derivate of folate) clears the renegade fats. The use of a cold-processed oil with a 4:1 ratio of Omega 6 to Omega 3 (e.g., sunflower to flax) helps restore the normal membrane function in the presence of a nutrient-dense diet with adequate minerals.

Common sense laws forbidding the medication industry from self-serving on a government board, the well known, but little discussed "revolving door," is a necessary first step towards stopping and reversing this neuro-degenerative tsunami. Consumer advocate Tim Bolen (www.bolenreport.com) has posted a several-part series on the monumental cover-up by the CDC with regard to the safety of Thimerosal, (mercury) in vaccines. He notes that this issue is really going to "heat up", due to the exposure of the exact participants of the faked studies allowing the on-going protection of mercury by the CDC in vaccines.

"Vaccinations in 1986 were $86 per child per year with eight companies manufacturing them. In 2011, the costs were $2,200 per child per year with 13 companies manufacturing them. America's infant mortality rate is one of the worst of all developed nations. Six out of 1,000 children born live in America will die before their first birthday."

"It is time for all of us to stand up and end our participation in the failed pharma based health care paradigm so we can take back our health and our liberty. If vaccines are safe and effective for everyone, then those who chose to get vaccinated have nothing to fear from those who chose not to get vaccinated. If vaccines are not safe and effective for everyone, then it is unethical for anyone to get vaccinated without their informed consent."

Barbara Lee Fisher
Health Liberty Revolution and Forced Vaccination, www. NVIC.org

Dr. Russell Blaylock states that vaccines to improve immunity are both antiquated and dangerous. As Anthony Morris, MD, past director of the Virus Bureau of the FDA states, "Vaccines do more harm than good." Vaccination is not Immunization, by Tim O'Shea, D.C., should become mandatory for fifth grade science reading; it describes the house of cards that this $60 Billion giant stands on.

The even bigger concern is the pollution to our external environment. As Ben Franklin stated, "the cost of freedom is responsibility." We are all to blame, because we have let complacency replace vigilance, and thus, have allowed this to happen.

We as a nation can and must deal with this now. Hopefully, you will participate in the healing process.

Costs:

As noted earlier, the costs are absolutely staggering for this condition with an estimated cost on average of more than $29,000 per person per year.

The cost of treatment that helped turn this boy around in our office was as follows:

New Patient Exam & Treatment: $325
Office Visits (six at $125): $750
Provoked Heavy Metal Test: $100
Supplements:

   Citricidal $22
   Prebiotic $25
   Probiotic $30
   DMSA $70

          Total: $1,222

"On November 18, 2010 the US government paid $1.5 million to Hannah Poling. The response from the HRSA (the HHS division that runs the Vaccine Injury Compensation Program) is that we don't compensate for vaccine induced autism, we compensate for vaccine induced encephalopathy.

So this fall, when the school nurse advises you and your child to drive by Walmart and get a flu shot, know that it is a full dose mercury vaccine she is talking about. And know that three quarters of the studies that looked at whether or not Thimerosal containing vaccines can cause autism, actually support the position that they do."

Gary Gordon, MD, DO, MD(H)

Clostridium Difficile infects as many as 7,000 hospitalized Americans per day, and treatment of those infections is a major cause of antibiotic-associated diarrhea.

In about one fifth of the cases, the bacterial spores spring to life after antibiotic treatment stops. After clostridium difficile recurs, over half of the patients may develop chronic and potentially fatal infections.

Novel therapy for C. difficile infections:
Infusions of donated feces may help those with recurrent infections.
Harvard Health Letter, Oct 2011

5. Drug-Resistant Clostridium Difficile Infection, Severe Abdominal Pain and Diarrhea

A two-year-old boy was first brought to our office in May for treatment of a Clostridium difficile (C. difficile) infection, which was non-responsive to multiple drug interventions.

His mother stated that in December, two months before this current problem started, he had been treated for an ear infection with amoxicillin. In February he developed severe diarrhea. A stool analysis was performed which showed the gram-positive anaerobic bacteria C. difficile.

This infection represents one of the major causative agents of colitis and diarrhea that may occur following antibiotic intake and is one of the most common hospital (nosocomial) infections around the world. In the United States alone it causes about 3,000,000 cases of diarrhea and colitis per year. The organism and its spores have been demonstrated everywhere in the hospital environment, including toilets, telephones, stethoscopes and the hands of healthcare personnel.

While patient-to-patient spread of environmental contamination can be one of the reasons for cross-infection in C. difficile-associated diarrhea and colitis, antibiotic therapy is the major risk factor for this disease. Although nearly all antibiotics have been implicated with the disease, the most common antibiotics associated with C. difficile infection are Ampicillin, Amoxicillin, Cephalosporin and Clindamycin. The most common manifestation of C. difficile infection is fulminant colitis (severe sudden inflammation of the colon), frequently associated with very severe complications. Medical therapy ranges from none for asymptomatic carriers to discontinuation of antibiotics for noncomplicated patients with mild diarrhea, no fever and modest lower abdominal pain. When severe diarrhea is present, and in cases of established colitis, patients receive the antibiotic Metronidazole (Flagyl) or Vancomycin for 10-14 days. Several clinical trials have shown 95% of the patients (with mild to moderate cases of C. difficile infection) respond very well to this treatment. Diarrhea is expected to improve one to four days with complete resolution in two weeks. Nonresponders require surgical intervention.

At two months of age this two-year-old's medical history was positive for bronchitis which he contracted shortly after receiving a whooping cough vaccine. His mother noted that his digestion was "really bad because his food comes in and goes out the same way." This problem was present a short time prior to medications, but had increased substantially since their use.

His mom noted that since the diarrhea and the diagnosis of C. difficile began, he had one 10-day course of Flagyl. The diarrhea returned after five days so he went on another dose of Flagyl for 14 days. Once again the diarrhea returned after five days so they put him on Vancomycin for 21 days. The diarrhea returned just ten days after stopping this. Currently they were eight days into the second dose of Vancomycin. His bowel movements on the medication were loose 1-2 times per day. Off the meds they were 10-20 times a day with blood and mucus. She noted her child's abdomen was tender and distended. He had no appetite and frequently experienced moderate to severe pain in his abdomen, which caused him to cry out. His mother, needless to say, was at her wits end and was having extreme difficulty dealing with her sick child.

Physical examination revealed a tired, lethargic two-year-old boy. Challenge revealed a pure right cranial stress MAP with a category two, right pelvic-spinal MAP, and a bilateral tarsal tunnel MAP. These were all corrected with painless respiratory adjustments.

Sensitivity testing revealed marked sensitivity to Vancomycin. Reflex testing revealed a positive leaky gut reflex, positive food and mold sensitivities as well as both small and large intestine lymphatic congestion. He was found to be sensitive to seven molds, which were negated with olive leaf extract (a natural antifungal). He was sensitive to three grains (rye, corn and buckwheat), cow's milk, grapefruit, eggplant, cucumber, soy, almonds and chocolate. He was advised to stay off these foods for several weeks. The reflexes over the small and large intestine were negated with a probiotic consisting of 16 friendly species, which he was to use once a day.

The patient was seen one week later with slight improvement. We followed up with structural corrections of a category one right pelvic-spinal MAP. Persistent abdominal reflexes for the small and large intestine were negated with the non-cultivating yeast Saccharomyces boulardii. The patient was instructed to use one 250 mg capsule per day and remain off the previous offensive foods. Follow-up phone calls revealed complete resolution of the patient's symptoms within one week after beginning this regimen. Being able to help this child completely recover so quickly was truly a blessing!

Discussion:

It is interesting to note that this child became sensitive to Vancomycin. I believe it points to the fact that, as Dr. Bruce Ames says about nutrients, there is a "sweet spot." With nutrients there appears to be a parabolic curve for optimal function. Evidently, pharmaceuticals may present a moving sweet spot, with time, that may create genomic imprinting, later leading to disease.[1]

"If you act to correct a problem without a theory about its cause, you inevitably treat only the symptoms."

David Kortan, *Agenda for a New Economy*

PAK™ testing for food has been shown to have a close correlation with IGG food testing.[2] The screening of patients for adverse drug reactions utilizing PAK™ has the potential to dramatically reduce our current third-leading cause of death, prescription drugs taken as prescribed.

The training of primary care physicians and nurses in this technology has the potential to stop this disaster. Each year, $75 billion is spent on prescription and non-prescription drugs.

According to a study published in the Archives of Internal Medicine, more than $76 billion is spent on preventable drug-related medical problems caused by improper medication use. Follow up studies have re-confirmed these results.

When community pharmacists team up with patients to help them focus on improving medication use, the health outcomes are phenomenal. One example is The Asheville Project in North Carolina, where they experienced lower healthcare costs, reduced sick days, and improvements in clinical areas like blood sugar, cholesterol and blood pressure. Training pharmacists to test patients for potential adverse drug reactions utilizing PAK™ muscle testing will create exponential benefits.

"Chiropractic manual therapy improves lung function and overcomes exercise induced short-term respiratory resistance."

Roger Engel, D.C.,DO, et al [1]

6. Severe Asthma

A four-year-old girl, Abby, was brought to our office for help with an extremely serious case of asthma. During the previous year this child had spent more time in the hospital in an oxygen tent than she had in her own home.

The prior weekend, my brother met them at a beach in Maine, and had asked the little girl to go in for a swim. She informed him that she could not go near the water because it could lead to another life threatening lung reaction. He insisted that the mother bring her to my office and treat at his expense, since her HMO did not cover chiropractic care for pediatrics, and he knew that this type of care could possibly be a help to her.

Her early medical history was unremarkable. The problem had begun three years earlier when they had just moved into a new home. I asked whether or not there was mold in the house. At that point the girl's mother chuckled and said, "Mold! We have mushrooms growing in the basement!"

Upon examination of Abby, several abdominal reflexes were present, suggestive of a mold overgrowth in the small intestine with a subsequent leaky gut and food sensitivities. Further testing revealed that she was sensitive to a number of molds. We found a natural antifungal, an extract of citrus seed, in a liquid form that was easy to take. A number of foods evoked a positive sensitivity reaction and we instructed her mother to avoid these as much as possible for three weeks.

"These data suggest that children with high intakes of vitamins C and E may be associated with a reduced prevalence of asthma."

K Nakamura, et al.
Public Health Nutr. 2012;Oct 1: p1-6.

This time period is necessary for the overactive immune system to quiet down. It takes three weeks for the antigen-antibody complex (white blood cells that have engulfed undigested food) to clear from the blood stream. The magnesium stretch test was positive. Repetitive testing created muscle inhibition, suggesting a need to up-regulate her essential fatty acid status.

Structurally Abby's musculoskeletal system was strained throughout. Challenge revealed a pure right cranial stress MAP, a category two right pelvic-spinal MAP, and a bilateral tarsal tunnel MAP. Extra pelvic-spinal complex lesions included: T3-6 and T9-12 anterior with ribs bilaterally lateral.

At the end of the first visit we reviewed everything that we had found, clearly explained the steps that they needed to take and assured her mother that I would be available at any time should Abby need to be seen. The mother needed this reassurance since the asthma attacks could strike at any time, and she was definitely wanting to change the treatment approach, as it was not working. At the same time she needed to know that she could rely on me to be available at a moment's notice because her intent was to remove Abby from the steady, heavy doses of pharmaceuticals that she was on. She knew that it would not be easy since the child's condition was so extreme.

In a model that adjusted for all risk factors for asthma, asthma was significantly more likely to develop in children receiving antibiotics in a dose-dependent manner.

Al Kozyrskyj, et al.
"Increased risk of childhood asthma from antibiotic use in early life"
Chest, June 2007; 131(6):1753-9

My phone rang at 2:00 a.m. five days later and Abby was having a severe attack. I immediately met her at my office, and after about one and a half hours of using a variety of calming therapies, successfully quelled the attack. One of the biggest helps at this point was finding a flower essence that strengthened her lungs and adrenal reflexes. This was a major turning point for both Abby and her mother, because a trip to the hospital and oxygen tent had been avoided for the first time.

From that point forward there were no more serious asthma attacks. Abby's condition improved steadily, and was noticed by all, including her HMO. They suggested she become their asthma poster child; however, her mother was quick to inform them that the cure credit was not theirs, and had, in fact, occurred naturally. Abby went on to excel at dance, and is asthma free to this day.

Discussion:

Asthma has a significant impact on pubic health. It is the most common chronic condition among children. It accounts for 25% of all emergency room visits (2M a year). According to one source,[2] "the prevalence of asthma is rising at a faster rate than any other chronic disease in America today." It is one of the most common diseases of childhood, affecting more than one in ten children. It also affects one in twelve adults. The incidence of asthma has doubled since 1980, and according to the CDC, 16 million adults and 7 million children are affected. In fact, it is on track to double again by 2020. In the review of the origins of asthma by Saglani and Bush, it is important to note that, "the roots of asthma are to be found in the first three years of life. By age three, the die is cast and lung function tracks life long.[3] In older kids, it is the number one cause of missed days at school and poor academic performance. It accounts for more than 14 million total missed days of school.

Each day eleven Americans die from asthma. There are greater than 4,000 deaths due to asthma each year, many of which are avoidable.[4] The death rate for children under 19 has increased by 80% since 1980!

Oxygen deprivation occurs with every asthma attack, and even mild attacks create hypoxia (decreased oxygen) to the brain, with adverse impacts on development, behavior, and academic achievement. The most common treatment for childhood asthma is the use of inhaled corticosteroid drugs. According to Dr. David Perlmutter,[5] German researchers have discovered that asthmatic patients who used inhaled corticosteroids had significantly lower levels of BDNF (brain derived nerve growth factor), the growth hormone in the brain that is critical for brain development. The memory center of the brain is the hippocampus, and this is damaged with long-term inhaled corticosteroid use.

The existing medical literature totally supports the treatment protocol[6-8] used to support and treat Abby. The identification and removal of antecedents (food and environmental toxins like molds), triggers (pro-inflammatory cytokines: antigen antibody complexes from a leaky gut), combined with dietary changes and the identification and elimination of nutritional insufficiencies (e.g., magnesium,[9,10] selenium,[11] pycnolgenol,[12] vitamin E,[13] vitamin C,[14] dihydroepiandrosterone [dhea],[15] conjugated linoleic acid [cla],[16] vitamin D [17,18,19]) must be adapted immediately to affect a different outcome. The cost effectiveness is an elephant in the waiting room of medical change.

Each course of antibiotics in children increases the risk of the child developing atopic disorders (allergy and asthma). One course of antibiotics increased the risk by 159%. Two courses of antibiotics increased the risk by 387%. Three courses of antibiotics increased the risk 415%, with some children being at an increased risk of 1,920%.[20]

The annual cost of asthma is estimated to be $18B. Direct costs are $10B, with the majority of this going to hospitals. Every day 5,000 people go to the emergency room, and 1,000 people are admitted to the hospital for asthma. The average length of stay (LOS) for asthma hospitalization is three days. Nearly half (44%) of all asthma hospitalizations are for children.

Further evidence that environmental triggers in the form of phthalates (plasticizers) found in house dust, have a strong association between asthma/allergy, has come from Swedish researchers working with their American counterparts at Rutgers University. These endocrine disrupters are everywhere (hair spray, additives, plastic toys, ice cube trays, nail polish, fragrance-containing soaps), and the only way they can come out is through sweat. Far Infrared Saunas are the best way to unload these.

According to the AMA, approximately 200 over-the-counter drugs contain acetaminophen. Research done by Dr. Barr at Columbia University found that if a woman used acetaminophen for more than half of the days in a given month, that "there was a significant increase (63%), in the risk of a new diagnosis of asthma."[21]

"Before turning to medicines, we should attempt to adjust the normal body constituents to match the needs for optimal functioning."
Linus Pauling's Orthomolecular (Right Molecule) Medicine

"Since oral antibiotics are frequently prescribed for upper and lower respiratory tract infections in children, an understanding of the relationship between antibiotic use and asthma is critical to clinicians and healthcare policy makers worldwide." [22]

A small study published in the May 2012 issue of *Annals of Allergy, Asthma and Immunology* reported that 89% of the asthma patients in the study were allergic to molds, pet dander or dust mites. This recent paper thus reinforces the premise of this case story.

The Microflora Hypothesis of allergic disease points out that the early-in-life commensal microbial intestinal flora is responsible for proper T cell immunologic maturation and function, and that early in life exposure to antibiotics alters gastrointestinal microflora and diminishes Th-1 responses and increases allergic airway disease. Antibiotic disruption of intestinal microflora impairs the gastro-intestinal barrier function leading to allergen penetration and subsequent inflammation.

Using nutrition to improve the immune system along with body alignment [23,24] is the evidence-based approach which must be quickly integrated.

The big challenge that lies ahead is to educate and empower patients about their healthcare choices. Viewing health as an actively created state is a view brought forward by Dr. Andrew Weil. Prevention with the emphasis on the patient as an integrated whole is the goal.

7. Recurrent Otitis Media

A five-year-old boy was brought in for treatment for recurrent middle ear infections. In the past year and one half, he had suffered two perforations of his left ear drum. This left him with slight hearing loss. One month previously, he had started to have right ear pain. This was treated with Augmentin. Claritin had also been used for the past three weeks for left ear pain. The Ear, Nose and Throat Doctor was ready to schedule a tube in his left ear. The child's only other complaint was sub-occipital headaches that occurred about once a month at the end of the day.

Physical examination revealed a healthy 5-year-old boy in no apparent distress. Posturally his right occiput was elevated by one inch, as was his left shoulder and iliac crest. His spine demonstrated a mild "S" scoliosis, left lumbar, right thoracic that straightened on forward bending. Both feet were severely pronated. Challenge revealed a category two right pelvic-spinal MAP and a bilateral tarsal tunnel MAP sprain. Extra complex lesions included T1-6, left with ribs left, T3-6 anterior with ribs bilaterally lateral, and C5, 6, 7, left right left (LRL). The left deltoid was 3/5, but became 5/5 with approximation of the left acromioclavicular joint, suggestive of a strain to this ligament. The occiput was laterally displaced to the left. The left clavicle was laterally strained as well with a left holographic mandible. The muscles relating to the following organs were inhibited bilaterally, suggesting a need to improve their function: stomach, liver, gallbladder, and small intestine. Additionally, reflexes were positive for a leaky gut and ongoing food and mold sensitivities.

On his first visit, we corrected the category two right pelvic-spinal MAP, the bilateral tarsal tunnel MAP, and the extra-category lesions, as well as the left lateral occiput, clavicle and holographic mandible.

Neuro-musculoskeletal sensitivity testing revealed multiple mold sensitivities, along with the following foods: oats, mushrooms, soybeans, wheat, cashew, cow's milk, chicken, broccoli, cantaloupe and chocolate. The patient was instructed in the use of a natural antifungal— Citricidal—and placed on a low sugar diet with restriction of the offending foods. We also recommended a probiotic to re-inoculate his good bacteria.

The patient was seen one month later and he was doing much better with the dietary changes. He had stopped the diet five days previously, and started getting fluid in his left ear. He also had a cough and runny nose. Posturally his head, shoulders and pelvis were level. We found and corrected a category one, right pelvic-spinal MAP, C5, 6, 7 LRL and a left lateral occiput, clavicle and holographic mandible. Therapy localization to the thymus was negated with an anti-viral so we suggested a tapering dose of this product. Re-neuro-musculoskeletal testing showed no molds and two foods: soy and wheat. We reduced the citricidal to three drops, twice per week, and reinforced the avoidance of wheat and soy.

> *"When a doctor recommends that you take a test or have surgery, ask whether the doctor would suggest that his or her spouse or children go through such a procedure. Contrary to popular belief, doctors can't cure everyone. So why cause unnecessary pain with surgery?"*
> Shigeaki Hinohara, 99-year-old author and physician

The patient was seen four months later with complete resolution of his ear problems. A category zero spinal MAP was found and corrected. All gastro-intestinal reflexes were normal. Repetition muscle testing was positive, indicating a need to increase his essential fatty acids. No tubes equals a happy patient!

Discussion:
Myringotomy (slicing the ear drum and inserting a drainage tube) is the second most common surgery for kids, after circumcision. In 2006—the latest year for which I could find statistics—700,000 of these surgeries were done, with 280,000 performed on children under age three. At $3,000 a surgery, this represents an average $2.1B a year.

This procedure is of questionable necessity. It may not be a permanent cure, for as many as 30% of the children undergoing myringotomy, with insertion of the ear tubes, need to undergo another procedure within five years. A 1994 study showed that 25% of the ear tube insertions were inappropriate. Dr. Stephan Berman, a pediatrician at the University of Colorado, believes "tens of thousands could now be considered unnecessary each year." He considers the high use of ear tube placement comparable to the overuse of tonsillectomies in the 1960s. Dr. Jack Paradise, professor of pediatrics at Children's Hospital of Pittsburgh and other independent studies found no lasting effects of lingering fluids in the middle ear in otherwise healthy children.

This procedure represents the most common reason for a child to undergo a general anesthetic, so it carries the risks associated with sedatives or general anesthesia. Other risks are cutting the outer ear, persistent discharge (otorrhea) 13%, a permanent hole in the ear drum with some hearing loss, increased risk of infection and more.

Paying attention to the web findings will net us big savings—big returns on investment. Clearing up the abnormal gut function with the Four R Program (remove, replace, re-inoculate, repair) eliminates inflammation in the small intestine, which reduces the production of extra secretions made in the naso-pharynx including the sinuses and inner ears. The introduction of a probiotic has been shown to decrease the need for antibiotics in children by 80%.[1]

The identification and elimination of cranial and pelvic-spinal stress MAPs may be elegantly performed. It has been our experience that placing the child over the mother's shoulder, using her other arm, while you use her arm (surrogate testing) to challenge the child, then using her other arm, while you use her arm (surrogate testing) to challenge the child, then using low force respiratory adjusting, is both quick and effective. In fact, many times the infant sleeps right through the entire procedure.

Another reason to approach treatment this way is the following: Recurrent otitis media increases the risk of a child developing ADD,[2,3] an effect that is not associated with hearing loss, but may result from the effects of antibiotics on the microbial ecology of the gut.

"Understanding human needs is half the job of meeting them."
Adlai E. Stevenson II

8. Blocked Naso-Lacrimal Canal

A 14-month-old boy was brought in for treatment. His mother noted that he had poor drainage from his left eye that left it consistently crusty. He'd also had several colds over the last six months, and had been referred by her pediatrician to a pediatric plastic surgeon for surgical correction of his blocked tear duct. She was interested in seeking a conservative approach first.

An otherwise healthy 14-month-old child presented with tears rolling from his left eye out of the bottom part of his lid, since there was blockage of the tear duct. Surrogate testing, utilizing the mother's arm, was used to specify necessary treatment. The child was treated five times over a six-week period, with complete resolution of the blocked tear duct.

Treatment consisted of the reduction of the pure left cranial stress MAP, a category two left pelvic-spinal MAP, and a bilateral tarsal tunnel MAP. Extra pelvic-spinal complex lesions included: C5, 6, 7 LRL and T1-3 left with ribs left.

The following muscles were balanced: bilateral spasm of the masseter, temporalis and pterygoids. The neck flexors were strengthened bilaterally as well as the left upper trapezius.

Discussion:

Tears are produced by glands in the upper, outer aspect of the eye and drain across the eye through an opening in the inner canthus—the naso-lacrimal canal—into the upper oral pharynx. Jamming of the orbital bones, in this case—internal frontal, external zygomae, as well as locking of the major vault bones (parietal descent, temporo-parietal bulge, bilateral spheno-basilar flexion)—leads to increased tension, then swelling and closure of the naso-lacrimal canal.

The dura mater, which invaginates all the cranial sutures and forms the tube that the spinal cord sits in ending on S2 and the tip of the coccyx, needs to be freed at both ends to allow balanced physiology. Correction of the pelvis, along with the compensatory vertebral spinal dysarthrias, as well as the correction of the cranial structural dis-relationships, allows for a more normal dural membrane physiological status. In this case, it allowed the return to normal function of the left nasal lacrimal canal. This conservative, cost-effective approach represents the best practice for the problem, and should be executed prior to more invasive techniques.

Costs:

The average cost to treat this problem surgically is between $1,000-$2,000 dollars. In 2003, there were about 70,000 of these procedures done (www.mymedicalcosts.com). It is unclear how many of these were for this exact type of problem. Having the cranial stress complex MAP reduced first by a qualified health professional represents the best practice since it is a fraction of the cost, without the inherent dangers of general anesthesia and surgery.

> *All works of love are works of peace.*
> Mother Teresa

9. Attention Deficit Disorder (ADD) and Attention Deficit Hyperactivity Disorder (ADHD)

An eight-year-old boy in second grade was brought in by his mother for evaluation and treatment for symptoms of Attention Deficit Hyperactivity Disorder (ADHD). He was easily distracted and had poor impulse control. He had difficulty sitting still and focusing. Additionally, he had a need to satisfy his tactile sensory system by touching everything. His school responded to his needs by evaluating him and creating an Individualized Education Plan (IEP). His mother wanted to avoid the use of psychotropic medications and treat him with a more natural approach.

Physical examination revealed an alert eight-year-old boy. His medical history was unremarkable except for the use of Singulair® 5 mg, bid (twice a day) for wheezing. Posturally, his left iliac crest was elevated by two inches, his right shoulder by one and a half inches, and his left occiput by one-half inch. Multiple muscles weakened after a quick stretch, which is suggestive of a magnesium insufficiency. Challenge revealed a right-left-left cranial MAP, a category two right, pelvic-spinal MAP and a bilateral tarsal tunnel MAP.

The muscles relating to his stomach (pectoralis major clavicular) were found to be bilaterally inhibited. This was suggestive of a lack of hydrochloric acid production. The quadriceps, which relate to the small intestine, were also bilaterally inhibited, suggesting nutrient mal-absorption and lymphatic stasis. Positive reflexes indicative of a small intestine mold overgrowth, a leaky gut, and on-going food and mold sensitivities were found. Repetitive muscle (aerobic) testing caused muscle inhibition, suggestive of a need to up-regulate his essential fatty acid metabolism.

On his first visit, all the aforementioned structural findings were reduced and the related muscles balanced. We advised the patient to use two betaine hydrochloride tablets with each meal to improve his stomach's digestive capability. Additionally, we had him use a powder mixed with water taken one half hour before meals to debride his small intestine of undigested food and mucous residues to enhance nutrient absorption. He was instructed to stimulate the lymphatic drainage of his small intestines on a 3-times-a-day basis for 10-15 seconds. He was advised to use 200 mgs of magnesium citrate per day, and one teaspoon containing a 4:1 ratio of Omega 6 to Omega 3 fatty acids daily (sunflower/flaxseed oil).

On his second visit, we structurally corrected a category one pelvic-spinal MAP and the typical attendant spinal dysarthrias. At this point we tested him for food and mold sensitivities. We found that he was sensitive to four molds and the following foods: wheat, millet, American cheese, carrots, chick peas, cashews, bananas, lemons, fructose and chamomile. We had him closely avoid these foods for three weeks. Additionally, we had him use olive leaf, a natural antifungal (two, twice a day), and avoid sugar and sugar-containing foods for three weeks.

On his third visit, one month later, the patient had marked improvement. He stated that his thinking was clear, and he no longer felt anxious, needing to move around a lot. His energy level was markedly improved. His teacher commented on his changed behavior, and improved grades. On this visit, we found and corrected a category zero right pelvic-spinal MAP. He was no longer showing a sensitivity to foods or molds. We reduced his olive leaf to two, twice per week, between meals.

Discussion:

The diagnosis of ADHD has increased in recent years by 400%. Coinciding with this is an increased use of prescription drugs to treat ADHD by 274%.

Four and one-half million children and adolescents in the U.S. have been diagnosed with ADHD. An estimated 2.5 million are taking medications for their conditions. The latest research suggested the potentially lethal dangers of prescription drugs. A study published in the American Journal of Psychiatry suggest certain stimulant medications used to treat ADHD may cause sudden unexplained death. Methylphenidate is the generic form of brand-name ADHD drugs, such as Ritalin and Concerta. Last year the American Heart Association (AHA) recommended children with ADHD undergo cardiac screening tests prior to taking stimulant drugs and called for research to assess the potential risk of sudden death.[1]

During the last two decades, over a dozen studies have shown that people with learning disorders, including ADHD, dyslexia and autism, either have signs of essential fatty acid deficiency (dry skin, hair, nails, frequent thirst and urination) or lower than normal blood concentrations of docosahexaenoic acid (DHA) and arachidonic acid (AA). A recent meta-analysis[2] of pooled data from the red blood cell and plasma/serum showed that red blood cell arachidonic acid and docosahexaenoic acid concentrations were significantly lower than normal.

Recent research[3] has also implicated that organophosphate exposure at levels common among U.S. children, may contribute to ADHD prevalence.

A very recent report[4] suggests that "a multimodal chiropractic method" (read PAK) that assesses and treats motor dysfunction, reduced symptoms and balanced the cognitive performance in a group of 157 children. Developmental delay syndromes (DDS) encompass the following conditions: dyspraxia, dyslexia, learning disabilities, and attention deficit hyperactivity disorder. The most common feature in DDS is motor impairments, and the muscle inhibitions found with manual muscle testing confirm this. Chiropractic manipulative treatment in children with DDS showed good improvements on psychometric testing evaluating cognitive function.

This DDS research was done in Switzerland by Dr. Michel Barras. In that country they are not allowed by law to use clinical nutrition, so all of these positive results in this case series report were achieved with the structural component of the

Web of Wellness only! This work must now progress to randomized control trials.

> "Now more than ever, it's important we take preventive steps to maintain our health, rather than wait to take action until we're diagnosed with a disease or have a serious health scare. Unfortunately, the psychiatry ield (along with nearly every other medical discipline) is almost totally controlled by the pharmaceutical industry. Obviously, pharmacology is useful with severe mental disorders, but the tragedy of contemporary psychiatry is that it no longer searches for the cause of such problems or tries to address them. Common causes include stress, poor diet and chemical dependencies, along with de iciencies of certain nutrients, hormones and neurotransmitters. By addressing these issues the integrative approach prevents, minimizes and remedies health problems. This is the healthcare reform we need."
>
> Dr Stephen Sinatra, *Heart Health and Nutrition*, May 2010

The cost to improve this case study was:

Office visit: (new patient)	$400
Follow-up visits (two plus initial food/mold neuro-musculoskeletal sensitivity test, and tests)	$350
Supplements:	
Sea Klenz	$30
Olive Leaf	$30
EFA Oil	$25
Magnesium	$20
Total:	$855

As Dr. Goodheart was fond of saying, "Find it, fix it, and leave it alone." Fixing the underlying problems in the Web of Wellness is not only evidence-guided medicine, but it is also safer and more cost effective. Don't all of our children deserve to be treated with this gentle approach?

10. Severe Constipation

One fall day I was helping a woman whose low back was strained and I asked her in passing about her children. She mentioned that her 12-year-old son, Steve, had never had a bowel movement. Curious, I inquired how he got by with this terrible condition. Once a week, in fact every Saturday morning, she would administer an enema. This process had gone on for 12 years!

Evidently the condition had started soon after birth and they had taken Steve to the most prestigious hospitals including Children's Hospital, Massachusetts General Hospital and UMass Medical School, without success. They had tried mineral oil and a number of other potential remedies to no avail. Thus the weekly enema ensued, due to all the previous failed attempts.

After hearing this story, I suggested that since the best medical minds on the planet had failed to cure the condition that perhaps he was suffering from an asymptomatic compressed disc in his low back affecting the valve at the junction of his small intestine leading to the large intestine. The medical community had certainly ruled out any pathology. To my knowledge, traditional medicine had no way of diagnosing a functional aberration of the ileocecal valve.

A few days later she brought Steve in for his first visit. When his ileocecal valve was pressed upward toward his left shoulder it caused a strong muscle to weaken. This is called a "positive challenge." It is a positive indicator for a closed or spastic ileocecal valve, which is exactly what I thought would have escaped the traditional medical paradigm. We found and fixed the counter-rotated lumbar spine with a compressed disc at L3/L4. This is where the nerve supply that controls the sphincter called the ileocecal valve comes from. This allows the contents of the 23 feet of small intestine to empty into the five foot long large intestine, where water is absorbed and waste is prepared for evacuation.

Steve had never experienced low back pain. He returned two days later for a follow up visit and reported having two bowel movements per day after his first visit. We treated him a second time, finalizing the balancing of his pelvis and removing the residual spinal dysarthrias (MAPs). He did not return for a follow-up visit.

The following spring his mother strained her back again and when I inquired how Steve was doing she remarked that he was cured and that he had two or three bowel movements daily. Just think of how many people can be helped when this therapeutic approach is fully integrated.

Discussion:

Ideally, every time we eat we should have a bowel movement. We see new patients all the time who move their bowels once a week or once every two weeks! The time from when we eat something to the time when we pass it is known as the transit time. The normal transit time is 20 hours, and the average American's transit time is 50 hours. We are one constipated nation! It has been estimated that 18% of the total population (or one in seven adults) has this problem. Thirty percent have had the problem for greater than 10 years.

Every newborn child deserves to be carefully screened and adjusted by a person skilled in PAK.™ This is the right (and best) thing to do, and we will receive an abundant return on investment if this is done. Let me give you another example.

Remember the story from the beginning of the book about the twenty-two-year-old paraplegic that was a high-forceps delivery? Just think of the suffering that can be avoided by systematically identifying and correcting people's stress MAPs. One win-win way we can do this is to create "centers of soft tissue excellence" in hospitals across the country. From discussions with emergency room physicians, about 30% of emergency room visits are for neck and back pain. Once fracture, infection, or cancer metastasis has been ruled out, the emergency room doctor's job is complete. At this point, the patient may or may not be given an anti-inflammatory medication, and is then referred back to their primary care physician. This is a huge dilemma, because this is often the beginning of a nexus of harm to the patient, through a volley of prescription drugs, without correction of the underlying cause.

Instead, a seamless referral from the emergency room to a "Soft Tissue Injury Clinic" in the same facility—to examine and correct the underlying stress MAPs—would eradicate the vast majority of chronic pain before it gets started. Armed with the tools of PAK™ and Functional Medicine, patients could be triaged and educated effectively. This would create a source of hospital income that is currently non-existent. From here the patient can be referred to a community-based health care center to provide ongoing care and support.

This very well may prove to be the ticket to lessening the extent of spinal cord injury. The thorough integration of PAK™ right into the emergency rooms themselves, to gently realign persons with acute spinal cord injuries, will result in much less paraplegia and quadriplegia. I say this for two reasons: first, it just makes sense; second, several years ago, I treated an emergency room nurse from Pennsylvania, and she related to me that in her 15 years in the ER, none of the spinal cord injuries resulted in paraplegia or quadriplegia. I inquired why, and she stated that the attending neurosurgeon worked hand-in-hand with a chiropractor who reduced the vertebral subluxations in the area of injury.

One relevant analogy: if you have an elephant's foot on your foot, you have several treatment options. You could take corticosteroids to reduce inflammation, which is the standard medical approach for spinal cord injury. You could remove the elephant's foot from yours (i.e., gently realigning the vertebrae), or you could do both. In this case, mechanical removal of the nerve interference to the ileocecal valve restored normal function instantly.

There are 12,000 plus new spinal cord injuries per year. Surrogate testing to determine the exact vertebral crush pattern, along with gentle respiratory adjusting to reduce the trauma is quick and non-invasive. My own experience with an acute spinal cord injury was the opportunity to treat a patient with an L4 burst fracture paraplegia, caused by a plane crash. Within a week of the crash the pilot called me and asked if I could take a look at him. At the time he was wheelchair confined and unable to walk. With just a couple of visits he regained his ability to walk. I believe that having this option available for these types of injuries would quickly lead to results that would be absolutely life-changing for this class of injury.

"The question is not 'can you make a difference?' You already do make a difference. It's just a matter of what kind of difference you want to make, during your life on this planet."

Julia Butterfly Hill
American environmentalist

11. Encopresis (Loss of Bowel Control) and Eczema

An eight-year-old girl was brought to our office for loss of bowel control. Three weeks earlier, the child had a three-day-bout of severe constipation. Her pediatrician treated the problem with miralax powder. Subsequently the girl was having bowel accidents two to three times a day. The pediatrician termed this loss of bowel control "encopresis" and informed the family that the symptoms could last up to two years. Her mother noted that her daughter's eczema had also flared up since this incident as well.

Physical examination revealed an alert, but distraught eight-year-old girl, 4'7" tall weighing 100 pounds. Posturally, her left iliac crest was elevated by one inch, her right shoulder by two inches and her left occiput by one half inch. Her spine demonstrated a mild "S" scoliosis—left lumbar, right thoracic—which straightened on forward flexion suggestive of a functional curvature.

Challenge revealed a category two and three right pelvic-spinal MAPs, and a bilateral tarsal tunnel MAP. This sets the individual up for nine compensatory spinal dysarthrias (C1, 2, 3 RLR; T10, 11, 12 RLR; L3, 4, 5 RLR) as a result of the sacral un-leveling (low sacral base right). The term category three, which was present, indicates a torque of the torso as a compartment with respect to that of the pelvis as a compartment. The subtle inter-compartmental torque of category three may have profound consequences as it not only creates a shearing and compression of all of the lumbar inter-vertebral discs, but also impairs the associated parasympathetic out flow to this region.

Examination revealed a positive magnesium stretch test suggestive of a functional magnesium insufficiency. The muscles relating to the following organs were bilaterally inhibited suggesting decreased function: liver, small intestine, large intestine. Reflexes were positive for a leaky gut and ongoing food and mold sensitivities.

Treatment consisted of the reduction of the category two/three right pelvic-spinal and bilateral tarsal tunnel sprain complexes. All inhibited muscles were facilitated. The patient was advised to use 200 mgs magnesium citrate, twice a day, olive leaf extract (a natural antifungal), and was advised to avoid sugars and sugar-containing foods for three weeks.

The patient was seen three weeks later for a follow-up visit. The mother noted immediate cessation of the encopresis after the previous treatment. Her daughter's eczema had also disappeared. Needless to say, everyone was happy!

Discussion:

The lumbo-sacral plexus emanating from the lumbar and sacral spinal areas innervates the colorectal neuro anatomy. Probably either the severe strain of the child trying to move her bowels (bearing down while twisting could create the category three) or the reflexogenic trauma of the laxative working created an aberrant viscero-somatic reflex, as the origin of the bowel dysfunction.

"Not only will men of science have to grapple with the sciences that deal with man, but—and this is a far more difficult matter—they will have to persuade the world to listen to what they have discovered. If they cannot succeed in this difficult enterprise, man will destroy himself by this halfway cleverness."

Bertrand Russell

Structure and function are inextricably interwoven. The pediatrician was informed of the turn around. She never picked up the phone to inquire what we had done nor comment on the positive results. This unfortunate non-sharing of health information outcomes and physician behavior is pervasive throughout the system.

This needs to change for everyone's benefit.

One potential idea to catapult positive change is as follows:
The creation of nationally accepted health condition/treatment algorithms from a least invasive first (Hippocratic Order of Therapy-HOT^{TM}) point of view. By transparently applying the Web of Wellness, regional groups of experts, divested of corporate interests, can meet to discuss and agree upon best treatment practices. The regional groups can meet nationally on a periodic basis. The general public can weigh in, as 330 million brains and sets of eyes provide that much more input into the end result we all want. Innovative ideas would be recognized and rewarded on a scale commensurate with their relative value. Coherent consensus by the entire country will radiate positive results.

The American Heart Association (AHA) recommends a reduced sugar intake. High intake of added sugars is implicated in the nationwide obesity epidemic, as well as increased risk for high blood pressure, high triglyceride (blood fat) levels and other risk factors for heart disease, stroke and inflammation. New guidelines published in AHA's journal "*Circulation*" recommends no more that 25 gm or 6 teaspoons of added sugar daily for women and nine teaspoons (37.5 gm) for men. Soft drinks and other sugar sweetened beverages are the number one source of added sugars in American diets. One 12 ounce can of regular soda contains about 8 teaspoons of sugar.

12. Fainting

A seven-year-old boy, Dan, was brought in by his parents, with a history of passing out after physical exertion. During the previous year he had three episodes of fainting after exercise. He had been brought to Children's Hospital, where they performed an echocardiogram and stress test. Both of these were normal. His blood pressure, lying and standing, was also normal.

His medical history was one of a normal vaginal delivery. He used no prescription medications. He had hit his head several times but had not been knocked unconscious. Dan was a baseball player and used a Centrum children's one-a-day multivitamin. Upon examination of his diet, it became apparent that he seriously enjoyed sweets.

Physical examination revealed an alert 7-year-old boy weighing 45 pounds. The paired muscles relating to his stomach, pancreas and adrenal glands were very weak. Since the pancreas and adrenals are key sugar-handling organs we surmised that his sweet tooth was creating blood sugar highs and lows resulting in the loss of consciousness post exertion. This was exacerbated by an inability to digest proteins, and absorb blood-sugar-controlling minerals like magnesium and calcium.

We supported the stomach with digestive enzymes. The adrenal muscles strengthened with ayurvedic adaptogens, so these were incorporated. The magnesium stretch test was positive, so we added some powdered magnesium, to be mixed with water for easy assimilation. We suggested a great reduction in sugar and candy intake. Dan has had no more episodes of passing out. PAK's quick, noninvasive techniques of talking to the body once again allowed balance to take place and symptoms to go away. No more rides in the ambulance to the ER for Dan!

Discussion:

Increased sugar intake takes its toll in other areas as well. In the past 30 years, the rate of adolescent forearm fractures increased 32% in boys and 56% in girls.[1] Over the past 20 years, there has been a dramatic increase in the consumption of carbonated soft drinks, with significantly contributes to bone loss. Soft drink consumption in girls averages 14 oz per day. Taxes for unhealthful foods are one way being considered to stem the tide of diet-related disease. Read my upcoming book *The Beacon: A Plan to Make America First in Global Health* for more detailed information.

"Intuition is the clear conception of the whole at once."
Johann Kasper LaVater

13. Chronic Drug-Resistant Throat Infection

A registered nurse who heard me lecture on the topic of PAK™ brought her 9-year-old daughter, Tracy, in for care. Tracy was on an antibiotic continuously for five years. As soon as she discontinued the antibiotic, a streptococcal infection would resurge in her throat, causing severe soreness, difficulty swallowing and a fever. Besides the above history, her medical background was unremarkable.

PAK™ examination revealed a pure right cranial stress MAP, a category two right pelvic-spinal MAP, and a bilateral tarsal tunnel MAP. Extra pelvic-spinal complex lesions included C5, 6, 7 RLR, T1-6 right with ribs right, and T3-6 anterior with ribs bilaterally lateral. Isolation and testing of her neck flexors revealed that all eight of them were inhibited.

Because the muscles at the front of Tracy's neck were turned off, the ones at the back of her neck were unopposed and as a result were abnormally tightened. This created a situation where all of the neck vertebrae were counter-rotated causing them to be compressed at the back, decreasing the nerve and blood supply and blocking the lymphatic drainage to the neck and throat tissues. This situation allowed the bacteria to thrive in this oxygen and nutrient deprived environment. The strengthening of Tracy's neck flexors, together with the reduction of the stress MAPs and at-home exercises cured this long-standing infection in two visits.

When aberrant human physiology is found and corrected, our wonderful immune system can function efficiently again, and fend off foreign invaders. Recent research has shown that immune organs, like the thymus gland, are innervated by the sympathetic nervous system, and that immunity is largely controlled by the sympathetic nervous system.[1] The thymus gland receives its sympathetic input from the nerves in the superior cervical chain to the T3 sympathetic ganglia. Studies have shown that there are spinal cord reflexes between the mechanoreceptors of the spine and the sympathetic nervous system. Incorporating the functional aspect of the Web of Wellness was all that was needed in this case. At any rate, the identification and removal of stress MAPs is primary. Fixing altered biomechanics normalizes physiology and immunity.

14. Allergies and Asthma

A seven-year-old boy presented for treatment with a constellation of conditions including allergies, asthma, poor immunity and constipation. His mother noted that for nine months of the year, her son had allergic symptoms resulting in watery and itchy eyes, a stuffy nose and frequent sneezing attacks. He had frequent fevers (103° F) and "stomach bugs." In the previous 15 months, he had nine fevers and they were treated with antibiotics. He had asthma, kicking up seasonally in August, coincident with ragweed pollen season. Historically, his bowel movements were once every three days as "he had a tendency to be too busy."

He had a history of allergies to grass, trees, weeds and outdoor molds. He also had a chronic cough one year previously, which went away with the use of high dose Flovent. The pediatrician had questioned reflux as a cause, but the medication made no difference. He used 5 mgs of Singular and 10 mgs of Claritin daily for one year. This cleared his itchy eyes and got rid of the lump in his throat. He used Flovent daily for the past one and one half years. His mother had recently (two weeks earlier) started him on Benefiber, which increased his bowel movement frequency to once per day. For the week prior to his first office visit, she started him on 200 mgs of magnesium per day as well. The visit was prompted by a desire to see if a solution, other than weekly allergy shots for several years, existed.

Physical examination revealed an alert, 4 foot tall, 50 lb, 7-year-old boy.

Posturally, his pelvis and head were level. His left shoulder was elevated by one and one half inches. His spine demonstrated a mild "S" scoliosis, left lumbar, right thoracic. This straightened on forward bending suggestive of a non-structural scoliosis. Both feet were mildly pronated. Challenge revealed a right major cranial MAP, a category two right pelvic-spinal MAP, and a bilateral tarsal tunnel MAPs. Extra-complex spinal dysarthrias included C5, 6, 7 RLR and T1-4 right with ribs right. Both psoas muscles were hypertonic, and the diaphragm was strained. Muscles relating to the small intestine and liver were bilaterally inhibited, suggestive of diminished organ function. Reflexes were positive for a leaky gut and ongoing food and mold sensitivities.

On his first visit, we corrected the cranial, pelvic-spinal, extra-complex spinal and tarsal tunnel MAPs. Next, we performed neuro-musculoskeletal testing which revealed the following: positive sensitivity to 10 molds (negated with citrus seed extract), wheat, cow's milk, peanut, onion, grape, grapefruit, chocolate and MSG. The patient was instructed to avoid the offending foods, follow a low sugar diet, and take two citricidal drops in water, twice a day on an empty stomach.

The second visit was three weeks later, and all of his allergy signs and symptoms were markedly improved. His bowel movements were twice daily. We found and corrected bilateral post-tarsal tunnel syndrome MAPs and a category one right pelvic-spinal MAP. Extra-complex spinal dysarthrias were found and corrected at C5, 6, 7 RLR and T4 anterior.

The patient was given foot strengthening exercises. A follow-up neuro-musculoskeletal sensitivity test revealed no mold and no food sensitivities. The citricidal drops were reduced to two drops in water, three times per week. We recommended a probiotic, UltraFlora Plus®, one a day on an empty stomach, and a medical Food, UltraClear® Plus ph, as a breakfast or a snack on a regular basis to up-regulate his liver function. We doubled his magnesium intake to 400 mgs per day, and suggested several hundred mgs of buffered vitamin C if he had any flare-ups. We recommended using fresh organic beets and beet greens several times per week. We instructed him in the use of lymphatic massage reflexes for the liver and small intestines, as well as across-the-board sugar restraint.

Six weeks later he returned for his third visit doing quite well. Two remaining complaints included a "lump in his throat" feeling without Singulair and a belly ache if he ate yogurt. The digestive related muscles and reflexes were normal. Structurally, we found and corrected a category zero pelvic-spinal MAP, and strengthened inhibited neck flexors.

The patient was not seen for eight months. At this time, his mother reported that his allergies had been better until the past week. His eyes and throat were constantly irritated and were worse at night. She noted he had experienced a mild fever of 101° F two days once a month since January (it was now May) that went away on their own.

"Kindness affects more than severity."

Aesop

Six months later, the symptoms of his allergies and asthma were completely gone. The lump in his throat was gone without Singulair! Her son was healthy and drug free.

Discussion:

Previous research[1] has confirmed that over 98% of allergy patients had vertebral misalignment. The authors believed that the symptom improvements with the correction of the vertebral misalignments were due to rebalanced function of the autonomic sympathetic nerves. The Takeda treatment approach used here was developed in 1994 at the University of Tokyo, Japan. Their Graduate School of Engineering, Department of Human Engineering, found that "It was necessary to give daily stimulation for at least three to six months to the autonomic nerves indirectly to obtain sure treatment effect."

The use of PAK™ and FM in this case avoided the use of weekly allergy shots, which may have gone on for years. Their combined effect in this case resulted in a positive outcome, with much reduced intervention compared to the Takeda method cited in the research. When you think about the costs in terms of time and money spent, and with that the many trips in a car and needles in the child's arm, treating the Web of Wellness is compelling.

"Any intelligent fool can make things bigger and more complex. It takes a touch of genius — and a lot of courage— to move in the opposite direction."

Albert Einstein

15. Habitual Stress Cough

A 12-year-old boy presented to our office with a dry cough of three months duration. The symptom had been diagnosed as a "habitual stress cough" by his pediatrician. He was also experiencing a moderate ache in his right buttocks, and weekly headaches at the top of his head.

Physical examination revealed a healthy 12-year-old boy, with an elevated left hip of two inches and an elevated right shoulder of one inch. His body was found to be in torsion, with a category two right pelvic-spinal MAP and a bilateral tarsal tunnel MAP. Additionally, his upper neck was strained, with his third neck (cervical) vertebra anteriorly displaced. This is significant because the respiratory center of the midbrain lies at this level of the cervical spine. Experience has shown, that a vertebra misaligned anteriorly at this level may cause respiratory symptoms, such as coughing, hiccups, dry heaves and/or difficulty swallowing. We used gentle respiratory correction of all the dysfunctional areas, and immediately his cough frequency went from two times a minute to one time every three to five minutes. A second visit one week later cleared the remaining symptoms.

Discussion:

This type of diagnosis is quite common in medicine today. Another example is "growing pains" in children. In my experience, there is inevitably an underlying cause, with related stress MAPs found. Children don't usually complain unless there is a reason. We must rally our leadership to promote the widespread teaching of medicine along the HOT™ paradigm—least invasive first— to reverse the decline of our health.

> *"First create a vision for what you would like to have happen, then commit 100% to that vision."*
>
> Marion Stoddert

16. Chronic Juvenile Migraines

A seven-year-old girl was brought to our office for the treatment of severe migraine headaches. Her parents noted that they had started several years earlier, around age four. Initially the headaches occurred two to three times a month, lasting one day, and over-the-counter headache medication helped. As time went by, the headaches became more severe, lasting several days. Her pediatrician referred her to a neurologist, who diagnosed the condition as juvenile migraine headache. She was given stronger and stronger medications, which initially seemed to help, but were now ineffective, causing severe drowsiness and inability to think clearly. She was missing quite a bit of school and her parents were concerned about her worsening condition.

Physical examination revealed an alert seven year old, 3' 8" inch female weighing 52 pounds. Posturally her right occiput was elevated by one inch, her left shoulder by one inch, and her left iliac crest by one inch. Challenge revealed a right-left-right cranial MAP; category two, right pelvic spinal MAP; and a bilateral tarsal tunnel MAP. Extra-pelvic spinal dysarthrias included: C5, 6, 7 RLR, thoracic one through three, right, with ribs right, thoracic three through five and nine through twelve anterior, with ribs bilaterally lateral.

Organ related muscles that were bilaterally inhibited included those relating to her small intestine, liver and gallbladder. The magnesium stretch test was positive. Reflexes were present for a leaky gut, congested gallbladder, and ongoing food and mold sensitivities.

Treatment on the first visit consisted of reducing the cranial right-left-right MAP, the category two right pelvic-spinal MAP, and the bilateral tarsal MAPs. The extra pelvic-spinal complex spinal dysarthrias and rib luxations were also reduced. The patient was instructed to use 100 mg of magnesium citrate, BID. She was also instructed in the use of a product to debride her small intestine of accumulated undigested food and mucous. A lipotrophic (fat mobilizing) product, consisting of beet greens in tablet form, was given to decongest the gallbladder. She was instructed to increase her intake of steamed greens and whole grains, as well as nuts and seeds, to better improve her magnesium status and liver function. She also received education concerning correct posture, neck and upper back stretching exercises.

One-and-a-half weeks later, on her second visit, the patient presented with level neck, shoulders and pelvis. She reported feeling better and experienced no headaches. On this visit, we found and fixed the following: a category one right pelvic-spinal MAP, a bilateral post-tarsal tunnel MAP, and thoracic three anterior, with ribs bilaterally lateral.

We performed neuro-musculoskeletal sensitivity testing, and found her to be sensitive to a number of molds and several foods including corn, wheat, sweet potatoes and chicken.

We placed her on a low sugar diet and had her use olive leaf extract (two per day between meals) as an antifungal. We advised her to avoid the foods to which she was sensitive.

She was seen three weeks later for a follow-up visit. She continued to be headache free and had stopped using her medications. She noted her energy level had improved and she was thinking much more clearly. Her postural analysis revealed a continued balanced neck, shoulders and hips. A category zero right, pelvic-spinal MAP was found and corrected. The muscles relating to the liver, gallbladder and small intestine were facilitated. Re-neuro-musculoskeletal sensitivity testing revealed no food or mold sensitivities. The patient and her parents were ecstatic to have her symptoms resolved.

Discussion:

In a recent article[1] on chronic migraine, reviewer Dan Murphy, DC made the following remarks:

> "Chronic migraine is a disabling form of primary headache. It is a disabling, under diagnosed, unrecognized, and under-treated disorder. Although most individuals with chronic migraine sought medical care for this disorder, the majority did not receive specific acute or preventive medications. Most chronic migraine sufferers treat their headache exacerbations with non-specific migraine medications. Although most consider their medications well-tolerated, a sizable proportion are dissatisfied with their acute medicines.
>
> 13.9% of chronic migraine patients had rebound headaches or medication overuse headaches. For medications, one or more over-the-counter medications are used by 82.6% of chronic migraine individuals. Non-steroidal anti-inflammatory drugs (NSAIDs) were used by 64.1% of the sample, ibuprofen by 45.2%, naproxen by 26.2% and aspirin, the most common, by 23.6%. Acetaminophen was used by 45.3%.
>
> Chiropractors were the third most consulted professionals at 36.2%. The professionals consulted for chronic migraine were: family practice doctors (80.1%), neurologists (41.6%), chiropractors (36.2%) and headache or pain doctors (26.9%).
>
> Nutraceuticals were associated with satisfaction levels rangeing from 40% (magnesium) to 58% (feverfew). They were well tolerated."

Research work by the world famous Nikolai Bogduk[2], BSc(Med), MB, BS, MD, PhD, DSc, DipAnat, Dip Pam Med, FAFRM, FFPM, has shown that all headaches have a common anatomy and physiology. All headaches are mediated by the trigemino-cervical nucleus, which is a region of grey matter in the brainstem and upper cervical spinal cord. A headache can be triggered by an aggravation of any of the nerves that flow into this nucleus. The nerves that go into this nucleus come from the upper three cervical nerves and cranial nerves 5, 7, 9 and 10.

Jesus said, "If you bring forth that which is within you, that which is within you will save you. If you do not bring forth that which is within you, that which is within you will destroy you."
From The Gospel of Thomas
(one of the Gnostic Gospels)

17. Hives, Drug Resistant

An 18-year-old man presented to our office with a history of severe hives that had been present for several months. They covered his entire torso, but were most pronounced on his chest and abdomen. He had been to his primary care physician, who referred him to a dermatologist. The dermatologist had prescribed Benadryl topically and a course of steroids. He initially responded to these; however, as the steroids were finished, the hives reappeared with a vengeance.

Physical examination revealed weakness of the muscles relating to the liver and gallbladder. Palpation of the gallbladder (Murphy's sign) was quite sensitive, suggestive of biliary stasis. I tell patients that their liver is the engine that cleans their bloodstream and the gallbladder is the oil filter that allows the engine to run smoothly. Additionally, the thoracic spine area between the shoulder blades, relating to the normal nerve supply to these digestive organs, was very much misaligned.

In trying to understand why such a young individual would have this condition, we asked some very pointed questions regarding his diet. It seemed as though his job involved a lot of driving and he frequently ate at restaurants. He absolutely loved french fries, which he ate daily.

For treatment, we gently realigned his skeletal frame and introduced substances to thin out his bile. These are called lipotrophic or fat-mobilizing substances, that consist of choline, methionine and inositol. They are found in beet greens. We had him avoid the consumption of fried foods and undergo a therapeutic cleansing of his gallbladder.

His hives disappeared shortly thereafter and have never returned.

Discussion:

Your liver gets the majority of the resting blood supply, and uses the majority of the nutrients obtained from our diet (after age 18) to make the molecules to detoxify our bodies. Eating fried foods of any type, on a regular basis, is asking for trouble. Acrylamides are carcinogens made by oils in the process of frying. Less is better, none is best. If you crave a fried meal on occasion, make it in your own home using only high-heat stable oils, such as coconut, grape seed, red palm oil, or ghee (clarified butter).

18. Arm Paralysis—Post Cervical Fracture

A 17-year-old young man, driving a Jeep Cheroke moving at 40 mph, was hit by a drunk driver pulling out of a bar parking lot, colliding with the rear corner of the jeep. The Jeep rolled a number of times and the beltless driver was ejected from the car. They rushed him to UMass Medical Hospital ICU. He suffered two skull fractures and a broken neck with a C5/C6 spine fracture. He had double vision in his right eye, bruised lungs and swelling of the brain. The fracture was surgically corrected at Brigham and Women's Hospital in Boston with metal plates. He then went to Shepherd's Center in Atlanta, Georgia, for one month of spinal rehabilitation. He had just returned to Massachusetts to start another rehab program.

His family brought him to our office with the chief complaint that he had lost the use of his left arm. Even after therapy, he was unable to move it at all. He presented with left-sided neck pain, which radiated to his left shoulder. It was worse standing and better when he elevated the area. The constant pain rated from a moderate 7 to severe 10. Other complaints included knee pain, double vision in his right eye and left sided frontal temporal migraines. He also had no feeling in the five fingers of his left hand. Medications included Ultran, Neurontin, Motrin and Darvon for pain.

Our examination revealed a Neck Disability Index of 52% with regards to his left arm, which is severe. He had no ability to move his left arm forward (0° of flexion). He could not move his arm away from his side (0° of abduction). He could extend his arm 30°, but there was no internal rotation at all. He had increased deep tendon reflexes in his left biceps and triceps. The sensory nerves into his left arm were greatly diminished. The large muscle at the top of his shoulder, his deltoid, had atrophied and was no longer functional.

The ranges of motion of his neck were greatly diminished and caused pain. His entire left ribcage was rotated to the left. The acromio-clavicular ligament (connecting the distal clavicle to the scapulae or shoulder blade) of his left shoulder was sprained ("separated shoulder"). All of the intervertebral discs surrounding the area of the lower neck that had been fractured and then surgically fused, both above and below the fusion, were extremely compressed between severely misaligned vertebral segments.

Challenge revealed a pure left cranial MAP, a category two-right pelvic-spinal MAP with a left EX illium and a bilateral tarsal MAP (right-lateral talus-external tibia, left medial talus, internal tibia). The left medial meniscus was stretched and compressed, creating severe left medial knee pain.

We utilized a combination therapy consisting of low force, respiratory assisted chiropractic adjustments to reduce the cranial, pelvic-spinal, and tarsal MAPs, as well as the extra pelvic-spinal complex lesions. Muscle balancing (strengthening inhibited and inhibiting hypertonic muscles) was performed throughout his frame. We manually tractioned the intervertebral discs that were not surgically fused, and utilized interferential current to facilitate the healing process.

"We believe in patient empowerment and aim to educate patients with information about all their treatment options so they can make the decision that is best for them."

Jeff Skler, DC
Director of Chiropractic Services at Cancer Treatment Centers of America Eastern Regional Medical Center, Philadelphia, PA.

Corrective stretching exercises were given, along with the generous use of moist cold, to lessen the post traumatic inflammation. He received deep muscle therapy—Therese Pfrimmer style—on a regular basis, to improve both blood flow, lymphatic drainage, and to reduce scar tissue formation. Nutritionally, we utilized a combination of antioxidants, essential fatty acids, vitamins and minerals.

Over the course of a year of intense work, all of his symptoms resolved and he regained complete use of his left arm.

Discussion:

In cases of severe trauma like this one, there is a need to address the function of the entire frame, in addition to the area requiring surgery. Utilizing a team approach to achieve this is essential!

The use of respiratory chiropractic adjustments and muscle balancing, along with key nutrients to facilitate soft tissue healing, lays the groundwork for improved global function. This is exponentially expanded upon with deep muscle therapy. Good deep muscle therapy, on a regular basis, along with good structural care, is a win-win for good health, as well as healing post-traumatically.

A systemic review of the literature[1] by J.W. Brantingham, DC, PhD, provides an evidence-based rationale for the appropriate use of manipulation, soft-tissue techniques, exercise and other therapy when treating shoulder complaints. According to the authors, "multi-modal treatment appears at this time to be the most efficacious approach for shoulder problems."

My friend and colleague, Dr. Eugene Charles, recently published a case report[2] involving the successful relief of a right arm paralysis, with the restoration of normal arm movement. His treatment was a multi-modal approach; treating the neuro-structural distortion pattern known as Parsonage-Turner Syndrome (PTS), also known as acute brachialneuritis, neuralgic amyotrophy, brachial neuropathy or neuritis of the shoulder girdle. The known incidence in the United States is 1.64 per 100,000 per year, with an unknown etiology.

One of the best ways to create a win-win in healthcare today is with the use of Soft Tissue Injury Clinics (STIC). This assessment and treatment process would consist of combined approaches of; PAK™ and pertinent Functional Medicine with assistance from chiropractors, massage therapists, acupuncturists and first-line therapists. From here, the patient would flow to the nearest community-based healthcare team. In many instances this will be the same team as the STIC.

"Approximately 60% of whiplash injuries are occult to magnetic resonance imaging (MRI) and include occult soft-tissue, intervertebral disc and ligamentous injuries, accounting for approximately 90% of injuries missed by MRI."

Vincenzo Giuliano, MD, et al. *Kinematic Cervical spine MRI in Low-Impact Trauma Assessment Seminars in Ultrasound, CT and MRI* June 2009; vol 30, number 3:168-173

This additional immediate service will help to stop the chronic pain epidemic at one of its root causes. The end results are good for everyone. Refer to the Five Star Plan in my upcoming book, *The Beacon: Making the United States First in Global Health.*

"Build for your team a feeling of oneness, of dependence on one another and of strength to be derived by unity."
Vince Lombardi

19. Recurrent Sinus Infection, Drug-Resistant

A fifteen-year-old girl was brought in by her mother for treatment of a constant, chronic sinus infection. For the previous three years, she had been living on antibiotics due to severe nasal congestion and post nasal drip, which created severe frontal headaches. She found that the use of an antibiotic relieved the pressure in her head, so that she could get by without headaches. If she discontinued the antibiotic, or tried to taper down, the headaches would return. Her mother was tired of her child living on antibiotics, with continuous low grade head pressure and allergy symptoms.

Physical examination revealed an alert, but distraught 5'7", 130 pound female. Posturally, her head was elevated on the right by a half inch, her right shoulder was elevated by one and a half inches, and her left hip was elevated by two inches.

Her medical history was positive for a fractured jaw she suffered in a fall from a bicycle at age 12. It was from this accident that she developed the sinus and allergy problems. She had been to a pediatric allergist, but the desensitization shots did not seem to work.

Challenge revealed a pure right cranial MAP, a category two right, pelvic-spinal MAP, and a bilateral tarsal tunnel MAP. Extra pelvic-spinal complex spinal dysarthrias were found as follows: C5, 6, 7 RLR; T1-8 right with ribs right; T2-6 anterior with ribs bilaterally lateral. Extremity lesions included a right carpal tunnel sprain, a right lateral ulna, and a right acromio-clavicular sprain/strain.

The paired muscles to the following organs were found to be inhibited, suggestive of a need to up-regulate their function: stomach, small intestine, liver and gallbladder. Reflexes were positive for a leaky gut, small intestine mold overgrowth, and ongoing food and mold sensitivities. The magnesium stretch test was positive, indicating a need for increased magnesium. Repetitive muscle testing provoked inhibition, suggesting a need to up-regulate her fatty acid metabolism.

On her first visit, the cranial stress MAP was reduced along with the category two right, pelvic-spinal MAP, extra complex spinal dysarthrias, and extremity areas. The temporalis and masseter muscles were bilaterally inhibited. Strain counter-strain techniques were applied to her internal pterygoid muscles and both frontal sphenoidal sutures were deimbricated. The patient was instructed in correct posture and related spinal exercises, and the use of moist cold for her right acromio-clavicular strain. She was advised to use betaine hydrochloride (2 per meal), 200 mgs magnesium glycinate, BID, and 600 mgs of EPA/DHA, BID. She was also given the sea klenz protocol to debride her small intestine of undigested food and mucous.

On her second visit, one week later, the patient noted noticeably less head pressure and congestion. Posturally, her head was level, her right shoulder was elevated by .75 of an inch, and her pelvis was level. A positive challenge, followed by correction, took place at the following areas: a post tarsal tunnel complex (bilateral), a category one right, pelvic-spinal complex, C5, 6, 7 RLR; T7-8 R with ribs right; T6 anterior with ribs bilaterally lateral.

Neuro-musculoskeletal sensitivity testing revealed multiple mold sensitivities (negated by olive leaf), and sensitivity to the following foods: chocolate, cow's milk, rice, corn and peanuts. The patient was instructed to follow a low sugar diet avoiding the offending foods and the use of olive leaf extract, 2 BID, on an empty stomach.

On her third visit, three weeks later, the patient had been able to stop the antibiotic, with no headaches or increased sinus pressure. At this point, we challenged and corrected a category one, right pelvic-spinal MAP. Neuro-musculoskeletal sensitivity testing positive, revealed one mold sensitivity and two foods: oatmeal and tuna. Challenge to the small intestine was negated with a probiotic strain of acidophilus. We advised one per day of this probiotic to re-inoculate her gut.

One month later, the patient was asymptomatic with regards to sinus pressure and headaches. The patient's leaky gut, food and mold sensitivities, as well as, musculoskeletal MAPs were now history, as was her dependence on antibiotics.

Discussion:

From a purely structural standpoint; there seems to be a direct correlation between sinus drainage and cranial function, but also, normal mid and upper thoracic spine function are necessary for proper sinus drainage. By slouching on soft couches and reading in bed, people jam their mid and upper thoracic vertebrae anteriorly. This predisposes a person to poor drainage of the sinuses.

Part of the reason may be the blocking of lymphatic drainage due to imbalances in the muscles running from the shoulder to the upper chest wall.

From the expanded picture of the Web of Wellness, there is the embryonic relationship of the naso-pharyngeal (sinuses) tissue and the small intestine. Chronic gut inflammation leads to congested sinuses, increased nasal mucous and congestion.

In cases like this, where treatment is going nowhere, there needs to be enforceable laws to keep a patient moving to other specialists. The lack of medical treatment oversight, and the prolonged drugging of a child like this, is a great example of the need for Professional Health Forums to generate "best practices" as soon as possible.

> *"It's confusing as to why kids with OCD are not given strep tests immediately?"*
>
> *"Well respected doctors at NIMH had theorized the link; isn't this exactly why taxpayers fund such institutions, to develop cutting-edge medical advice?"*
>
> *"Unlike with law—there is no central repository of medical information."*
>
> Beth Alison Maloney
> *Saving Sammy: Curing the Boy Who Caught OCD*

In the recent book, *Saving Sammy: Curing the Boy Who Caught OCD*, Beth Alison Maloney makes us aware of several key points. In this book, she depicts her heart-wrenching experience with a chronic undiagnosed strep infection (misdiagnosed and improperly treated as Obsessive Compulsive Disorder [OCD]), in her middle son. The term PANDAS is an acronym for Pediatric Autoimmune Neuropsychiatric Disorders Associated with Streptococcal Infections. Her persistent fight for the true cause leading to a cure makes this book an astonishing, wake-up call.

As an attorney, Maloney brings up one important point that needs to be acted upon immediately. She notes that, unlike the law profession, there is no central repository of medical information. There is a complete lack of coordination between physical health and mental health providers. She states, "I also found it confusing that children were not routinely given strep blood tests the moment they exhibited OCD behaviors. Well-respected doctors at the National Institutes for Mental Health (NIMH) had routinely given strep blood tests the moment they exhibited OCD behaviors. Well-respected doctors at the

National Institutes for Mental Health (NIMH) had theorized the link. Isn't this exactly why taxpayers fund such institutions, to develop cutting-edge medical advice?"[1]

> *"In the old days doctors didn't reach for medications. First, they used natural remedies like baking soda and vinegar. Drug companies don't cure you. They make you go from one medication to another."*
> Anonymous patient

The director of NIMH, Thomas Insel, posted a piece called, "Microbes and Mortal Illness," August 13, 2010. In this article, he states that in this century the field of microbiomics, which is the mapping of the microbial environment of the human organism, "may transform the way we think about human physical and mental development. It is already clear that 90% of 'our DNA' is microbial, not human. 'We' are, in fact "super-organisms" made up of thousands of species, many of which are being identified for the first time."

Although microbiomics have proven important for understanding Type I Diabetes[2] and Obesity,[3] it has not yet become a focus for research on mental illness. Two independent studies[4,5] in the past year have fueled credibility for the PANDAS concept. "Do infectious agents influence the development of autism, anxiety or mood disorders? This remains a frontier area for NIMH research. The increasing evidence linking strep infection to OCD in children suggests that microbiomics may prove an important research area for understanding and treating mental disorders."

> *"What began as an investigation to help me diagnose mercury-related symptoms in my patients, grew into another diagnosis—that of a broken, misused, and abused regulatory system. In 2005, our regulatory system is still trying to keep up with the polluters, and our healthcare team is still in the dark when it comes to environmental toxicants."*
>
> Jane M. Hightower, MD, *Diagnosis: Mercury.*

20. Severe Mercury Poisoning

A 19-year-old man presented for treatment of a constellation of symptoms including: frontal headaches, numbness and tingling of his hands and feet, inability to concentrate, poor memory, hyperesthesia (increased sensitivity to touch) of his abdomen, fatigue and depression.

He noted that these symptoms had been gradually worsening over the last one and a half years, but recently had gotten so bad that he had to discontinue his college courses. He had also lost 30 pounds, due to loss of appetite. His primary care physician ran extensive blood chemistries, which were all within normal limits. The subsequent psychiatric referral sent his parents in search of someone with a clinical nutrition background, as they intuitively knew this problem was biochemical.

Physical examination revealed an anxious, distraught 6-foot-tall 160 pound, 19-year-old male. Postural analysis revealed an elevated right occiput by one inch, right shoulder by two inches, and left iliac crest by two inches. Challenge revealed a right-right-right cranial stress MAP; a category two right pelvic-spinal MAP, and a bilateral tarsal tunnel stress MAP. Extra pelvic-spinal disarthrias included: C5, 6, 7 RLR; T1-7 right with ribs right; T3-5, T10-12 anterior with ribs bilaterally lateral. Paired muscle inhibition was present for the following organs: stomach, pancreas, liver, gallbladder, small intestine and large intestine.

The thymus and spleen related muscles were also bilaterally inhibited. Reflexes were positive, suggesting ongoing food and mold sensitivities, a small intestine mold overgrowth and a leaky gut. Repetitive testing was positive for essential fatty acids, as was the magnesium stretch test.

Further questioning of the patient revealed that all of the symptoms occurred after moving into a rental house located on a small pond, next to a textile mill. Given his young age, the normal lab work, and the extreme dysfunction of his digestive and immune systems, I suspected an environmental poison. Urinary testing of heavy metals had already been done. It had not shown anything so I suggested we repeat the test after provocation with a chelating agent.

On his first visit, we reduced the cranial MAP, the category two right, pelvic-spinal MAP, and the bilateral tarsal tunnel MAPs. Additionally, we reduced the extra pelvic-spinal complex spinal dysarthrias and rib subluxations.

We started him on supplement program which included two betaine hydrochloride with each meal, 200 mgs of magnesium glycinate BID, 1000 mgs of EPA/DHA and the Sea Klenz protocol to debride his small intestine of undigested food and mucous.

On his second visit, 10 days later, we reviewed the results of his provoked heavy metal urinalysis which indicated a severe mercury exposure. Evidently, the pond next to the textile mill where he had lived was outgasing mercury vapors.

"With more than five thousand tons of mercury bellowing into the air annually world wide, we cannot allow industry to proceed as if pollution cases no harm to the environment."

Jane Hightower, MD
Diagnosis Mercury—Money, Politics and Poison

We began a program of (dimercaptosuccinic acid) DMSA 200 mgs/TID for three days on, two weeks off. This was done for a three-month period.

We also found and corrected a category one right, pelvic spinal MAP and a bilateral post-tarsal tunnel MAP. Neuro-musculoskeletal sensitivity testing revealed a number of molds sensitive to olive leaf. Th e food sensitivities included: rice, corn, beef, potatoes, chocolate and cow's milk. He was placed on a low sugar, anti-fungal diet, and instructed to stay off both the food sensitivities and fish, to avoid further mercury exposure.

Three weeks later his symptoms had receded by 50%-60%. His headaches had disappeared, his mood was better and the intense sensitivity of touch to his abdomen was going away. At this point, the molds had cleared up but we still kept him on olive leaf extract daily (at a quarter of the original amount). His food sensitivities on the second round of testing revealed: wheat, chicken and cow's milk. Since the cow's milk was persistent, we added a lactobacillus acidophilus culture, as it had been my clinical experience that dairy sensitivity will usually go away with the build-up of this bacterial strain. We also found and corrected a category zero right pelvic-spinal MAP.

Over the course of the next few months the patient stuck to a program of a low sugar diet, moderate progressive resistance exercise, spinal stretching and light cardiovascular exercise (walking). Th e chelation protocol was maintained. Retesting four months later, revealed a marked mercury reduction. His symptoms had been reduced globally by 90%, and he had gained 20 pounds. I suggested he continue on another few months of chelation.

Five years later, he came to our office for a tune-up. He was happy, healthy and the proud owner of a very successful roofing company.

Discussion:

Mercury, along with lead, cadmium and arsenic, are toxic heavy metals, released with the burning of coal. We globally burn about 27 billion pounds of coal per day. These heavy metals are spewed into the air where they then enter into our ecosystems. As of August, 2008, mercury was the second leading cause of stream impairment throughout the United States. (USEPA 303{d} list.) Methylmercury is a neurotoxin that is biomagnified in aquatic food webs; carnivorous fish, wildlife and humans that consume fish, are potentially at greater risk of exposure to methylmercury.

A neurotoxin is a chemical that poisons the nervous system. An excitotoxin[1] is a chemical that causes a nerve cell (neuron) to fire repetitively until it dies. Mercury, aluminum, formaldehyde and glutamate are excitotoxins. There are really no safe limits for these poisons. This is especially true for children, because their brains are developing, and methylmercury interferes with a cell's ability to divide.

"The USDA office of Inspector General recently revealed that all three government agencies responsible for setting safe residue levels for pesticides, heavy metals and veterinary drugs in beef products failed to do so for over 20 years."

Wenonah Hauter, Executive Director, *Food and Water Watch*

The effects can be permanent. Chronic and low-end exposure, in utero, shows up later in school, in the form of reduced performance on some tests of language, coordination and intelligence. "Adverse cardiac events and other neurological and psychiatric effects are still being investigated."[2]

Researchers have estimated the impact of lower IQ, from power plant mercury emissions, for the lifetime of the individual, in regard to diminished productivity alone. For the cost of exposed children in the United States, the loss was estimated to be about $8 billion annually.[3] This only represents the tip of the iceberg, as 7 to 10 percent of the U.S. population is at risk of over-exposure to mercury![4]

Chronic low-grade poisoning in adults has shown statistically significant correlations between mercury consumption and symptoms, as follows: muscle stiffness, dysesthesia (abnormal sensations, especially the sense of touch), hand tremor, dizziness, loss of pain sensation, muscle cramps, upper arm muscular atrophy, joint pain, back pain, leg tremors, ringing in ears, muscular atrophy, chest pain, palpations, fatigue, visual dimness and staggering. These symptoms were described by Japanese researchers[5] looking into their lesser poisoned mercury patients. For men only, symptoms with statistical significance were thirst and difficulty with urination. Those in women only were muscular weakness, urinary incontinence, forgetfulness and insomnia.

Dr. Hightower notes that her patient population had various combinations of the above complaints, as well as: headache, hair loss, trouble thinking and performing complex tasks, memory loss, insomnia, gastrointestinal upset, abdominal pain, excessive salivation, trouble with concentration, trouble with word finding, excessive sweating, fatigue, depression, metallic taste and nausea.[6] Her patients also had diseases and conditions with which mercury had been previously correlated, including: atherosclerosis, myocardial infarctions, strokes, auto-antibodies, neuropsychiatric complaints and infertility. According to her research, the best review of the literature, with respect to the dilemma in the realm of trade-off between eating fish and an increased risk to heart problems, comes from a study of Finnish men.[7] Men with hair mercury levels of 2.03 mcg/g and greater (equivalent to about 8 mcg/1 in whole blood), had an increased risk of heart disease, heart attack, and risk of death by about 1.6 times compared to those with hair mercury levels of less than 2.03 mcg/g. The lowest risk of heart disease was found in those with the lowest mercury levels, and an elevated level of the good omega-3 fats in their blood.

> *"Animals exposed to both aluminum and mercury may have 30%, 60% or 90% more deaths than if their exposure had been limited to only one toxic metal. When you recall that most of us have toxic lead, cadmium, arsenic, iron, uranium and other metals in our bodies, the overall picture is frightening.*
>
> *Most U.S. citizens are operating with abnormal levels of estrogen, progesterone and testosterone, so they cannot optimally remove these metals."*
>
> Dr. Howenstein

The FDA's action level for fish is still at 1 mcg/g, which does not protect those who consume either the higher-mercury-content fish (swordfish, shark, king mackerel, tilefish, large tuna, sea bass, grouper, pike, large halibut), or those who consume a higher quantity of fish.

This level is "not adequate and is not enforced. There is something wrong with the system, when a serious problem with a food item is evident enough that it gains warnings from the FDA, yet physicians across the nation, from the private doctor's office to the American Medical Association, typically do not know much, if anything, about it." [8]

"For the medical establishment to play an effective role in these decisions that ultimately affect our patient's health, environmental medicine and nutrition need to become part of a medical school education. The healthcare team needs to be involved in understanding environmental issues, learning how these issues may affect the health of patients, and bringing the importance of environmental factors to wider attention when we see their significance at the front lines." [9]

"People in medicine have an important role to play, but to cope with the range of issues surrounding pollutants such as mercury, it takes public awareness and concern, reform of regulator process, scientific investigation free of outside influence, and willingness of industry to take some action for the common good. None of us can possibly know everything. But there is much we can discover from mercury's history and its effects on its victims, and from listening to each other." [10]

The Mercury Study Report to Congress was released in December, 1997. Congress required the EPA to fund the National Academy of Sciences (NAS) to review the literature and the RFD (a dose of mercury under which no harm is expected). In 2000, the NAS came out in support of the EPA's RFD: 0.1 mcg/ kg of body weight/day. A person consuming this amount of mercury would have an estimated blood level of 4-5 mcg/1. This amount threatens the coal-mining and fishing industries.

Until the revolving door between government and big industry is finally closed and locked; by us, the citizens of this country, and all the people in the world, we will continue to be poisoned on a daily basis. The mercury-neurological harm nexus has been covered up by FDA's Deputy Commissioner Joshua Sharfstein. He withdrew the FDA's website warning that dental mercury can cause permanent neurological harm to children and unborn children. When the Republicans ran the FDA, to their own credit, they put this warning on the FDA website: "Dental amalgams contain mercury, which may have neurological affects on the nervous system of developing children and fetuses."

Caution on liver and kidney consumption-2011-12 State of Maine Hunting and Trapping Laws and Rules, p.21.

The Maine Department of Inland Fisheries and Wildlife and the Maine Center for Disease Control and Prevention recommend that the liver and kidneys not be eaten because of possible contamination with the heavy metal cadmium.

Recent studies have shown smaller amounts of cadmium in liver tissues from Maine deer and deer, elk and antelope from other states. Maine health officials recommend that deer liver consumption be limited to 0.8 pounds in one sitting and 1 to 1.5 pounds per week. Human symptoms of acute cadmium poisoning include severe nausea, vomiting, diarrhea, muscle cramps and salivation. There is no known health risk from eating moose meat or deer meat.

The past FDA Commissioner, Margaret Hamburg, worked in the Clinton Administration and then went on to become a director of the dental products colossus Henry Schein. She earned a quarter of a million dollars a year for the few hours it takes to be a director. Corporations do this knowing the other party will come back in power, and then they can call in these favors. Upon becoming Commissioner, Dr. Hamburg owned between $250,000 and $500,000 of Henry Schein stock. Her next in command, Deputy Commissioner, Joshua Sharfstein, got the message that there was more at stake than honesty in government. Sadly, he heads up a new FDA "transparency task force." President Obama has been embarrassed by both Margaret Hamburg for bringing back revolving door government and Joshua Sharfstein for deciding not to reduce the use of mercury in oral healthcare. This is not science, but commerce. The FDA does not allow mercury in products for dogs and horses, but children and pregnant women are fine.

"Believe nothing, no matter where you read it, or who said it, no matter if I have said it, unless it agrees with your own reason and your own common sense."

Buddha

21. Post Extraction Trismus—Lockjaw

A fourteen-year-old girl presented to our office with her mother, after an oral surgery resulted in lockjaw (trismus). Evidently, following the extraction of four wisdom teeth, this patient could no longer open her mouth. She was told her only option was to eat through a straw for the next several months.

Physical examination revealed a 5' 2"tall, 120 pound, fourteen-year-old female. When asked to open her mouth, she was only capable of creating a 2-3 mm movement prior to her jaw motion locking. Normal mouth opening is three of your fingers sideways in your mouth. I doubt she could have even gotten a straw to fit between her teeth. Palpation of her temporo-mandibular joint muscles revealed marked hypertonicity and tenderness to the masseter, temporalis and pterygoid muscles bilaterallly.

Posturally, her occiput was elevated on the left by one inch, her right shoulder by two inches, and her right hip by one inch. Challenge revealed a left-left-left cranial MAP, a category two right, pelvic-spinal MAP, and bilateral tarsal tunnel MAPs. Extra pelvic-spinal complex spinal dysarthrias included C5,6,7 LRL; T1-5 left with ribs left; and T3-5 anterior with ribs bilaterally lateral. All of the left cervical facets were imbricated. Bilateral inhibition of the thyroid and adrenal muscles were present suggesting a dampening of her neuro-endocrine axis. The muscles related to her digestive and immune organs tested within normal limits.

During the first visit, the lower jaw opening initially went from 2-3 millimeters, to fifteen millimeters with inhibition (using golgi tendon organ stimulation technique), of the masseter and temporalis muscles bilaterally. Since her jaw opening was still extremely restricted, the pterygoid muscles had to be approached indirectly, since, by process of elimination, they were the only ones not treated that could create the present situation.

The technique known as the spondylogenic reflex technique provided me with the exact tool needed at this point. This brilliant innovation of Dr. George Goodheart's took an interesting observation by the Swedish neurologists, Jiri and Vaclav Dvorak,[1] and turned it into a practical application. The Dvoraks systematically injected the capsular (facet) joints at the posterior vertebral motor units with a saline solution. Once injected, they proceeded to palpate muscles throughout the body until they found ones that were exquisitely tender to palpation. They did this for the entire spinal column, mapping out the specific relationship between the vertebral embryonic origin of every muscle in the body. These pioneers mapped out an embryonic system that persists throughout life, called the spondylogenic reflex system. Goodheart read this fascinating work, and as only he could do, managed to turn it into a way to facilitate improved health. He found that if the posterior motor unit of a vertebral motor unit was bent upon itself (known as a holographic or intra-osseous subluxation) then unbending the segment normalized the function of the related muscle group.

In this case, the affected muscle groups were the lateral and medial pterygoid muscles. The related spinal segments are the fourth and seventh thoracic vertebrae, which were found to have a holographic subluxation on the side of cervico-thoracic strain (in this patient the left transverse process and spinous process were bent towards each other). I unbent the vertebrae, and then tapped them gently 30 times to activate proprioceptive memory of the correct position. The patient could now open her mouth three centimeters. All this profound release took place in the first treatment visit.

We now corrected the cranial MAP, the category two right, pelvic-spinal MAP, the tarsal tunnel MAPs, and the extra complex spinal dysarthrias. We instructed her to use moist cold on her temporo-mandibular joints.

The patient was treated the next day. Her posture revealed an elevated left occiput by one half inch, right shoulder by one inch and a level pelvis. We corrected category one right, pelvic-spinal MAP, and C5, 6, 7 LRL extra pelvic-spinal complexes. The spondylogenic reflex pattern was still found to be present, so it was repeated. The frontal sphenoidal sutures were also bilaterally de-imbricated. The patient now had a normal three finger-wide mouth opening. Her smile was priceless!

> *"Today's child of six years of age already has chemical levels that it used to take us until our forties to accumulate."*
>
> Sherry Rogers, MD
> *Total Wellness*, Feb 2012, p.3

Discussion:

Improved communication between professionals needs to be facilitated to create best practices. Lack of inter-professional communication creates stagnation, and diminishes patient outcomes.

Having a healthcare team-concept mentality, where the patient sits in the center, is the ideal that must be achieved. The World Health Organization has recently added Interprofessional Education (IPE) to its global health agenda. Mandatory interprofessional shadowing experiences is a mechanism to be used by chiropractic institutions to address this.[2] Not a bad baby step in the right direction. Creating patient-centered healthcare will make practicing medicine more fun and valuable for everyone.

> *"Come Senators, Congressmen, Please heed the call*
> *Don't stand in the doorway, Don't block up the hall*
> *For he that gets hurt*
> *Is he that has stalled*
> *The battle outside is raging,*
> *They'll soon shake your windows, And rattle your walls*
> *The First one now, will later be last, For the times –*
> *They are a changing!"*
>
> Bob Dylan

22. Crippling PreMenstrual Syndrome (PMS)

A twenty-year-old female presented to our office for help with severe premenstrual abdominal pain since the start of her period at age 11. She noted that she experienced severe pain (9/10) in her lower abdomen for the first two to three days of her period. She noted that she occasionally got relief with strong pain medications. She had previously tried acupuncture, and it gave her relief for two years. The pain had then returned, and she did not respond further to acupuncture or herbal treatments. She noted she had mild low back pain that worsened with exercise, or if she carried something heavy. A recent abdominal ultrasound was within normal limits. For the past two years, she moved her bowels once every two to three days.

Physical examination revealed an alert 20-year-old female with a stated height and weight of 5' 9" tall, 130 pounds. Her past medical and family histories were both unremarkable for major trauma or illness. Posturally, her feet were moderately pronated. She had an elevated left iliac crest by one inch. Her shoulders and head were level. Her spine demonstrated a mild S-curve, left lumbar, right thoracic that went away on forward bending; suggestive of a non-structural scoliosis. The magnesium stretch test was positive, and repetitive muscle testing provoked inhibition, suggesting a need to up-regulate her fatty acid metabolism. Challenge revealed a right-right-right cranial stress MAP, a category two, three right external pelvic-spinal MAP, and a bilateral tarsal tunnel MAP. Paired muscle inhibition was noted for the following organs: stomach, liver, gallbladder (Murphy: positive) and small intestine. The thyroid and adrenal paired muscles were also inhibited, along with a positive ligament stretch test, indicative of an imbalance of her neuro-endocrine axis. Extra pelvic-spinal complex vertebral subluxation complexes included T2,3,4 LRL and T8-10 anterior with ribs bilaterally lateral. Challenge was positive to the L2/3 to L5/S1 inter-vertebral discs; non-weight bearing. Challenge was positive for a closed ileocecal valve.

The first visit treatment consisted of the reduction of the cranial, pelvic-spinal and tarsal tunnel MAPs. All of the extra spinal-pelvic lesions were reduced, and the lumbar discs were manually tractioned. Interferential therapy was utilized as well. The patient was instructed in the use of moist cold, a balanced diet; and the use of magnesium glycinate (200 mgs BID), EPA/ DHA (1 gm/day), and betaine hydrochloride (2/meal).

The patient was seen for the second time four days later, and was sick with
a sore throat. We found a marked bilateral inhibition of the thymus-related muscles,
which were negated with Lauricidin, so we suggested she use 500 mgs of this, three
times per day, until the sore throat symptoms cleared. We found and corrected
a category one right pelvic-spinal MAP, and a bilateral post tarsal tunnel MAP.
We taught her the lumbar inter-vertebral disc exercises, tractioned, then applied
interferential therapy to her low back.

A few days later the patient was seen for her third visit. She was moving her
bowels twice a day and no longer had any low back pain. We found and corrected a
category zero right, pelvic-spinal MAP. The lumbar discs were negative to challenge.
We tested the triple zinc supplement she had been using and found that she was
sensitive to it, so we suggested she discontinue that.

The patient was seen one month later, and she noted that her period had
passed with very little pain, on just the first day. She continued to feel better and was
extremely happy with the outcome. We found and corrected a category zero right
pelvic-spinal MAP with C5, 6, LR. We instructed her in the use of a multi-vitamin/
mineral and suggested she continue with magnesium and EPA/DHA.

A follow-up call several months later revealed that her chief complaint had
completely resolved. This treatment approach; reduction of MAPs, upregulation of
the digestive, hepato-bilary tree, and providing key nutrients with attention to a
clean diet and life style, is very powerful medicine. Balancing the Web of Wellness
with the tenets of PAK™ and FM provides the keys to eradicate crippling PMS.

From a biochemical point of view, just before menstruation the liver has to
conjugate (prepare for elimination) increased amounts of progesterone and rising
amounts of estrogen. By leveraging a womans's web to do this, the body excretion of
these hormones on a monthly basis occurs smoothly with very little, if any,
symptomatology. PMS will become a thing of the past.

23. Amennorhea

A 22-two-year-old female presented to my office, due to lack of a menstrual period for over six months. She noted she had undergone hormone treatment, and had multiple examinations from her gynecologist, but still had no period. She had previously undergone care at our office for some musculoskeletal challenges, and noted afterwards that she, "was still in doubt that Dr. Maykel could start a menstrual cycle."

Physical examination revealed an alert 5'5" 120 pound female. Posturally, her head, shoulders and hips were level. Challenge revealed a pure right cranial stress MAP, a category two right pelvic-spinal MAP, and a bilateral tarsal tunnel MAP.

The magnesium stretch test was positive. The muscles relating to her female reproductive organs (gluteous medius and maximus, piriformis) were bilaterally inhibited. Therapy localization to the pineal reflex point, facilitated these muscles, suggesting a potential cause and effect.

The cranial stress MAP was reduced, along with the pelvic-spinal MAP and bilateral tarsal tunnel MAP.

> *"Molecules do not have to touch each other to interact.*
> *Energy can flow through ... The electromagnetic field ...*
> *Proteins may be semi-conductors."*
> Albert Szent-Gyorgyi

The patient phoned the next day to say that she got her period. Follow-up visits over the years provided the evidence that her periods occurred normally for years after this one intervention.

Discussion:

This scenario has occurred dozens of times in my office. In fact, up-regulation of the signal from the neuro-endocrine axis to the ovaries (reduction of the cranial stress MAP) can create the onset of a menstrual period within minutes.

With regards to fertility in general, we have seen many female patients unable to conceive, do so, after a few sessions of stress MAP reduction. On the other end of the spectrum, recent research[1] points to the fact that pregnancy-related lumbo-pelvic pain (PRLP) is quite common (estimated to affect between 48% and 66% of pregnant women). Active chiropractic treatment resulted in clearly significant improvement in disability in 73% of patients, and 82% of patients experienced clinically significant improvement in pain.

Recent research [2,3,4] has proven that the connective tissue system functions as a liquid crystal conductor conveying information much faster than the speed of neural transmission. Electromagnetic fields are a mechanism of biological signaling implicated in healing.[5] It is my observation that cranial stress MAP reduction upregulates the pineal gland allowing it to fully function as the master neurendocrine transducer amplifying the intelligence of the electromagnetic field.

"Public servants don't represent the people anymore. They represent their own fortunes, their own interests. How far down the list of their priorities does serving the people come? I'd say it's usually right down there with cleaning out the garbage. That's abuse of power on top of deceit—on top of lots of cash."

Jim Steffman
Shadow of DEAth

24. Gastro-Esophageal Reflux Disease (GERD)

A 26-year-old school teacher, Jim, was referred to this office for treatment of gastro-esophageal reflux disease (GERD). His chief complaints consisted of burning in his upper throat and throughout his chest area. He noted the pain was sharp and deep, ranging from a three (mild) to an eight (moderately severe). He noted it caused a "lump in his throat" and "choked him up". He noted that it was worse lying down and relieved with sitting up or standing. The condition had started four years previously, but had gotten increasingly worse over the past month. He had used Aciphex once a day for four years.

Jim also noted a history of a "sour stomach" for the first two hours after waking up. This caused an upper abdominal pain, made worse by eating late at night, and improved after a bowel movement. He noted that he also felt bloated less than one hour after eating, and that this had been going on for one year.

His past medical history was negative for any major surgeries or trauma. He noted that a gastroenterologist worked him up and performed an upper gastrointestinal (GI) series prior to prescribing Aciphex. Jim also noted that he had been tired a lot over the past two years, and occasionally got dizzy when he stood up quickly. He usually slept eight hours without problems, except for occasionally being woken up with reflux symptoms. Over the past six months, he had the feeling of losing his center of balance and felt disoriented. Jim scored 56 on the Medical Symptoms Questionnaire, which is relatively high considering his age.

Physical examination revealed a category two right pelvic-spinal stress MAP and a grade two sprain of the right sacroiliac ligaments and a concomitant strain of the lower thoracic spine. There are three degrees of injury to ligaments: Grade one is a stretch and is considered to be a mild sprain. Grade two is a moderate injury with a stretch and some tearing of the ligament. And grade three is a serious and frank rupture of the ligament usually requiring surgery. In this case Jim had a grade two injury to his right sacroiliac joint and ligament (posterior and external). As a result of this degree of injury, his body responded by having his psoas muscles tighten up to help stabilize the sacroiliac joints from the front. The psoas muscle starts from the front of the last thoracic vertebrae and all the lumbar vertebrae, crossing the pelvis in front of the sacroiliac joints, where it inserts on the lesser trochanter of the femur. It flexes the hip and is the muscle you don't want to contract when doing abdominal workouts, bending the knees takes this muscle out of the picture when doing abdominal crunches.

If the psoas tightens up, it pulls the diaphragm down, causing the stomach to ride up through the opening for the esophagus. This is termed a hiatal hernia. This creates a mechanical component that leads to gastro-esophageal reflux disease.

"When they call the roll in the Senate the Senators do not know whether to answer 'Present' or 'Not Guilty'."

Theodore Roosevelt

At the lower end of the esophagus (upper end of the stomach) is the lower esophageal sphincter, which is supposed to lie flush with the diaphragm. Mother nature intended it to be this way, so that the diaphragm would reinforce the sphincter, allowing it to function better, preventing reflux from the stomach.

It should be understood that with a grade two sacroiliac sprain and concomitant psoas muscle spasm, there is also a misalignment of the lower thoracic spine and ribs that may initiate and propagate further digestive difficulties.

Examination of his gastrointestinal tract related muscles revealed bilateral weakness of those related to his stomach, pancreas, liver, gallbladder and small intestine. Reflexes were also positive suggestive of a leaky gut, and ongoing food and mold sensitivities.

We suggested the use of two betaine hydrochloride with each meal to support his stomach digestive capabilities. We also recommended lifestyle changes to improve his digestive processes. For starters, we had him hydrate his gastrointestinal (GI) tract with two 8-ounce glasses of filtered water, taken 10 minutes prior to eating. This was followed by little to no water or other liquids (just what he needed to help swallow his food) for at least one and a half to two hours after his meals.

Structural treatment consisted of the reduction of cranial, pelvic-spinal and tarsal tunnel MAPs. The right psoas muscle was in marked spasm. His last three thoracic vertebrae were found to be anteriorly displaced, as well as counter-rotated. We corrected these musculoskeletal misalignments and reduced his diaphragm strain. The right psoas muscle spasm was reduced with a specific tool of PAK™, called muscle spindle and golgi tendon technique. This is a simple method of rearranging the specific neurological set points in a muscle. In this case we dampened, or turned down the psoas, as it had tightened up to act as a backup, to help stabilize the right sacroiliac joint, whose ligaments were partially torn. With the patient standing we pulled his stomach down and to the right, at the peak of exhalation to separate it from the diaphragm, which in effect reduces the hiatal hernia. We utilized the body's physiological motion to leverage the hiatal hernia correction. Thus the mechanical setup for reflux was now corrected as this lower esophageal sphincter was now flush with the diaphragm.

After the first visit the patient decided to discontinue the Aciphex on his own. He noticed no increased problems with his reflux. On the second visit we finished stabilizing his pelvis and un-rotating his spine. We strengthened his right rectus and oblique abdominals, and once again performed the hiatal hernia mechanical correction. On this visit we had him start to utilize a cleansing product for the small intestine, and we gave him the neurolymphatic points to rub for this organ system, as well as for the diaphragm.

On his third visit we tested for mold and food sensitivities and instructed the patient in the avoidance of the immune offensive foods, as well as in the use of an antifungal supplement and dietary changes. He was given corrective spinal exercises.

For one reason or another, there was a failure to follow up, due to this patient's busy life, and a year went by before we followed up with a phone call to see how he had been doing. He was 100% improved as of those three visits, and continued to be totally reflux free.

Discussion:

The global neuro-musculoskeletal stress compensation sets people up for the structural cause of reflux and GERD. Once the sacroiliac joints are sprained (category two pelvic-spinal complex), the psoas muscles tighten and pull the diaphragm down, causing the stomach to herniate up through the esophageal opening in the diaphragm. Normally, the lower esophageal sphincter aligns with the diaphragm, keeping the valve closed all the times, except for when it is supposed to open after a swallow. When there is a hiatal hernia or diaphragm strain, the lower esophageal sphincter rises above the diaphragm, weakening the valve and increasing the chances of reflux.

It has been estimated that 25% of people 50 years and older have a hiatal hernia, so this is a big problem! The medical treatment of this condition includes the use of acid suppressing substances. This has created "a large franchise built on a convenient deception."[1]

> "In 2012 Congress will be busy raising money from commercial interests so they can keep their jobs. There won't be much time to change anything about mis-allocated public budgets, unfair tax rules, undeclared costly wars and job-depleting trade policies, that, if fixed, would increase employment and public investment."
> Ralph Nader

At $13.5B, the current sales of acid blocking drugs (H$_2$ blockers and proton pump inhibitors) represents a huge threat to the health of our nation. Shutting off acid production not only prevents the absorption of key nutrients; like all of the essential amino acids, vitamins (e.g., A, E, B12, B1, B2, B3, and folic acid), but also all of the essential minerals, except sodium and potassium. Recent research has demonstrated that prolonged use leads to a 200% increase in hip fractures, and nocosomial (hospital-caused) pneumonia (a bacterial infection of the lungs), which is a huge problem accounting for 17% of hospital-acquired infections. This helps keep people in hospitals longer, and pushes medical costs through the roof, not to mention killing 50% of the people who develop this disease while on a mechanical ventilator.[2]

The concept that the stomach routinely makes too much acid flies in the face of "more than a century's worth of scientific research. Over 90% of the time the real culprit is likely, underproduction of stomach acid."[3] The production of hydrochloric acid takes six times more energy to manufacture than any other compound in the human body. Hydrogen and chloride have to be concentrated by the stomach's proton pump to achieve a pH of two, which then signals the pyloric or distal stomach sphincter to open.

Both stress and aging suppress our body's ability to manufacture enough hydrochloric acid. As far as stress goes, there are two major ways that the stomach's acid production is hindered. One is due to "stress-on" sympathetic overdrive of the autonomic nervous system. Most people have an overactive sympathetic and underactive parasympathetic nervous system imbalance. The parasympathetic nervous system, at its exit from cranium (via the vagus nerves), is responsible for digestive enzyme production, and a forward peristaltic wave in the GI tract. The end result of a cranial stress MAP is diminished vagus nerve function, especially in the presence of the second major stress, a lack of key nutrients. Zinc is one mineral that promotes tissue healing, and is depleted by both not enough acid, and also exposure to plasticizers, which are 10,000 times more prevalent, by molecular weight, than any other carcinogens. This is another stress-depleted mineral in high demand and short supply. Although this mineral is a key factor for over 200 body enzymes, there is no storage mechanism for it in the body, so it is clearly needed, and must be supplied by zinc-rich foods. The sympathetic dominance slows, stops or reverses the normal peristaltic wave which also diminishes the body's nutrient absorption.

Recent research has added to the evidence-body of chiropractic benefit in the management of chronic adult dyspepsia. The authors note that chronic dyspepsia has a low incidence of self-resolution and a natural history of deterioration. "This pilot study demonstrates that patients with a clinical complaint of dyspepsia might benefit from conservative chiropractic management in terms of both symptomatic relief and decreased use of palliative pharmaceutical interventions."[5]

Cost Comparison:
The costs for the medications to control heartburn or GERD on a monthly basis run about $26 a month ($312/year) for over the counter Prilosec to $210 a month ($2,520/year) for Nexium.

This patient spent $725 at this office as follows:

New patient exam and treatment :	$400
Follow up office visits: (2 @$125)	$250
Supplements:	
Betaine Hcl	$15
Sea Klenz	$30
Olive Leaf Extract	$30
Total:	$725

Increased tone of the sphincter at the end of the stomach (pyloric) further contributes to this condition. The decline in stomach acid secretion with advancing age has been well documented. The number of people with no or low acidity (also called hypochlorhydria) increases with age from a low of 4% at age 20 to 75% after age 60.[4]

To get an idea of the prevalence of the impact of stress on our society, the National Institute of Diabetes and Kidney Digestive Diseases stated that 60 million people, or one in five, experience heartburn at least once a month, and 2 million daily. The only medical condition known to cause increased stomach acid production is called the Zollinger-Ellison Syndrome. This is listed as a rare disease by the Office of Rare Diseases (ORD) at our National Institutes of Health, and affects only one in one million people.

There is a wide range of serious disorders related to low stomach acid including: accelerated aging, malnutrition (due to mal-absorption), allergies, bronchial asthma, depression, bacteria overgrowth of the stomach and small intestine, pernicious anemia, stomach cancer, gallbladder disease and a host of autoimmune diseases.

You need to pay attention to promote healthy aging with non-invasive therapies. Getting a tune-up, at the very least on an annual basis, is a good idea to maintain a healthy Web of Wellness for yourself.

25. Cervical Herniated Nerve Plexus (HNP) and Left Arm Pain

A 38-year-old male presented for treatment of an inter-vertebral disc herniation in his neck, at C5/C6. He noted that this gave him a grade 10 pain (on a scale of 0-10 and 10 being extreme) in his left deltoid, biceps, lateral forearm and thumb. The pain had been constant for a two-week period. He stated that the condition was a direct result of repetitive trauma at work. He drove a semi-trailer truck for a major food manufacturer.

In January of the previous year he had pain in his left lower neck that radiated laterally and to his shoulder. He was given a cortisone injection in his neck and that made the pain go away. In August the pain started again, so he started physical therapy again. He noted he had six weeks of physical therapy, with no good results. They did not do traction until the end of that period. He then had a cortisone injection and they actually severed his spinal membranes causing cerebrospinal fluid to leak out. This had happened two weeks earlier, and since then he had extremely severe daily headaches. He was taking six to eight 350 mg Percocet tablets per day.

His past medical history was positive for a herniated disc at L5/S1 (lower back), which was surgically repaired in 1980. Regarding his present case, he had consulted with a neurosurgeon who wanted to perform surgery and had advised him to seek some conservative therapy first.

His past history was negative for any accidents or infectious diseases. He noted the pain was worse at night and first thing in the morning. His family history was positive for rheumatoid arthritis and grand mal seizures in his mother and his father had a history of osteoarthritis, increased blood pressure, increased cholesterol and he had a history of cluster migraine headaches (see later chapter on Horton headaches).

Physical examination revealed an alert 38-year-old male, 5'11", 165 pounds. Cervical rotational ranges of motion were bilaterally restricted by 30° with pain; flexion was full, but increased the pain into his left arm. He also had decreased left lateral bending, with increased pain into his left arm.

The magnesium stretch test was positive, suggestive of a need to increase his magnesium intake. Multiple muscles weakened upon repetitive testing, indicative of a need to improve his essential fatty acid metabolism. His entire body was misaligned from head to toe. Challenge revealed a pure left cranial stress MAP, a category two right-external pelvic-spinal stress MAP and a bilateral tarsal tunnel MAP. Extra pelvic-spinal complex biomechanical lesions included T1 through 8 left with ribs left. This caused an un-leveling of his neck's foundation, setting the stage for the herniated disc and subsequent left arm pain and dysfunction.

We cleared all of these aberrations, supported him with stomach digestive enzymes (as indicated by weak stomach muscles), magnesium and essential fatty acids. We instructed him in a balanced, whole foods diet with correct portions of proteins, fats and carbohydrates. We instructed him in the use of moist cold as well.

After his first visit, the numbness was completely gone from his left thumb. Percocets were now six per day and he was sleeping four hours at a stretch. He felt strength in his left arm starting to come back.

On his third visit the pain had lessened in his left biceps, the numbness was leaving his left hand and the overall pain factor was reduced by 20-30%.

He was completely off the pain meds by his fifth visit. At this point the neurosurgeon canceled the impending neck surgery. She was going to fuse the fifth and sixth cervical vertebrae together with a metal plate. Twelve visits and nine weeks later he was back to full time work with a few restrictions. He treated once or twice a month for three months and by April he was completely better. He has an active life today, where he snowboards and drives a semi-trailer truck on a regular basis.

Discussion:

The total cost to treat this patient in my office was $1,100. The insurance company told him that my fees were excessive. The neck surgery the neurosurgeon canceled would have cost $40,000. HOT™ medicine with a full spectrum approach, can save us hundreds of billions of dollars if instituted on a wide scale basis immediately.

Based on the best available evidence, the risk of serious complications or death is calculated to be 400 times greater for the use of non-steroidal anti-inflammatory drugs (NSAIDSs) than for the use of cervical manipulation in the treatment of similar conditions. An article published in the medical journal "Spine"[1] compared the risks for cervical spine manipulations, use of NSAIDs, and cervical spine surgeries. Hurwitz, et al. report an average risk of vertebrobasilar accident, major impairment or death as 7.5 per 10,000,000 manipulations. They further report an average incidence rate of serious gastrointestinal event (bleeding, perforation, or other adverse reaction resulting in hospitalization or death) from the use of NSAIDs as 1 per 1,000 subjects. They report an average incidence rate of neurological complication or death from cervical spine surgeries as 11.25 per 1,000.

It is now known that stroke from vertebral artery dissection occurs in a genetically predisposed group of people that have fibromuscular dysplasia. Axial rotation has been shown to be the motion that has the greatest potential for this phenomenon to occur. The use of respiratory adjusting, with no axial rotation, will render this rare event extinct.

26. Anemia, Allergies, Asthma; Chronic Back, Chest and Low Back Pain; Recurrent Yeast Infections, Anxiety, Insomnia, Polycystic Ovary Disease, Bilateral Plantar Fasciitis, Hiatal Hernia and Heartburn, and Moderate PMS

A 34-year-old female presented for treatment of allergies, asthma, and chronic mid-back, chest and low back pain. She was referred by her massage therapist, Peter Churchill. She also had a 15-year history of chronic recurrent vaginal yeast infections that occurred once every three or four months. She noted that two years earlier she began having right subscapular pain that radiated into her anterior chest wall. She noted the pain was deep, sharp (10/10), constant, and it was progressively worsening with radiation into her neck and shoulders. Her right arm was weak and she experienced tingling in it on an intermittent basis. She had moderate (4/10) deep, right buttock pain for 11 years which was relieved for short periods of time with massage therapy.

She had a history of chronic asthma and had used Singulair® for the past year. She noted that two years previously her lung capacity was decreased by 50% by spirometric evaluation. Due to a hiatal hernia and gastritis, she had been on Prilosec for the previous two years. She also had used Klonopin for chronic chest pain, anxiety and stress for the previous two years. This had begun after being involved in a motor vehicle collision which wrenched her spine and also created a bilateral plantar fasciitis. She had been taking Ambien to get to sleep for the last 18 months. She dealt with moderate edema in her arms and legs on a weekly basis. She lost her left ovary due to an ovarian cyst at age 17. She had been on birth control pills for the previous 16 years to help control polycystic ovary disease. She was told not to think about having children, due to the fact that her remaining ovary was cystic. They had also found and removed a tumor from her left breast, which fortunately, was benign. Motrin was used on a daily basis to control pain.

She noted an allergy to several medications including: penicillin, erythromycin and sulfa drugs. She was also sensitive to dust and mold so she used Claritin® on a daily basis. She was employed at a dot com company doing secretarial work, and worked very hard as a spin instructor to stay fit.

Physical examination revealed a 5' 2" inch, 120 pound female. Posturally, her head was level, her right shoulder was elevated by one inch, and her left hip was elevated by one inch. Her spine demonstrated a moderate "S" scoliosis; left lumbar, right thoracic. It straightened on forward bending, except for an elevated left erector spinae by one inch, from T12 to L5. The left foot was mildly pronated, and the right foot was severely pronated.

Challenge revealed a pure right cranial stress MAP, a category two right external pelvic-spinal MAP, and a bilateral tarsal tunnel MAP. Extra pelvic-spinal complex spinal dysarthrias included the following: thoracic T1-6 right with ribs right; C5, 6, 7 RLR; T6-8 and C4-6 anterior right with ribs right. Challenge was positive to the C4-6 and T7-9 inter-vertebral discs indicative of soft tissue compressive trauma. The magnesium stretch test was positive, as was repetitive test muscle inhibition, suggesting a need to improve her essential fatty acid metabolism.

Bilaterally inhibited muscles related to the stomach, pancreas, liver, gallbladder and small intestine were found. The stomach was strained up through the opening for the esophagus (a hiatal hernia). Reflexes were positive suggesting ongoing food and mold sensitivities, a small intestine mold overgrowth and a leaky gut.

Recent lab work showed several abnormalities. Her fasting blood sugar was 75 (ideal is 85). Her total protein was 6.6 (ideal is 7). Her red blood cell count was 4.0 (low normal is 4.2).

On her first visit all positive challenge stress MAPs were reduced: cranial, pelvic-spinal and tarsal tunnel. The extra pelvic-spinal complex vertebral subluxation complexes were also reduced. The cervical and thoracic inter-vertebral discs were tractioned manually, and interferential therapy was used post manipulation to reduce pain and promote healing. She was instructed in correct posture and the correct use of moist cold over the key areas of soft tissue injury. We began a Seaklenz protocol, had her use 200 mgs of magnesium glycinate twice a day (BID), and 2 gms of EPA/DHA.

"I can think better. I am more intuitive.
The difference is quite remarkable."

Ada Shaw
Documentary Film Producer Commenting on getting a "Tune-Up"

Her second visit was the next day. We found and reduced a category one right, pelvic-spinal complex, a bilateral post tarsal tunnel complex, and T1-4 right with ribs right; T7-9 anterior right with ribs right.

On the third visit one week later, the patient reported a 50% reduction in her spine pain. At this point, we screened all of her medications for neuro-musculoskeletal sensitivity testing, and found that she was sensitive to Singulair®, Prilosec and Claritin-D. We found and corrected a category zero right, pelvic-spinal MAP, and T3-4 anterior left with ribs left; T7-8 right with ribs right, and C5-6 LR. The T6-8 inter-vertebral discs were found in a torque challenge indicating that they were 60% decompressed. The discs were manually tractioned and she received interferential therapy.

"We stand at a critical point in human cultural evolution. Going back to the old normal where peace is just an interval between wars is not an option; what we need is a fundamental cultural transformation.

As Einstein said, we cannot solve problems with the same thinking that created them. We must transform from a system of domination to one of partnership. Spiritual courage is a much more deeply rooted human courage. It's the courage to stand up against injustice out of love."

Riame Eisler
Yes!

On her fourth visit, one week later, her overall pain was reduced from a 10 to a 4. Neuro-musculoskeletal sensitivity testing was performed and revealed sensitivity to four molds which were negated with olive leaf extract. She was sensitive to both her laundry detergent and fabric softener, as well as, the following foods: fructose, chocolate, peanuts and wheat. She was instructed to avoid the offending foods, observe a low sugar diet, and take olive leaf extract, (two-twice a day) between meals. The thoracic 6-8 inter-vertebral discs were now 80% better (positive flexion challenge). Traction and interferential therapy were, again, applied to the discs.

One month later on her fifth visit her pain was now a two. She was sleeping well without Ambien and experienced no more anxiety. The plantar fasciitis had cleared up. At this point she informed us that she had not used Motrin or Singular for several weeks. Her asthma and allergy symptoms had remarkably cleared up. We found and corrected a few spinal dysarthrias. The thoracic 6-8 intervertebral discs were found flexion-torque, so they received traction and interferential therapy. Neuro-musculoskeletal retesting revealed no molds and no food sensitivities, so we cut back her olive leaf to two, 3 times per week on an empty stomach.   *154*

During the ensuing year she gradually got stronger and healthier. She was rear-ended at one point, and this required a few visits to heal the injuries she sustained. In the meantime, her anemia, allergies, anxiety, insomnia, heartburn, PMS and chronic musculoskeletal pain vanished. Best of all, she met and married a lovely young man, and now has two beautiful children.

Capitalism—What Went Wrong
"America had a remarkable 150 years during which workers enjoyed a steadily rising standard of living (1820-1970). The amount of money an average worker made kept rising decade after decade when measured in "real wages": that's the money you earn compared to the prices you have to pay."

Richard Wolff, UMass Economics Professor Emeritus
Capitalism Hits the Fan: The Global Economic Meltdown and What to do About It.
Published 2009

27. Severe Dry Heaves and Endometriosis

A woman in her early thirties, Judy, was referred to our office by another kinesiologist for treatment of a severely disabling and unusual condition, chronic severe dry heaves. Judy would have "good days and bad days" with this condition. On a good day; the dry heaves, which were strong, loud and totally uncontrollable, would be present in the mornings and go away after about 10-20 minutes after waking. Also, on a good day, they would come back after lunch, lasting 15-20 minutes. On a bad day, they would not stop at all and she was unable to function. This happened one to two days per week. As a teacher of severely handicapped children, this condition severely disabled her and was ruining her life.

It began as a severe case of bronchitis when she was 27 years old, which was treated with amoxicillin. As a result of this condition and treatment, two things subsequently happened; (1) she became depressed, (2) she developed a yeast (candida) infection that affected her inner ears and started endometriosis. This condition caused severe pain throughout her body on an ongoing basis. The pain was migrating and would move from her head to her stomach or tongue or fingers. Her primary care physician could not figure out what was wrong with her. He ended up referring her to an OB/GYN. This doctor performed a laparoscopic examination of her abdomen, which is how the diagnosis of endometriosis was made. She went to several ear, nose and throat specialists and they could not come up with a diagnosis as to why her inner ears were constantly blocked.

Several months after this occurred, she was water skiing and took a bad fall, straining her left hip. It was after this fall that she began having the dry heaves. As a result of the hip injury, she started treating with a professional applied kinesiologist, who referred her to our office for a second opinion since he could not help the problem, which was now escalating way beyond control.

Physical examination of Judy revealed a pure right cranial stress MAP. Her temporo-mandibular joints were severely strained with a tremendous amount of tension, not only in her jaw musculature but also in her upper neck muscles. A category two right pelvic-spinal and bilateral tarsal complex stress MAPs were also present.

Additionally we found that the muscles related to her stomach, small intestine and liver were weak on both sides of her body, suggestive of diminished function of those organs. Reflexes were positive, indicative of a leaky gut along with food and mold sensitivities. We put her on a natural antifungal and a low sugar diet. Additionally we had her avoid the offending foods for one month.

Structurally speaking, she had a very unusual displacement of her upper neck vertebrae. There are seven cervical or neck vertebrae. The top one is called the atlas, like Charles Atlas, the muscle man who is often pictured holding the world (or head in his hand). The midbrain or medulla oblongata extends into the cervical spine as far down as the fourth segment. Judy's third vertebra was found to be anteriorly displaced. The forward mal-position of the third cervical vertebra was stressing the respiratory center in her midbrain (the intermedial nucleus of the medulla). Adjustment and stabilization at this specific segment (in addition to the rest of her body) stopped the dry heaves; they were completely gone, giving this beautiful woman her life back.

The key to relieving the dry heaves was correcting the forward displacement of her third cervical vertebra. The upper ribs, cervical spine (neck), jaw and cranium (22 skull bones) are known as the stomatognathic system. Every part of this closed kinematic chain affects every other part. In this case, Judy's bite was off; when her upper and lower teeth came together, they did not interlock (intercuspate) or align correctly. This is called malocclusion. Ideally, when the upper and lower teeth contact one another, they should not only firmly lock together, but also create no torsion of the jaw joints at the same time.

"This produced the expectation that in the US every generation would live better than the one before it and with hard work you could deliver a better standard of living for your kids.

The end of this trend represents quite a trauma to the working population. It's the end of the nation that a better future is the reward for hard work. The trauma is worsened by the fact that there is no discussion of it. No way to share the experience because most of the population literally believes that it hasn't happened."

Richard Wolff

When Judy clenched her teeth together firmly while touching her jaw joints, it weakened a strong muscle on both sides which is indicative of a malocclusion. Because of this, we sent Judy to one of our healing team members, Dr. Gary Wetreich (prosthodontist extraordinaire), to evaluate and correct her malocclusion. He also made her a splint to wear at night, to disocclude (open up) her rear molars. This is done to prevent the jamming of the cranial bones and destruction of the teeth, which can occur when people clench or grind their teeth at night. Once Judy had this done, it added great stability to her neck and helped to lock in the correct alignment of her neck by balancing her stomatognathic system.

The patient was instructed in the use of a natural antifungal and a mold reducing diet. She was also told to avoid the foods that her immune system was reacting to. Over the course of her first three months of care, her ears cleared up and all of the migrating pains gradually disappeared. The symptoms of her endometriosis never returned.

28. Mononucleosis and Sciatica

A 27-year-old professional tennis player presented at my office for the treatment of sciatica. He was Swedish, and was in the United States visiting with a friend who referred him to our office. He noted that he had a constant right, grade two sciatica (9/10) for the past three weeks. When I asked him if he had injured himself playing tennis, he informed me that he had been unable to play tennis for the last six months, due to a severe case of mononucleosis, that left him with no energy.

Physical examination revealed an alert 5'9" tall, 170 pound male. Posturally, he had an elevated right occiput by one inch, left shoulder by two inches, and left iliac crest by two inches. Challenge revealed a pure right cranial MAP, a category two right external pelvic-spinal MAP, and a bilateral tarsal tunnel MAP. Extra pelvic-spinal vertebral lesions included: C5, 6, 7 RLR; T1-6 right with ribs right, and T3-5 anterior with ribs bilaterally lateral. The sacroiliac compression test was positive on the right. The straight leg raise test was positive on the right at 25°. There was marked spasm and inhibition of his right quadratus lumborum, gluteus maximus and piriformis muscles.

The patient's thymus related muscles (infraspinatus) were bilaterally inhibited. They were facilitated with the patient's insalivation of monolauren, indicating that this might improve his immune system. The magnesium stretch test was positive. Other paired muscle weaknesses, suggesting organ dysfunction, were positive for his stomach and small intestine.

Treatment consisted of the reduction of the right cranial MAP, the category two and three pelvic-spinal MAPs, and all the extra pelvic-spinal complex biomechanical lesions. We then reduced bilateral tarsal tunnel MAPs, the lumbo-sacral spinal muscles were percussed and the T12 to base of right calf were treated with fifteen minutes of interferential therapy. The patient was instructed in the use of moist cold,as well as corrective lumbar disc and pelvic diaphragm exercises. He was also instructed in the use of a sacro-iliac belt.

He was advised to use 500 mgs of monolauren, three times per day, after an initial loading dose of 1000 mgs. We also recommended two betaine hydrochloride tablets per meal to improve stomach digestive function. This would increase both his protein digestion and alkaline mineral absorption. Two hundred milligrams of magnesium glycinate was recommended twice per day.

The patient was seen the following day, and when asked how he was doing remarked that he had just finished playing four hours of singles tennis. He was totally ecstatic at both his physical lack of pain and his huge energy level increase. We found and corrected a category one right, pelvic-spinal MAP and bilateral post tarsal tunnel MAPs.

"Since the 1970s American employers have enjoyed record profits—but the wage earned by the majority of workers hasn't changed. In real terms, adjusted for inflation, what a worker makes in 2011 is about what the same worker made in 1978.

Americans have committed to an incredible number of work hours per household to try to achieve a rising standard of living."

Richard Wolff

Discussion:
It has been my professional experience that the use of monolauren to

destroy the Epstein Barr Virus (EBV) is phenomenal. Lauric acid is a naturally occurring fatty acid found in nature in both mother's breast milk and coconuts. It is capable of preventing the EBV from assembling a cell wall, so it can be destroyed by our immune system. The lack of this knowledge is profound, as evidenced by a recent Duke University Health Newsletter, in which they stated that there is no known cure for EBV.

I have used this product for over twenty years and it inevitably turns around those infected with mononucleosis within 24 hours. The fact that this virus has been identified as a causative agent in hypertension, makes the dissemination of this knowledge all the more important.

One of the greatest challenges in medicine is how to approach immune system dysfunction. More specifically, the question of whether a patient is sick primarily due to a bacteria or a virus.

The thymus gland and its related muscle, the infraspinatus, represents one potential avenue to help resolve this pertinent clinical question.

Usually the patient is given an antibiotic. This is routine, even for virally-caused illness like a cold. Most likely this occurs due to a combination of trying to meet patient expectation, and lack of a convenient differentiation tool, coupled with physicians' lack of training in the use of natural antivirals.

When a patient presents at this office with a bilaterally weak infraspinatus muscle, indicating a weakened, stressed thymus gland, we routinely check it and see if it is strengthened with the introduction of various antivirals into the energy field of the body. If it does, their use has led to many very successful outcomes. Once this understanding is widely disseminated, with supportive scientific research, the overuse of antibiotics will no longer be a problem. This will give doctors and patients a one-up on the plethora of viruses in today's world.

"The other thing the American working class has done since the 1970s to keep their consumption rising is take on debt. American workers started to borrow money on a scale that had never been seen before in any country. So the current crisis really began in the 1970's, when the wages stopped rising, but its effects were postponed for a generation by debt. By 2007, the American working class had accumulated a level of debt that was unsustainable. People could not make the payments."

Richard Wolff

29. Chronic Recurrent Torticollis -Heel Height and Health are Related

A childhood friend of mine presented for treatment at my office for a recurrent stiff neck, also known as a wry neck or torticollis. I had just graduated from chiropractic college and opened my doors to practice. He told me that he had to get adjusted at a chiropractic office two to three times a week to deal with this terrible problem. When I asked how long this had been going on, he indicated it had been years. He was in a rock and roll band, playing guitar and singing. Every time he played, his neck gradually stiffened up, and then locked up. After a few hours, he would end up in excruciating pain. Something else had to be wrong.

Physical examination revealed a 5'11" 175 pound healthy 24-year-old male. He presented with acute severe neck pain. His head was locked in a 45° left-sided rotation with his neck bent to the right at a 45° angle. Visually, his left occiput and left shoulder were elevated by 2 inches, and his left hip by one inch. Challenge revealed a category two right pelvic-spinal MAP with a bilateral tarsal tunnel MAP. Extra pelvic-spinal lesions included a left lateral occiput, T1-7 left with ribs left, and C5, 6, 7 LRL. His left clavicle was also laterally displaced. Muscle testing revealed marked weakness of all of his left neck flexors (anterior, middle, posterior scalene, and sternocleidomastoid). There was marked bilateral hypertonicity of his temporo-mandibular joint muscles (masseter, temporalis and pterygoid muscles). All of his right cervical facet joints were imbricated, and the cervical 4-6 intervertebral discs challenged positive for compression in a non-weight bearing position.

I corrected the category two right pelvic-spinal MAP and the bilateral tarsal tunnel MAPs. I gently reduced the thoracic vertebrae and ribs, then unlocked the lower cervical vertebrae, right facets, left clavicle and occiput. After facilitating his left neck flexors, and inhibiting his right sternocleidomastoid, I manually tractioned his neck. He now stood up with level occiput, shoulders and pelvis looking straight ahead. He immediately felt much better.

Still puzzled as to the real cause of this recurrent nightmare, I further queried him about his profession. He told me that he always wore a "Rod Stewart type" boot with a three inch heel. A light immediately went off in my head. At this point I placed the two Dejarnette pelvic blocks (tools used to un-rotate sprained sacroiliac joints) on the floor with the high ends against the baseboard of the wall.

'They were exhausted financially, exhausted physically by all the hard work and exhausted psychologically because the family had been torn apart by everyone working.
The sitcoms of the 1960's showed happy middle-class families, but many sitcoms today show struggling families. Americans are 5% of the worlds population, but we consume 65% of the world's psychotropic
drugs, tranquilizers and mood enhancers. We are a people under unbelievable stress."

Richard Wolff

I then tested a few large shoulder muscles, and found them to be facilitated (strong). Next, I had him put his back against the wall, and asked him to back his heels up on the blocks until they approximated the height of the boots he wore while playing. He actually backed all the way up the blocks before signaling to me that this was the correct height (about a 3" heel elevation). I retested the previously facilitated shoulder muscles, and to my amazement, they were all totally inhibited. I had him gradually move down on the blocks, a half inch at a time, while retesting a muscle at each lower heel elevation until he had intact muscles again.

This occurred at one and one half inches of heel elevation. I recommended that he did not exceed the 1.5" heel height. He followed my instructions, and never had a stiff neck again.

Discussion:

In trying to understand what had happened, I theorized, there was a fixed point of heel elevation that a person's nervous system can tolerate. Beyond this fixed point, which is usually between one to two inches, every single muscle in a person's body weakens. I believe that this is due to a tethering of the spinal cord. It can only be stretched so far before it becomes dysfunctional. I named this tipping point "the calcaneal tolerance factor." I obtained a U.S. patent for the testing of a person's maximum heel height, and manufactured a metal wedge for doctors to use to test this, called the "Heal Helper." It has proven useful through the years, especially with women who wear high heels. Everyone should know what their maximum permissible heel height is, because once exceeded you are definitely an accident waiting to happen.

'This isn't a typical business cycle. This is the culmination of a 30 year postponement of what happens when 150 years of real-wage increase comes to an end. As a society, we have been unwilling to think critically about capitalism and it shows. Another reason this crisis is so different is that it's coping at the end of a long period of denial. Capitalism is unstable and goes in cycles—today the majority of graduate programs in economics have no courses on business cycles at all."

Richard Wolff

30. Recurrent Vaginal Yeast Infections/Chronic Left Subscapular Pain

A 32-year-old female presented for treatment of intermittent, chronic left subscapular pain, which worsened with increased physical activity and the lifting of heavy objects. She had awakened with the pain several weeks earlier, worsening as the day went on, and persisting since then. She noted that moist cold packs helped. She had a history of monthly vaginal yeast infections since the birth of her first child, nine years earlier. Recently, her OB/GYN doctor suggested Monistat, twice a week for two weeks prior to her period. She noted that she had done this for the past two months and it "seemed to help."

Her history was positive for asthma diagnosed at age eight, which flared up with colds and allergies. She noted environmental allergies to cats and dogs. She was also sensitive to mold and dust mites. Her allergy symptoms were definitely worse in the fall. She moved her bowels once every 2-3 days, and occasionally went as long as five days.

Physical examination revealed an alert, 32-year-old female, 5' 6" tall, weighing 108 pounds. Posturally, her left iliac crest was elevated by one inch. Her spine demonstrated a very mild "S" curvature, left lumbar, right thoracic that straightened on forward bending suggestive of a non-structural curve. A right-left-left cranial stress MAP was found.

Her left deltoid was inhibited (3/5) and became facilitated (5/5) with approximation of the left acromio-clavicular joint, suggestive of a sprain to this ligament. There was marked inhibition of the left wrist muscles (opponens pollicis and digiti minimi), which strengthened with bending her neck to the right, suggestive of a compression of the cervical discs, and restricted neurological outflow to her left wrist and arm.

A category two right pelvic spinal MAP was present. Extra-pelvic spinal category listings included: T1-7 left with ribs left, T2-5 anterior with ribs bilaterally lateral, and C5, 6, 7 LRL. The muscles related to her stomach, liver, gallbladder and small intestines were inhibited, indicating mal-digestion and mal-absorption problems. Positive reflexes were present indicative of both a leaky gut, and on-going food and mold sensitivities.

The thyroid and adrenal related muscles were inhibited bilaterally. This, in conjunction with a positive ligament stretch test, is indicative of a dampening of the neuroendocrine axis.

"We've produced a generation, maybe even two generations, of economists who think economics is about celebrating capitalism and greatness, instead of assessing its strengths and weaknesses.

Capitalism is an institution, like our public school system or our healthcare system. Why is it taboo to ask whether the way we organize the production and distribution of goods and services is meeting our needs?"

Richard Wolff

Multiple facilitated muscles became inhibited after being stretched, indicative of a magnesium insufficiency. Her initial treatment consisted of the reduction of her cranial stress MAP, bilateral tarsal tunnel MAPs, category two right pelvic-spinal MAP, and the extra category listings previously noted. The patient was instructed in correct posture, to prevent thoracic spine re-injury, and the use of moist cold to heal her strained left acromio-clavicular ligament.

Nutritionally, she was instructed to use betaine hydrochloride, two with each meal, and magnesium citrate 200 mgs, two times per day, and a product to thin her bile containing lipotrophic substances. Additionally, we had her use a product to debride her small intestine of undigested food remnants and mucous.

She was seen one week later. She felt much better after her first visit, and could now sleep on her left side. She received corrective care as a category one right, pelvic-spinal MAP, thoracic 5,6 anterior with ribs left, and bilateral post tarsal tunnel MAPs. We performed neuro-musculoskeletal sensitivity testing and found numerous molds and food sensitivities as follows: corn, oats, wheat, peanuts, sesame, mozzarella cheese, beef, yogurt, white potatoes, turkey, lemon, MSG and chocolate. We instructed her in the use of a low sugar diet, and had her use olive leaf extract, a natural antifungal, two, two times a day on an empty stomach.

The patient was seen three weeks later. She felt less bloated, had more energy, and had no yeast infection for the first time in nine years. Re-neuro-musculoskeletal stress test revealed no molds, and one food sensitivity to wheat. The patient also noted 2-3 bowel movements daily since her first adjustment.

The patient has been seen for annual tune-ups, with no flare ups of her previously chronic yeast infections. In our experience, these results for chronic yeast infections are routine occurring hundreds of times. This should be the first line of therapy for this condition for multiple reasons; clinical efficacy, minimal intervention, cost effectiveness and safety.

> *"There's a certain market fundamentalism in the US that equates capitalism with freedom. Yes, employers are free, in this system, to stop raising the workers wages. How do you talk about freedom to the 20 to 30 million Americans who currently have no job?*
>
> *The proportion of the unemployed who have been without work for more than a year is greater than we have seen in decades. There's no question that this crisis is more severe than any other since the Great Depression, in terms of longevity of unemployment."*
>
> Richard Wolff

31. Rheumatoid Arthritis/Electric Blankets

A 32-year old female presented to our office for help with a crippling arthritic condition that deformed her hands. She noted that her knees were starting to get painful, and that the overall quality of her life was quite diminished. She had been diagnosed as having rheumatoid arthritis.

Physical examination revealed a 5'5", 140 pound female. Postural examination revealed a level head, level shoulders and hips. Challenge revealed no cranial, pelvic-spinal or tarsal tunnel complex MAPs. All of the paired muscle groups associated with her digestive, immune and endocrine systems were intact.

Observation of her hands revealed severe clubbing and swelling of all the joints in both hands. There was a moderate to severe flexion contracture deformity present in all of her digits. This condition had a gradual onset beginning three years previously, and was progressive, worsening over time.

At the end of the exam, I informed the patient that I was unable to find anything structurally or obviously functionally wrong with her. In an effort to try to be of some use to her, I suggested she give some serious thought to anything she may have changed in her lifestyle prior to the symptom onset years earlier.

Two days later she phoned back and informed me that she had purchased an electric blanket a few months before her symptoms had begun. She noted that she used the blanket every night because of the warmth it offered her. I suggested she return to the office and bring the blanket.

A few days later the patient returned with the electric blanket. I had her lay on her back on an adjusting table. The patient was extremely robust with all of her muscles graded 5/5. I then put the blanket on her, first not plugging it in. All of the patient's muscles then tested 3+/5, which is a moderate weakness. This was apparently due to the effect of the blanket's wire configuration on her energetic field. I then plugged the blanket into the electric outlet and retested multiple muscles. With the blanket turned on, all of her muscles were pathologically weak, 3-/5.

I refer to enlightening times such as these as "kinesthetic moments." I suggested she discontinue the blanket use and substitute a down comforter. She did so and returned five months later for re-examination. When I looked at her hands, they were totally normal.

Discussion:

This exact scenario happened with another female patient with severe rheumatoid arthritis of 15 years duration. It too cleared up and went away entirely with the cessation of the use of the electric blanket. Our bodies are electric and need an electromagnetic stress-free environment to heal themselves while we sleep.

> *"From the '70s, profits in business went through the roof because of stagnant wages. Economic shifts enabled CEOs to stop raising worker's wages yet keep getting more out of them. It was at this point that US corporations began to pay their CEOs out-of-whack sums of money, plus multi-million dollar bonuses at the end of each year and huge stock options.*
>
> *You're giving 5-10% of the people an enormous boost of income while everybody else gets nothing."*
>
> Richard Wolff, *Capitalism Hits The Fan*

Recently, Dr. Stephan Sinatra[1] has written about the anti-inflammatory healing properties of earth-grounding in his new book, *Earthing*. Dr. Sinatra feels as though this is the most important breakthrough in medicine in the last 40 years. The earth's electromagnetic field, fueled by 7,000 lightening strikes per day, is negative. All of the free radicals our bodies produce are positive. Walking barefoot, sleeping or studying with an earth-grounded mattress cover or foot pad will negate these positive ions. Several of my patients have already reported back to me their experience of better sleep patterns, lower blood pressure and lessened pain and swelling throughout their bodies. According to the Optimum Health Brochure, "Earthing may: improve the symptoms of inflammation-related disorders, reduce or eliminate chronic pain, improve sleep, increase energy, moderate nervous system activity, thin blood and improve circulation, relieve muscle tension, reduce jet lag and accelerate recovery from strenuous athletic activity." The book and related products (bed, computer mats) are available at 800-228-1507.

As far as convenience technologies go, not all of them have a positive impact on our health and well being. Utilizing PAK™ testing demonstrates clearly that there are certain technologies that one must use with caution or not at all. These are microwaved food or liquids, electric blankets, chlorinated water, fluoridated water and toothpaste, genetically modified foods, car seat heaters, high fructose corn syrups and all processed foods to name a few.

The use of the earthing tools helped to bring clarity to something I had seen repeatedly, but couldn't put my finger on its cause. One very common energetic stress MAP created by our lack of contact with the earth's magnetic field. As a result of our modern day fast paced lives we may go for long periods of time without earth contact, especially in the northern climates in the winter. This results in an imbalance in the kidney and bladder meridians with too much energy in the kidney meridians (psoas muscle spasm) and not enough energy in the bladder meridian (all muscles on the entire back of the body, head to toe). This promotes the all too commonly seen slumped forward posture in the frail and elderly. This imbalance goes away with placing one's feet on the ground. Adjacencies with balance and reflux issues abound.

"Thirty years ago the US was one of the most egalitarian societies in terms of wealth. Now, we have the greatest disparity between rich and poor of all the industrial nations.

The wealth inequality in the US has occurred due to an explosion in the value of the stock market in the last 30 years."

Richard Wolff

32. Chronic Insomnia and Tension Headaches

A 33-year-old female presented for the treatment of a severe sleep disorder, of 20 years duration. She also had a list of neuro-musculoskeletal aches and pains, including daily tension headaches, neck and low back pain. She noted trouble both falling and staying asleep. A good night's sleep consisted of three hours of continuous sleep. She had tried a variety of both pharmacological and nutritional approaches, to no avail. Some of the items she tried included Nexium, Lunesta, valerian, tryptophan and essential oil of lavender.

Physical examination revealed an alert but distraught 33-year-old female. Posturally, her right occiput was elevated by one half inch, her right shoulder by two inches, and her left iliac crest by one and a half inches. Challenge revealed a left-right-right cranial complex stress MAP. The muscles of mastication (temporalis, masseter, internal pterygoid) were hypertonic bilaterally.

A category two right pelvic-spinal complex MAP was also found, along with bilateral tarsal tunnel MAPs. Extra-pelvic spinal complex lesions consisted of T1-6 right with ribs right, and C5, 6, 7 RLR. All of the cervical facet joints, (these form the exit holes or windows where the nerves leave the neck to control the shoulder, arm, and hand muscles) as well as the blood supply to the thyroid and parathyroid glands were jammed together. We use the term imbrications to describe the wedging together of sliding/gliding joints. Her cervical facet joints were imbricated bilaterally at all levels. The magnesium stretch test was positive.

Initial treatment consisted of the reduction of the cranial complex stress MAP. Clinical observation has shown that the normal function of the motion of the cranial vault up-regulates the function of the neuroendocrine axis, or where your brain folds in upon itself and becomes the endocrine system. This takes place in the middle of the brain and includes the pineal, pituitary, and hypothalamic endocrine glands. These glands are known to be your body's master endocrine control center. For example, these glands control your sleep-wakefulness cycles (or your circadian rhythms), reproductive cycles, stress-handling capabilities, and your structural integrity. In fact, it has been stated that the neuroendocrine axis has a direct influence on one hundred physiological set points, including our perception of pain, body temperature, and clotting characteristics to name a few. I have found that up-regulation of this functional area is key to making all of the other body corrections hold firmly, making the tone of the ligaments holding the joints in alignment more like steel and less like rubber.

"Between 1934 and 1940 the federal government under Roosevelt created and filled 11 million jobs. It put people back to work and gave them a decent income so they didn't lose their homes. Roosevelt made the wealthy in this country pay for the effort. He raised taxes on companies and the rich to obtain the money to hire all the unemployed."

Richard Wolff

I gently realigned her feet, knees and pelvis, and corrected all of the rotated vertebrae and ribs. In the process, I un-jammed (de-imbricated) all of the cervical facet joints on both sides of her neck, and balanced the muscles in all areas of the correction.

The patient was instructed to use 400 mg of magnesium citrate per day. She was taught correct spinal posture, and neck and low back stretches. The patient was treated on three occasions a few weeks apart, with full resolution of her sleep disorder (she now sleeps eight hours a night with no interruptions), tension headaches, neck and low back pain. This patient has been treated periodically for various other injuries over the last ten years, so I have had the clinical opportunity to observe the complete resolution of both the chronic sleep disorder and tension headaches. Needless to say, she is a great advocate of PAK™.

Discussion:

Sleep debt has been shown to hasten the onset of diseases like type II diabetes and obesity, and to reduce immunity. According to the National Institutes of Health consensus statement, about 30% of American adults have some symptoms of insomnia within a given year, while approximately 10% have associated symptoms of daytime functional impairment. 30% of the people over age 50 experience some degree of insomnia, which may come as no surprise as melatonin levels decrease dramatically with aging.

In this case, functional restoration of the neuroendocrine axis most likely facilitated the return to balance of this patient's ability to sleep in a normal manner. When it gets dark outside, the pineal gland secretes melatonin, which eventually causes a person to fall asleep. Inadequate stimulation of this gland by lack of cranial motion, may reduce its production of this key hormone, and thus create down stream problems. This treatment should be the very first line of therapy for sleep disorders, as it is simple, cost effective and non-invasive.

A recent case report published by Dr. Scott Cuthbert and Dr. Anthony Rosner, described the successful removal of anxiety and insomnia with MMT (manual muscle testing) utilized as a guide to the appropriate interventions. The patients long-term anxiety and insomnia (as well as frequent headaches) were resolved in six visits, over three weeks.[1]

"The world as we have created it is a process of our thinking. It cannot be changed without changing our thinking."

Albert Einstein

Discussion:

An estimated three out of four adults suffer from tension headaches.[1] This makes them the most common of all headaches. According to this source, there are more than 300 types of headaches, but only 10% have a known cause. The others are known as primary headaches; (no known cause), tension-type headaches being one of the major primary headaches.

After relieving hundreds, if not thousands of patients with tension-type headaches, I feel as though I can argue against their arising from "an unknown" cause. The facet joints at the posterior aspect of the vertebral motor unit have a pain sensitive meniscus that can be the cause of head pain. They have historically created such head pain that neurosurgeons have cut the nerves to these facet joints (in a procedure known as facet rhizotomy) in an effort to abort the pain. The functional causes of head pain are created by both cranial and pelvic spinal stress MAPs.

"When you advocate taxing corporations and the rich, you're not talking socialism or communism. You're talking about re-creating a chapter of our history in which a president, enabled by a powerful trade union movement, led the country in a radically different direction.

President Obama repeatedly compromises with the Right and ignores or throws minor concessions to his core constituents."

Richard Wolff

33. Carpal Tunnel Syndrome

A 35-year-old female presented for treatment of problems with her right hand. In the previous six to twelve months, she had experienced a gradual onset of numbness. It was specifically located in the second and third metacarpal and occasionally in the first metacarpal (finger). She reported loss of grip strength. The patient had been using a wrist support, which helped at night, and Advil with Motrin had been recommended. The next steps were to be cortisone, followed by surgery, if necessary.

Her past history included an automobile accident 16 years earlier, in which she rear-ended another car, resulting in injuries which occasioned the loss of her four upper central incisors.

The patient reported a moderate to severe right orbital headache, occurring one to two times per week. It usually came on as the day progressed, and was relieved by aspirin. She noted occurrences of pain in her upper right arm (in the anterior deltoid), reflecting into her biceps area.

She was employed as a quality control inspector, pulling down 10-15 pounds of ceramic decals and shifting from right to left on a regular basis. She was also involved in shipping and receiving, and sometimes pushed a cart of several pounds at the end of the day.

Physical examination revealed an alert 35-year-old, 5'6" 138 pound female. Auscultation of the tempormandibular joint was negative for a click bilaterally. The mandible showed a mild "S" path of motion with a normal width of opening. The masseter, temoralis and pterygoid muscsles were bilaterally hypertonic. Challenge revealed a left-left-right cranial stress MAP, a category two right pelvic-spinal MAP, and bilateral tarsal tunnel MAPs. Extra pelvic-spinal lesions included C5, 6, 7 RLR, T1-5 right with ribs right and T3-5 anterior with ribs bilaterally lateral. The cervical 4-6 inter-vertebral discs challenged positive (very compressed) in a non-weight bearing position.

There was a positive Phalen's and Tinel's Test on the right (orthopedic tests used to identify a carpal tunnel syndrome). Cervical ranges of motion were within normal limits. Cervical compression caused pain in her right wrist. The strength of the right opponent pollicis and digiti minimi muscles improved dramatically with the patient laterally bending her head to the left. This suggested a double crush injury, where the nerve to the wrist muscle is compromised both at its exit from the neck and its course through the wrist (carpal) tunnel.

Carpal Tunnel is among the most common hand surgeries. A number of experts believe that release surgery is performed too often. "Aggressive" conservative treatment; such as splinting, physical therapy and anti-inflammatory agents are recommended first. Certain factors, like diabetes and high blood pressure, may reduce the chances for success, increasing the need for a second operation.

It is important to note that both of these conditions are also related to low magnesium. So embracing the concept of identifying and correcting primary nutrient deficits should be at the forefront of our therapeutic endeavors. Once again, the FM's model's system-based approach is real healing medicine.

Over the years we have had resounding success applying the approach used with this patient (re: carpal tunnel) on hundreds of patients. At a fraction of the cost ($1,500 vs. $7,000 for surgery = 80% savings), the opportunity for vast cost savings is apparent when you look at the big picture (500,000 surgeries at a cost of $7,000 each, costing a total of $3.5 billion dollars a year). It's time to efficiently integrate an internal referral system to achieve this. Soft Tissue Injury Clinics (STIC) in conjunction with all Emergency Rooms will create a robust healthcare system. They will also create tens of thousands of new jobs.

34. Alopecia Arreata

A 42-year-old male presented for treatment of a condition that manifested as clumps of his black hair turning white and then falling off his scalp, exposing silver dollar patches of bare scalp. He also had half of his moustache turn white and fall off his face. This problem had started about one week previously. His medical history was unremarkable for any significant illness. He used no medications.

Physical examination revealed an alert 5'11", 175 pound male. Posturally his right occiput, right shoulder and left hip were all elevated by one inch. Challenge was positive for a pure right cranial MAP, a category two right, pelvic-spinal MAP and bilateral tarsal tunnel MAPs. Extra pelvic-spinal complex lesions included: C5, 6, 7, RLR and T1-5 right with ribs right.

There was paired inhibition of the muscles related to the following organs: stomach, small intestine, liver and gallbladder. The reflexes were positive for a small intestine mold overgrowth, leaky gut, and ongoing food and mold sensitivities. The magnesium stretch test was positive, as was repetitive muscle testing, suggesting a need to up-regulate both his magnesium and essential fatty acid status.

On his first visit, we reduced the right cranial stress MAP, the category two, right pelvic-spinal MAP and the bilateral tarsal tunnel MAPs. Additionally we reduced the extra pelvic-spinal complex spinal lesions and balanced the related muscle inhibitions.

The patient was instructed to use two betaine hydrochloride tablets with each meal, 200 mgs magnesium citrate BID, and 1000 mgs of EPA/DHA complex per day. He was placed on the Sea Klenz program to clear his small intestine of built up undigested food and mucous.

He was seen several days later and he remarked that his hair had stopped falling out. We found and corrected a category one right, pelvic-spinal complex and a bilateral post tarsal tunnel complex sprain. Neuro-musculoskeletal sensitivity testing revealed sensitivity to several molds and the following foods: wheat, rye, potatoes, eggs, beets and citrus. He was advised to avoid the offending foods, to follow a low sugar diet, and use the antifungal olive leaf extract (two, twice daily on an empty stomach).

I referred him to a dermatologist, Dr. Alan Dattner, who confirmed the diagnosis. He injected the areas of large hair loss with a steroid as a precaution against further loss.

The patient was seen three weeks later and all of his hair had started to fill in with no further areas turning white or falling out. We found and corrected a category zero right, pelvic-spinal MAP. Neuro-musculoskeletal sensitivity retesting revealed no molds and a few food sensitivities: chocolate, rice and apples. He was instructed to reduce the olive leaf to 2-3 times per week on an empty stomach.

One month later the patient presented with a full head of black hair and a full mustache. He was ecstatic, as he had been previously informed that he would probably either lose all of his hair or have a patchy head of bald spots amidst gray and black hair.

Discussion:

Autoimmune diseases are an epidemic now in the United States. According to Donna Jackson Nakazawa in her book, *The Autoimmune Epidemic*, nearly 24 million Americans are suffering from an autoimmune disease, "yet nine out of ten Americans cannot name a single one of these diseases." Eighty percent of these are women. The economic burden, at more than $120 billion dollars per year, is staggering. The National Institutes of Health state that more people have autoimmune disease than the 9 million Americans with cancer, and the 16 million with coronary disease. Spreading to almost every industrialized nation, the world has dubbed it ,"the Western disease." Dr. Russell Jaffee recently stated that "more than half of all American adults, and a rapidly growing proportion of young people, experience some type of autoimmune condition."[1]

According to researcher Delisa Fairweather, PhD, at the Bloomberg School of Public Health's, Department of Environmental Health Sciences Division of Toxicology, it is the innate immune response through overactive mast cells, and not the adaptive immune response that goes out of control leading to autoimmune diseases. She has "concluded that the human immune system can become so besieged by unrelenting contact with a toxic barrage of viruses, chemicals and heavy metals, that it's practically forced to run amok.[2]

When the innate immune system meets a constant onslaught of potentially dangerous challenges, be they infections or toxic substances, it behaves like a car whose accelerator is stuck at 80 miles an hour and whose breaks aren't working."[3]

Environmental triggers can be viral. For example, John Harley says, "Epstein-Barr Virus has been shown to trigger Lupus."

At Massachusetts General Hospital (MGH), Dr. Denise Faustman, Associate Professor of Medicine at Harvard Medical School and Director of the MGH Immunology Laboratory, may be on the verge of developing a cure for Type I Diabetes. The culprit is auto-reactive T-cells that escape from the bone marrow. They are compromised with the cytokine TNF alpha. When killed, the body is capable of regenerating the insulin-producing cells and reversing the disease entirely. This has the potential to impact the treatment of other autoimmune diseases like: MS, Chrohn's, Hashimoto's, Sjogren's Syndrome and Lupus.

"Major shareholders and their boards of directors use profits to buy political power needed to undo reforms the mass movements manage to win.

This is a deep and long lasting crisis with global impact. Although I cannot predict whether a tipping point has been reached, I am glad that the questions of whether capitalism continues to serve people's needs is now on the minds of millions worldwide. That's a long overdue development."

Richard Wolff

When the paradigm is changed in a way that affects others in the field negatively, it upsets a lot of people. Industry calls it "disruptive technology." When the immune system is pushed to turn haywire in one area, it's more likely to go haywire in many areas.[4] So a person with one autoimmune disease is predisposed to developing sequential autoimmune diseases. If Fairweather and her colleagues' discovery is correct, that autoimmune disease, when stimulated through the mast cell interaction, does not require any genetic predisposition, this problem could potentially affect every person. The thinking is that 25% of Americans (or 75 million), carry a genetic pre-disposition to autoimmunity, and that this would be the ceiling or upper level of possible incidence. When the immune system is overloaded with chemicals, non-nutrient dense foods, dyes, preservatives and heavy metals, everyone is a potential target.

Every one of us has to dismantle the offenders and build a lifestyle to minimize the immune corruptors. The integrity of the gastro-intestinal tract is "inextricably linked to what's transpiring elsewhere in the body."[5] We know that "the autoimmune process can be arrested if the interplay between genes and environmental triggers is prevented, by re-establishing intestinal barrier competency."[6]

Lowering inflammation and stress, utilizing antioxidants, essential fatty acids, vitamin D, white tea, bodywork, and detoxification in a Far Infrared sauna (on a regular basis), all add up to a good medium for such prevention.

Let's create a healthy world, now. Albert Einstein said "the most important decision you ever have to make is whether you live in a friendly universe or a hostile one." He also stated that "the world is not dangerous because of those who do harm, but because of those who look at it without doing anything".

"Every part of our economic history over the last 30 years would have been radically improved if we'd had a different way of organizing our enterprises—not the top-down, undemocratic and bureaucratic arrangement of corporations today, but a more cooperative collective, community focused method that is democratic at its core."

Richard Wolff

35. Car Seat Heaters

A 44-year-old male who had been a patient for several years presented with acute left neck, mid-back and low back pain of several days duration. One of his jobs/hobbies is being a professional photographer of natural beauty. Usually he presented with this type of full-body pain after he had just returned from some beautiful remote area like Antarctica, Africa or Iceland, stretching himself beyond limits for days on end, carrying heavy camera equipment, and filming for long hours in contorted positions. But this time was different. He had been home for some time.

Physical examination revealed a 6' tall, 170 pound male, in acute distress. Posturally, his left occiput was elevated by one inch, his left shoulder by two inches, and his left hip by one inch. Challenge revealed a pure left cranial stress MAP, a category two right pelvic-spinal MAP, and bilateral tarsal tunnel MAPs. Extra pelvic-spinal complex lesions included the following: C5, 6, 7 LRL, T1-7 left with ribs left, T3-6 anterior with ribs bilaterally lateral, T10-12 anterior with ribs bilaterally lateral, and sacral base extended with L5 anterior.

The magnesium stretch test was negative. All of the bilateral muscles relating to his gastrointestinal and immune system were intact. Shock absorber test for mineral balances was normal. Repetitive muscle testing was normal, suggesting good essential fatty acid status.

The cranial stress MAP creates a positive pineal reflex, as this is the part of our endocrine system that is motion-dependent for normal function. I tell people that their pineal gland is their GPS. It lets them know where they are located in space. In this case, the pineal, thyroid and adrenal reflexes were all positive as a downstream affect of the cranial stress MAP.

We reduced the cranial, pelvic-spinal and bilateral tarsal tunnel complex MAPs as well as all of the extra pelvic-spinal lesions. After balancing the related inhibited muscles, we percussed all of the muscles in the areas of involvement, and then applied interferential stimulation therapy to the cervical-thoracic and lumbo-pelvic areas.

After this, we had the patient walk around for a few minutes, and then cleared up a category one pelvic-spinal complex, and a bilateral post tarsal tunnel sprain complex. I refer to this sequential treatment protocol as "compressed treatment," since you can achieve the equivalent of several weeks of traditional physical medicine in a shortened timeframe.

He was now starting to feel much better, but I still wanted to figure out the cause of this episode. I had been treating him and his family for several years, and he had done everything that I suggested along the way to feel better.

"Sanity is a madness put to good use."
George Santayana

Originally, he was brought in by another patient and friend due to injuries sustained in a car accident. He had been at a full stop, reaching over to get something in his glove box, when a car rear-ended him at 50 miles an hour. He ended up at my office after being in severe pain for several years, seeing many other doctors, trying many different therapies, and using many kinds of pain medications with no results.

All that was history, and along the way, we had him visit our team member, Dr. Gary Wetreich, DDS. Dr. Wetreich, a prosthodontist, and former student of the renowned Dr. Nathan Allen Shore, DDS., is unsurpassed when it comes to creating a perfect bite. He is assistant clinical professor at Harvard School of Dental Medicine and is the course director of the Advanced Postgraduate Prosthodontic Complex Treatment Planning and Applied Occlusion.

The treatment process is known as occlusal equilibration. When the upper and lower teeth meet, they are supposed to interlock (inter-cuspate) without interference, at the same time the ends of the mandible (jaw bone) have to be perfectly seated in their articular beds in the skull (the temporal fossae). This process is a key part of healing that has major systemic effects—for several reasons. The temporomandibular joint (TMJ) is sometimes called the most important joint in the human body, because it has input into 90% of the motor and sensory parts of the brain. It is innervated by the trigeminal nerve, which continues to descend down the entire spinal canal to the level of the twelfth thoracic vertebrae, and at any of these levels, out from the spine, is capable of causing remote phantom pain which may be reflexively experienced in the jaw. Thus, the 'great imposter' is another name attached to the TMJ.

That said, one of the causes of a cranial stress MAP is the clenching and grinding we do at night. The teeth have to be sharpened so they inter-cuspate without interference. The next step is to have a small splint made to wear at night that dis-occludes the rear molars, preventing trauma to the teeth, and not allowing any significant forces to build up in the jaw muscles that could jam the cranial sutures.

Since the patient had been through this process, I asked if he had been good about using his splint at night. He had been using it, so I was still stumped. Since he had experienced no head trauma, no acute infections, used his splint, and had excellent nutrition, with no signs of magnesium or essential fatty acid need, the only other thing that I knew could jam his cranials and start the neuro-musculoskeletal cascade he demonstrated was exposure to an abnormally strong electromagnetic field.

He said that he kept his cell phone away from his head, and did not use an electric blanket. The next question was whether he used a car seat heater. His reply was "yes"—he did a lot of driving, and loved to drive with the seat heater cranked up as high as it could go. Bingo!

Some of our latest technological advances are fraught with hidden dangers. (See appendix: "A Short List of Technologies to be Wary of").

We took a walk out to his vehicle and had him get in the driver's seat and start the engine. He opened the driver's window, and I checked his pineal reflex at the back of his head; it was not active. I had him turn on the car seat heater; upon retesting, the pineal reflex was now positive. There was the answer to my question.

That was several years ago, and I now routinely add this information to my patient coaching statements, which included what "not to do" to stay healthy. My understanding is that one of the many functions of the pineal gland is that of letting us know where we are located in space—so it is extremely electromagnetically sensitive. My advice is, if you live in a frigid area of the world, and are lucky enough to own a car with a seat heater, to do the following: start the car, let the seat warm up for a few minutes without you in it, and when you get in turn it off immediately. Your body will thank you by running more smoothly.

36. Thoracic Outlet Syndrome (TOS)

A 54-year-old female presented for treatment of thoracic outlet syndrome, a condition diagnosed a week prior by a medical doctor. Her complaints consisted of right-sided neck pain that "radiated posterolaterally and left." She rated the pain as a 10 and described it as "achy and sharp." She actually circled the entire row of pain adjectives on our intake form: ache, burning, stabbing, pins and needles; and filled in cold, discolored, stiff and swollen as well as throbbing of hands, and no strength under "other". These symptoms were constant and had started five years earlier. They were more intense for the last two years, and were increasing. She noted that the burning in her hands would go away if she stood up, and certain postures would sometimes lessen the symptoms.

Her second chief complaint was that of a hot tongue that had been constant for two years. She noted that it had started after antibiotic therapy. The tongue appeared cracked, caused her eating "to be different" and the only thing that made it better was not thinking about it. This condition was self-rated as a 7/10.

The third chief complaint was the loss of strength in her hands and wrists. Additionally, both ring fingers were locking up in flexion as "trigger fingers." All of her fingers felt "thick and heavy." These symptoms were worsened with exposure to cold, and she had experienced them "for ten years or more." She noted that a series of cortisone shots three years earlier had not really helped, "especially when they injected the median nerve in her left wrist." This constellation of symptoms was also rated as a 7/10.

Her fourth chief complaint was an achy, stabbing pain, with pins and needles, that ran from her low back and buttocks to her right ankle. This pain also centered across the lumbo-sacral spine, greater on the right than the left. She noted this pain as a 7/10 and "intermittent", but it was "more on than off." Her body position was the only thing that made it better.

The next complaint was that of vertigo, which had started six years earlier. She noted that it caused a "fuzzy, confined feeling" along with nausea and confusion." She would wake up with an "exploding" pain over her right mastoid-occiput areas. This had started about one year ago, previously occurring two to three times a week, and currently happening twice a month.

She had used anti-inflammatories and muscle relaxants for the last five years. Included in her regimen was naproxen (375 mgs/day) and tranadine (2 mgs/day) to relax. She also used Concerta (54 mgs/day) for two years to improve her ADHD symptoms. She also used a multi- vitamin/mineral, chondroitin and glucosamine sulfate product for 10 years.

Her past medical history included the delivery of two healthy boys both by C-Section when she was 27 and 29 years of age, tonsillectomy at age 16, and four impacted wisdom teeth removed at age 18. She crushed the distal phalanx of her left thumb at age 21 in a car door. She was rear-ended twice; once at age 46, and a second time one year later.

These accidents exacerbated her neck and back pain, and led to a change in the patterns of her thought process. She had an inguinal hernia repair at age 48. She had developed a long term infection (six to seven months) following a tissue biopsy from an Ob-Gyn visit. Several rounds of antibiotics were used prior to a D and C which she had two years earlier. The patient noted she enjoyed walking 4-5 miles a day but had to discontinue this exercise regimen due to increased spinal pain.

Diagnostic imaging studies were performed with the following results: Lumbar spine films taken in January of 2001 revealed a mild to moderate decrease of all lumbar discs. Moderate lateral canal stenosis was present throughout. Cervical spine films taken at the same time revealed no fracture, with a straightening of the normal forward cervical curve with no reversal.

Lateral canal stenosis was mild on the left at levels 2-5, and moderate on the right from 3-6. A cervical MRI done a few months later revealed a bulging disc at C5/6 and once again noted the flattened or straight cervical curve, with no reversal. follow up MRI was done in February of 2007 with no significant cord abnormality, and no evidence of thoracic outlet syndrome. A chest MRA (magnetic resonance angiograph) was performed two weeks later. This imaging revealed mild to moderate compression of the left subclavian artery with abduction, and moderate to severe compression of the left subclavian vein with abduction. It was after this study that they had recommended the removal of her left first rib to relieve the thoracic outlet syndrome.

Physical examination revealed an alert, but distraught 54-year-old female with a stated height of 5'3", weighing 103 pounds. Posturally, her left iliac crest was elevated by two inches, her right shoulder was elevated by two inches, and her head was level. Her spine was essentially straight.

Challenge revealed multiple cranial structural dis-relationships (a right-left-left MAP). There was a category two right-external pelvic-spinal MAP. Extra-pelvic-spinal complex vertebral biomechanical lesions included the following: T1-8 left with ribs left, T2-5 anterior with ribs bilaterally lateral, T10-12 anterior with ribs bilaterally lateral, C5-7, LRL with all left spine facets imbricated. Non-weight bearing compressed intervertebral discs were found at the lumbar 3-5 and cervical 4-6. Approximation of the left acromioclavicular ligament facilitated the left mid-deltoid suggesting a sprain to that ligament.

Bilateral tarsal tunnel MAPs were present. Muscle testing revealed a 3/5 weakness with the approximation of the thumb and little fingers (the opponens pollicis and digiti minimi muscles, bilaterally). This weakness went away with the bending of her head on her neck toward the opposite side (this opens up the holes where the nerves exit from the spine into the shoulder and head) which suggested the presence of a "double crush" injury: crush one on the nerve at its exit from the neck, and crush two at its passage through the carpal tunnel at the wrist. Myotomes tested positive for the C5 and C7 levels bilaterally.

Other significant findings included bilateral weakness of the muscles related to the following organs: stomach, pancreas, small intestine, large intestine, thyroid and adrenals. Multiple muscles weakened after a quick stretch, suggesting a magnesium insufficiency. Positive reflexes were found suggestive of both a leaky gut (mold overgrowth) and ongoing food and mold sensitivities. Shock absorber test was positive, suggestive of a need to increase trace minerals for ligament strength, so we recommended an improved multivitamin/mineral formula.

On her first visit, we reduced the cranial pelvic-spinal and tarsal tunnel stress MAPs. Both carpal tunnel sprains were reduced, with muscle work applied, as needed, to normalize function. The patient was instructed to use moist cold on the areas of disc compression, as well as her right sacroiliac and left acromioclavicular joints. She was instructed in the correct use of a sacroiliac belt.

Nutritionally, her diet was fairly well balanced, so we suggested the use of a better multivitamin/mineral (2/meal), hydrochloric acid (2/meal) and 200 mgs of magnesium glycinate (twice/day). We started her on Sea Klenz to debride undigested foods and mucous from her small intestines.

On her second visit, five days later, her pelvis and head were level, right shoulder high by .75 inches. She noted she felt pretty good all over, feeling only slightly achy for the past two days. We found and corrected a Category I right pelvic-spinal stress MAP. Only two extra-complex lesions were found; T5 and 6 left with ribs left. Cervical facet joints were bilaterally imbricated at levels 4-7. The patient was given exercises to stretch and strengthen her cervical and lumbar spinal discs, as well as her pelvic diaphragm.

The patient was seen on her third visit one week later. The hand and arm burning had gone from a 10 to a 2. Her whole body pain was reduced from 7 to a 4. Her wrist strength was coming back. Category zero right pelvic-spinal MAP was found and reduced.

The cervical and lumbar discs compression were 60% and 80% decompressed respectively. Neuro-musculoskeletal stress testing revealed marked sensitivity to a number of molds and foods, so the patient was instructed to use a natural antifungal (olive leaf extract), and put on a low sugar diet. Additionally she was instructed to avoid the following foods: corn, wheat, oats, mushrooms, cashews, white potatoes, shrimp, tomatoes, cauliflower, cherries, green peas and lemons.

Three weeks later, the patient's mold sensitivities were no longer present. The olive leaf was reduced to two, twice per week, on an empty stomach. She was found sensitive to the following foods: rye, wheat, cow's milk, beet, cauliflower, peach, brewer's yeast, chamomile and chocolate. At this point, we advised her to consider a gluten-free diet, due to the positive testing of wheat and rye. Examination and correction involved category zero right pelvic-spinal MAP. She noted her overall symptoms were 50%-75% better. Her left hand, where the cortisone shot hit the median nerve one year previously, was still very numb.

On her next visit one month later she demonstrated continued improvement with no more suboccipital pain. The burn was completely gone from her right hand. She had described a few episodes of right hip and leg pain while getting in and out of her car, and challenge revealed a category three right pelvic-spinal complex with increased compression of the L3-5 intervertebral discs. Her last three lumbar facets were also deimbricated. We instructed the patient in the use of high dose pancreatic enzymes on an empty stomach, to alleviate both the cracked and burning tongue and pressure sensitivity in her digits.

Two months later the patient was seen for her sixth visit and was ecstatic, as her hands were "95% better." All of her pain syndromes were markedly decreased, and she felt "1000 % better overall." At this point, she wanted to start walking daily again. We advised the use of alpha lipoic acid (as she had been craving sweets), and had her restart nutrients specific of healthy cartilage.

The seventh visit was three months later, and she was "feeling fantastic." She had been off both wheat and sugar, and had lost 8 pounds. Her balance was better, and she felt more grounded. We recommended the use of grape seed extract to help desensitize her hands to cold. Structurally, we found and corrected a category zero pelvic-spinal stress MAP, with a sacral base and L5 anterior. She was now doing cardiovascular exercise a few times a week, and felt, once again, in control of her life.

37. Vertigo—Sub-Occipital Headaches

A 42-year-old female presented for treatment of moderate to severe vertigo and sub-occipital headaches. Eight months earlier, while at a formal dinner party, she was walking down a flight of stairs, when she tripped, catching her evening gown on her high heel. She lurched forward, and avoided falling by running very fast down the remaining six stairs. She hit the wall at the bottom of the stairs head first, with her wine glass lodged between her head and the wall, breaking her nose. She lost consciousness and suffered a severe concussion. Her neck was severely sprained. She developed short-term amnesia and "noises in her head", for which she was treated with "tranquilizers." For three weeks after the injury, she had severe right-sided abdominal pain, never definitively diagnosed, despite re-hospitalization. One week after the accident, she experienced "labrynthitis," and couldn't sleep, owing to a feeling of falling down while in the recumbent position. Since then she had to sleep in a chair, sitting up.

Her chief complaint was moderate to severe vertigo, worse lying down, and particularly with looking up (head in extension). The vertigo was characterized by a "sensation of spinning around in a circle, like being on a carousel, going from right to left." There was a constant mild pain at the back of her cervical spine. Neck stiffness and immobility were present, but had improved with physical therapy. She had moderate sub-occipital headaches. Sleep was grossly disturbed by the presenting problems, and she had been unable to participate in competitive tennis. Her prior medical history was unremarkable, except for multiple drug sensitivities.

Physical examination revealed a distressed, 5'7" tall, 140-pound female. Posturally, both feet were moderately to severely pronated. Her left iliac crest, shoulder and occiput were all mildly elevated. Her spine demonstrated a mild "S" scoliosis, right lumbar, left thoracic, that straightened on forward bending, suggesting a non-structural curvature. There was a severe flattening of the thoracic kyphosis, from T3-T6. There was a 10 point systolic drop in blood pressure, from lying to standing, suggestive of moderate hypoadrenia. The mandible demonstrated a moderate "S" path of motion on opening and closing. The right temporomandibular joint (TMJ) was positive for a click on opening. Challenge revealed a right-left-left cranial stress MAP, a category two right pelvic-spinal MAP, and a bilateral tarsal tunnel MAP. Non-weight bearing inter-vertebral disc challenges were positive from C3/4 through C5/6, suggesting severe neck compressive trauma. The atlas (C1 vertebrae), was anteriorly displaced. Challenge also revealed bilateral sterno-clavicular, acromio-clavicular and carpal tunnel sprains.

Cervical ranges of motion all caused pain at the cervico-thoracic junction, while all ranges were normal, except for left and right rotation, which were diminished by 5 degrees each. Hyperesthesia was noted in the right C3/4, and anterior T2 dermatomes. Muscle testing revealed a 3/5 weakness of the following neck muscles: bilateral anterior, middle and posterior scalene as well as sternocleidomastoids. The following myotomes were positive for the upper extremity: right C5 deltoid, left C5 biceps, left C6 wrist extensor, left C7 finger flexor and bilateral T1 interossei. The Freeman Wyke Test was positive bilaterally, indicating balance problems due to upper cervical mechanoreceptor strain.

Cervical spine films taken at the time of the initial hospitalization revealed a severe hypolordosis of the cervical spine, with no reversal. There were moderately decreased inter-vertebral disc spaces seen at C5/6 and C6/7. Moderate right lateral canal stenosis was noted at C3/4 and C6/7, and on the left at C4/5, 5/6 and 6/7. Mild osteoarthritic degenerative changes were seen from C4 through C7.

Muscles were bilaterally inhibited for the following organs: stomach, small intestine, liver and gallbladder. The magnesium stretch test was positive. Repetitive testing showed multiple muscle inhibitions present, suggesting a need to upregulate her essential fatty acid metabolism.

The initial diagnoses included: cervical acceleration/deceleration syndrome with vertigo secondary to acute post-traumatic occipital-atlantal sprain strain, C3/4 through C5/6 inter-vertebral disc syndromes and moderate hypoadrenia.

Initial treatment consisted of the reduction of the cranial, pelvic-spinal, and the bilateral tarsal tunnel complex stress MAPs. The extra pelvic-spinal corrections included: C1 anterior, C5, 6, 7 RLR, T1-5 right with ribs right and T3-5 anterior with ribs bilaterally lateral. The C3 to C6 inter-vertebral discs were tractioned and treated with interferential electric stimulation. All of the cervical facet joints were bilaterally de-imbricated. Her neck flexors were facilitated (up-regulated).

The patient was taught how to utilize moist cold and the correct posture and spinal stretching exercises as her treatment progressed. We reviewed the components of a healthy diet, and advised the patient to use two betaine hydrochloride tablets with each meal, 200 mgs of magnesium glycinate two times per day, and two grams of EPA/DHA daily.

Substantial improvement was noted after 15 treatments over a six-week period. Three months after initiating care, she was able to play competitive tennis again, without vertigo. To facilitate stability, I referred her to Dr. Gary Wetreich so that he could occlusally equilibrate her bite and make her a night guard to prevent future cranial stress MAPs.

Discussion:

The main patho-physiology in this patient related to the jamming and anterior displacement of the atlas, in addition to the stress MAPs. This resulted in increased noxious (pain) afferents from the atlanto-axial mechanoreceptors. Correction and stabilization of this structural problem, along with strengthening the supportive musculature, resulted in cure.

Vertigo is a huge problem in the elderly, affecting 40% of those over 65. I believe that one of the largest causes of upper cervical strain, besides trauma, is postural abuse of the neck. This occurs for two major reasons: reading in bed or while reclined in a recliner, and falling asleep sitting up. Even though these common problems are referred to as "benign positional vertigo," there is nothing benign about this.

I have seen many patients with chronic severe vertigo cured in a very short treatment window. This definitely represents a best practice for this condition when the vertigo stems from the upper cervical spine and not the middle ear (see Appendix: A Prescient Point of View on Balance, p. 258).

"Real wealth indicators of the health and well being of our children, families, communities and natural systems reveal terminal systemic failure."

David C Kortan, *Agenda for a New Economy*

38. Bell's Palsy

A 57-year-old male presented for treatment wearing large, dark glasses and a turtle-neck sweater pulled up to "hide" his "horrible face." His chief complaint was a one week history of "lopsidedness" and swelling of his face. This came on rapidly, three hours after chewing a "very thick crusted pizza while eating quickly." He could not "puff up" his cheek or elevate his right eyelid. He had a sensation of numbness through his chin and the right side of his face. There was difficulty chewing. Other complaints included weeklong episodes of heartburn every 3-4 months, recurrent frontal headaches, and chronic low back pain. Eighteen months prior to his first visit, he slipped and fell, aggravating his right acromio-clavicular joint (shoulder). There was no history of any fever or other antecedent illness. The diagnosis of Bell's Palsy was made by a neurologist and a course of steroids begun.

Physical examination revealed a distraught 5'9" tall, 180 pound 57-year-old male. Posturally, his occiput was elevated on the right by one inch, his shoulders were level, and his left iliac crest was elevated by two inches. The mandible exhibited a mild "S" on opening and closing. The masseter, temporalis and pterygoid muscles were bilaterally hypertonic. Challenge revealed a pure right cranial stress MAP, a category two right pelvic-spinal MAP, and a bilateral tarsal tunnel MAP. Extra pelvic-spinal dysarthrias included the following: C5, 6, 7 RLR, T3-5 anterior with ribs bilaterally lateral and T1-3 right with ribs right. Approximation of the right acromio-clavicular joint facilitated the right deltoid muscle, indicating a sprain of the right acromio-clavicular ligament (a separated shoulder). Other inhibited muscles included the right subclavius, right sternocleidomastoid, and right pectoralis major clavicular. The left sternocleidomastoid was hypertonic.

Challenge revealed positive non-weight bearing inter-vertebral discs at C4-6 and L3-5. The right clavicle was laterally sprained, and all of the right cervical facet joints were imbricated. This patient had a palsy of the seventh cranial nerve, causing a paralysis of the muscles on the right side of his face and an inability to close his right eye. His chronic headaches were related to chronic inter-vertebral disc syndromes from C4-6. In addition, his chronic low back trouble was related to his category 2, 3 right external, pelvic-spinal stress MAPs.

Treatment on the initial visit included the reduction of the right cranial stress MAP, the category 2, 3 right external, pelvic-spinal MAP, and the bilateral tarsal tunnel MAPs. The extra-pelvic spinal complex areas were adjusted as follows: C5, 6, 7 RLR, T1-3R with ribs right, and T3-5 anterior with ribs bilaterally lateral. All of the cervical facets were de-imbricated. The cervical 4-6 inter-vertebral discs were manually tractioned. All of the related neck, shoulder, jaw and low back muscles were balanced. The right occipito-mastoid suture was opened up with a move known as an inspiration assist. Interferential was applied to the facial nerve, from its cranial exit to the right peri-oral area, as well as, to the cervical 4-6 inter-vertebral discs; and from the mid-lumbar spine to the base of the sacroiliac joints.

He was similarly treated three times over a four-day period, resulting in 80% improvement. Two days after the last treatment, he was completely asymptomatic and has remained so.

Discussion:

It is my contention, after successfully treating several dozen cases of Bell's Palsy, that this condition arises primarily from a crush-stretch injury of the facial nerve. The stomatognathic system has been described as a kinematic chain, and is composed of the: clavicles, cervical spine, cranium, TMJs, the first three ribs (origins of the neck flexors), and all the associated musculature. It indirectly includes the pelvis and other spinal areas, owing to the mechanics of the dural membrane system. The dura invaginates the sutures and lines the skull. It consists of a series of three tubes that the spinal cord sits in as it travels down through the spinal column, ending in its connection to the second sacral segment and tip of the coccyx.

In the true "double crush" concept, a nerve is rendered more vulnerable to injury if there is another injury (or "crush") at another site along its course. The "crush" injury can result from nerve compression, excessive stretch, or peripheral neuropathies from systemic illnesses, such as, diabetes, alcoholism, etc. The patient in this story demonstrates this concept.

Despite the ambiguity and controversy over the etiology of Bell's Palsy in the literature, there is ample evidence of inflammation and/or compression of the facial nerve as a "final common pathway" for the disorder. Therapies that would resolve these factors are, therefore, rational. Steroids can be expected to have anti-inflammatory effects; and therefore, reduce swelling, and can be expected to help. Their use, however, has not been convincingly demonstrated. Surgical decompression can be helpful, but is technically difficult and fraught with complications, and is appropriately reserved for extremely severe cases.

Correction of the derangement in the stomatognathic system, in this case, was accompanied by rapid and permanent resolution of the clinical picture. Although the patient was treated early in the course of this illness, the speed of his recovery, and the small number of treatments is notable. Alleviation of the structural problems which either create the pathology, predispose it to viral infection, or hinder healing, should be applied early on to shorten the course of the disease and to lessen the severity of the illness.

The facial nerve arises in the brainstem, passes through the internal auditory meatus, and courses through the petrous temporal bone. Jamming of the occipitomastoid and sqaumosal sutures surrounding the temporal bone (due to a

TMJ imbalance secondary to a lateral occiput) compresses and fixes the nerve at its exit through the stylomastoid foramen, and forms the first "crush". After exiting, the nerve immediately gives off motor branches to the stylohyoid and digastrics (posterior belly) muscles. An imbalanced TMJ may cause spasm of these muscles, which together with a posterior and laterally displaced occiput and clavicle would, in turn, exert traction on the already crushed seventh nerve. This "stretching" of the nerve is like a second "crush", but can be more accurately referred to as a crush-stretch injury.

In the present case described, in the prior shoulder injury, the patient attempted to stabilize himself during the fall using his right outstretched arm. This may well have resulted in a laterally-displaced clavicle, separated shoulder, lateral occiput, right holographic mandible, and spasm of the hyoid musculature. The subsequent stress on the TMJ, from eating pizza, was more than he could compensate for, and the "crush-stretch" injury became symptomatic.

The importance of correcting all of the injuries—a global approach—is apparent, for failing to do so leaves the nerve in a vulnerable condition, and relapse can be expected with greater frequency. There are more than 60,000 cases of Bell's Palsy diagnosed each year in the US.[1, 2] Approximately 15% of them (9,000 people) will have persistent facial nerve dysfunction and related impairments in quality of life.[3] Medical treatment consists of anti-inflammatory and anti-viral medications. The identification and elimination of the cranial and pelvic-spinal MAPs along with the related shoulder and cervical joint biomechanical lesions represents true First Line Therapeutics.

39. Gallstones—Right Upper Abdominal Pain

A 55-year-old male presented to our office for treatment of severe right, upper abdominal pain. He noted that the pain was worse after eating fatty foods. An abdominal ultrasound had shown several large gallstones in his gallbladder. He was scheduled to have his gallbladder surgically removed in another week, and sought an alternative, as he was petrified of the consequences of a surgery gone wrong.

Physical examination revealed a healthy, but anxious 5'10" 185 pound male. Gentle palpation of his right upper quadrant, with the patient lying on his back with his knees bent, evoked pain on inhalation. This test is known as Murphy's Test, and is indicative of congestion in the gall-bladder. The popliteus muscles were bilaterally inhibited: these are the gallbladder related muscles.

At this point, I recommended the patient perform a liver gallbladder flush.

This procedure originated with the Lahey clinic and was evidently their protocol before the advent of surgery. I learned this from a medical colleague, Dr. Dwight McKee, who thoroughly experimented with it many years earlier, and shared stories of its efficacy. In practice, I have routinely used it when clinically indicated. It is known in Eastern Medicine that the liver rules the ligaments.

In an effort to stabilize my injured patient's neuro-musculoskeletal problems I have utilized this procedure with excellent results. Lab analysis of the stones showed them to be mostly pure cholesterol, with an occasional bile stone.

Preparation included the use of 15 drops of phosphoric acid in water twice per day. This displaces any calcium from the gallstones, should there be any. The patient is urged to drink plenty of organic apple juice, as the malic acid in the juice also displaces calcium. Steamed beet greens, and/or beet greens tablets are also advised, as they contain ingredients that are lipotrophic (fat mobilizing).

After four days of preparation, the patient performed the flush. This consisted of the following: After a normal breakfast and lunch, the patient skipped his evening meal. He mixed two tablespoons of Epsom salts (magnesium sulfate) in 4 oz of water and drank this at 6 pm. This relaxes the smooth muscles lining the gastrointestinal tract, including those lining the gall-bladder, and the common bile duct (the tube from the gallbladder and pancreas to the lining of the small intestine.) Three hours later, he drank 1 cup of virgin olive oil and went to bed, being previously instructed to favor sleeping on his left side, to let gravity aid in the process.

The next morning he self-administered a warm-water salt enema. This consisted of one and one half quarts of body temperature spring water, with 2 tablespoons of sea salt dissolved in it. The salt is important, because it makes the solution iso-osmotic with the blood, so that the water is not absorbed. To provide extra contraction to the gallbladder, one cup of black organic coffee is added to the salt water mixture. After getting this solution in his large intestine, he laid on his left side, back, and then right side for five minutes each. After this, he evacuated the solution, and noticed a mass of green stones.

He called the next day to say that he had just eaten one half pound of bacon, and was pain free! At $5,000 a procedure, a reversion back to the use of this technique as a first line of therapy would be a proactive step.

This "oil change" procedure is not only effective from a fiscal standpoint, but its effects on the Web of Wellness are profound. Once the liver's detoxification outflow is unblocked, not only is a person's digestion of fats improved, but also bowel regularity, ability to hold chiropractic adjustments and best of all, the rise in overall energy is enormous. Think about the following for a moment: Researchers have discovered that when bile outflow is blocked from the hepato-biliary tree, and "backs up" in the body it has been found in women's breasts. It has to go somewhere. Since these products are highly carcinogenic, they most likely act as triggers for breast cancer. The incidence of male breast cancer is also on the rise.

Having performed this procedure routinely on myself, and through the feedback of some thousands of patients over several decades, I can honestly say that the side benefit of increased energy is remarkable. It has to be one of the best anti-aging secrets known to man. All people would be therapeutically served to have Murphy's sign checked and corrected on an annual basis.

Discussion:

Gallstones are present in about 30% of the population in the U.S. Weight loss, then weight gain, called "weight cycling" can double a man's risk for gallstones.[1] Obesity, insulin resistance, "hyperinsulinemia" and metabolic syndrome are related to various gallbladder diseases, including gallstones, cholecystitis, polyps and cancer of the gallbladder.[2]

According to the CDC, in 2005 about 325,000 gallbladders were removed, at an average cost of five thousand dollars per surgery. These costs totaled 1.6 billion dollars. Perhaps all primary care physicians could spend a couple of minutes to palpate their patients' gallbladders with the Murphy test and then instruct their patients in how to perform this simple procedure. This would lessen overall healthcare costs and may show positive collateral cost lowering by preventing other related problems like heart disease, constipation, skin problems, cancers and fatigue. Dr. Frank Shallenberger has noted that people who have had their gallbladders removed still form stones inside their livers. The livers ability to form bile is a complex process, aided by the use of vitamin C and phosphatidyl choline.

> *"The balance of omega-6/omega-3 fatty acids is an important determinant in decreasing the risk for coronary heart disease, both in the primary and secondary prevention of coronary heart disease."*
>
> Artemis Simopoulos, MD
> President, The Center for Genetics, Nutrition and Health,
> Washington, DC.

> *(Whether or not you absorb these fats depends on how well your gallbladder functions. Remember– you are not just what you eat, but digest, absorb, detoxify and eliminate.)*

Prevention includes daily exercise, avoidance of fried foods, cutting back on animal fat, high-fat dairy, refined foods and sugar.

> *"For the internet is the only tool we can rely upon just now. For at least the next five years, it will be the one tool that gives grass-roots movements an edge...*
>
> *For now, there is enormous credibility that comes from authentic engagement.*
>
> *We can build that engagement one click at a time."*
>
> L. Lessig

40. Torn Medial Meniscus

A 45-year-old businessman presented to my office for evaluation and treatment of right knee pain. He needed crutches to ambulate, and he had a brace on his right leg that extended from his right mid-thigh to his right mid-calf. Evidently he was golfing a few weeks earlier, and had twisted his right knee while following through on a drive. His primary care physician prescribed anti-inflammatories and ordered an MRI. The MRI demonstrated a tear in his medial meniscus, and he was scheduled for surgery. A friend of his, a patient of mine whom I had helped to avoid a similar surgery, referred him to our office.

Physical examination revealed a very fit 5'9" 200 pound male. Posture analysis revealed a level head, an elevated right shoulder by one inch, and an elevated right iliac crest by two inches. Both of his feet were moderate to severely pronated. Challenge revealed a right major cranial stress MAP, a category two left pelvic-spinal MAP, and bilateral tarsal tunnel MAPs. The left tarsal tunnel complex sprain was the common type, with a lateral talus and an externally-rotated tibia; the right one was the more uncommon variety, with a medial talus and an internally-rotated tibia. His right medial meniscus challenged positively in a posterior-medial direction. The right tibialis posterior muscle was inhibited (3/5), along with his right lower inner thigh muscle (vastus medialis inferior).

The paired muscle groups relating to his adrenal glands were bilaterally inhibited. Blood pressure in his right arm lying on his back (supine) was 120/80, dropping to 110/80 standing, suggestive of decreased adrenal gland function. The magnesium stretch test was positive as was repetitive muscle test inhibition, showing a need to improve his essential fatty acid status.

On his first visit we reduced the cranial, pelvic and tarsal tunnel MAPs. The right medial meniscus was specifically repositioned, and the aforementioned medial knee and ankle muscles were facilitated. Interferential current was pulsed through the right medial knee to reduce pain and promote healing. He was instructed in the use of moist cold. He was advised to use magnesium, 200 mg ; EPA-DHA 1 gm— both twice per day; and an adrenal support product containing adaptogens (ginseng, cordyceps and rhodiola). He walked out of the office without using crutches or the brace.

He returned for a follow-up visit one week later and said he felt 90% better. We found and corrected a category one left, pelvic-spinal MAP and a bilateral post tarsal tunnel MAP. The right medial meniscus still challenged positive in a posterior-medial direction, so that was reduced again and treated with interferential current.

He never had the knee surgery, and has been fine since, with no further knee symptoms.

Discussion:

This condition represents the most common knee injury. According to Emedicine.com, about 850,000 of these surgeries are performed per year. The surgery arthroscopy charges range from $5.4 to $12.6 thousand dollars. So at the low end of costs we have got a $3B bill.

In this case, costs to cure the patient were $530 as follows; about one twelfth of the direct medical costs plus indirect medical costs (from lost work due to the surgery) are not included:

Initial Exam and follow-up visits:	$450.00
Supplements :	$80.00
Total:	$530.00

More specifics on the underlying pathomechanics of the most common knee injuries can be found by referring to the tarsal tunnel stress MAPs in my upcoming book *Stress MAPS*.

41. Profuse Sweating

A 51-year-old male presented for treatment of "unbearable sweats" of 20 years duration. He noted that he never felt well. He would go two days with no sweats and then would sweat profusely, wetting through his clothing up to two times a day. He noted that the problem was exacerbated with hot weather and relieved with the use of a fan, and cold weather. Sometimes in the winter months it was so bad that he would open his sliding glass doors and stand at the entryway, with just a t-shirt on, letting subzero wind blow on him from the front, with a fan at his back, to try to relieve these horrible sweats.

This patient also had several other issues. He complained of mild dizziness when getting up or down too fast. He suffered from a broken sleep pattern of 30 years duration. Usually in bed by 12:00, he would awake three times before 7:00 a.m. averaging only five or six hours of sleep total. He was tired a lot, with his energy fluctuating up and down. Calf cramps at night contributed to this as well. About two times a month, he would suffer an "emotional crash", lasting one to two hours in duration. Digestive problems including bloating immediately after eating, generalized abdominal bloat and heartburn (severe with water intake) also plagued him.

His medical history revealed several fender benders. At the age of 27 he was run over by a train, and lost the lower half of one of his legs. He had difficulty walking because the calf of his remaining leg would cramp up. As a type II diabetic, he had been on Metformin 500 mg three times a day for several years. He had undergone cardiovascular surgery for stent implantation in one of his coronary arteries. He had used Lipitor for two years, but had to discontinue it due to aggravation of abdominal pain and bloating. Overall he scored 132 on the Metabolic Symptoms Questionnaire; any score over 50 is considered problematic. He noted that his primary care physician "was stumped" after ruling out thyroid and liver issues.

Physical examination revealed an alert, 5'10", 260 lb male. Posturally he had a level pelvis with a mild left lumbar, right thoracic scoliosis. His one foot had a tarsal tunnel MAP. He had a category two right pelvic-spinal complex stress MAP. In addition to all of the usual compensatory related vertebral misalignments throughout his spine, he had four of his mid-back vertebrae jammed forward with the related ribs fixated.

Examination of his endocrine reflexes was positive for his pineal and hypothalamus. The muscles relating to his thyroid and adrenal glands were weak on both sides, suggestive of diminished function of those endocrine glands. Additionally, the magnesium stretch test was positive, signifying a need for increased intake of that mineral. He had a pure right cranial stress MAP. Once these were corrected the thyroid and adrenal related muscles immediately strengthened. The pineal and hypothalamic reflexes also disappeared.

"We still agree about certain fundamentals: that it is a republic that we inherited, that it ought to be responsive to "the People alone"; that this one is not.

We are united in the view that this republic can do better."

L. Lessig

Several digestive related muscles were weak bilaterally including the stomach, small intestine and large intestine. A positive reflex was found suggestive of a leaky gut. The patient was given betaine hydrochloride, to take two with each meal to improve stomach acid function, and started on the Sea Klenz program to clean out the build-up mucus and undigested food in his small intestine, with the aim of improving his assimilation of nutrients.

The patient returned three weeks after his first visit, totally ecstatic, announcing that he had not experienced any more sweats in the previous two weeks, for the first time in 20 years.

The brain actively sits in a hammock of ligaments called the dura mater (or tough mother). These ligaments line the inside of our 22 cranial bones and extend downwards as part of a series of three tubes that line the entire spinal cord. Our spines have three curves that act as a resilient shock absorber, giving our spine about twenty times more strength and resiliency than a straight column. These curves flatten subtly on inhalation, and reform with exhalation. The functional reality of cranial movement, although well documented, is, for the most part unrecognized (not actively treated) in modern medicine. This subtle movement or rhythm pumps cerebrospinal fluid (CSF), which is an ultrafiltrate of venous blood. CSF is formed in the middle of the brain, in structures called ventricles, travels around the brain, and then down the spinal cord, where it goes out the nerve roots, and actually perfuses the organs that they innervate. This is how the nervous system feeds itself with oxygen and glucose, and it acts as a conduit for the transmission of neurotransmitters, which help in the communication between the nervous, immune and endocrine systems.

In the middle of the brain, the brain folds in upon itself and forms the endocrine system. There are three major glands here (pineal, pituitary and hypothalamus) whose function is up-regulated by this micro-movement/rhythm of the cranial-sacral system. It is my opinion that with the unlocking of the cranials, and the subsequent up-regulation of the hypothalamus, (which functions as the dipstick that monitors our internal temperature regulation) this patient's problem was fixed.

42. Post Surgical Foot Drop/Low Back Pain

A 57-year-old male presented for treatment of low back pain, and a left foot drop of one and a half years duration. His low back pain was mild to moderate (3-4/10) and was mostly located in the left lumbosacral and sacroiliac areas. He noted springtime allergies that affected his eyes and nose, for three years duration. He also noted occasional leg muscle cramps at rest.

His medical history was remarkable for a partial dissectomy on the left side of L4/5, performed two years previously. He had worked for years as a navigation officer on a jet fighter. He would never know what the pilot was going to do, and was subject to a lot of intense G-forces as the plane changed direction to move through space. Over the years, this repetitive trauma led to the herniation of his L1/2 disc, necessitating the surgery to remove free fragments of disc material lodged at the L4/5 level. Two months prior he had begun a diabetic medication along with a statin to lower his cholesterol. He had used aspirin, a multivitamin, omega 3 fats, garlic and vitamin C for many years. He walked and/or swam daily for 30 minutes. Due to his left foot drop, he had to wear an L-shaped brace inside his left shoe to prevent tripping. He had used this brace for the past year and a half.

Physical examination revealed a pleasant, alert 57 year old, 6'1", 182 lb male. Posturally, his left iliac crest was elevated by two inches, and his left shoulder by one half inch. His head was level. His spine demonstrated a mild "S" curvature, with a left lumbar, right thoracic curve that straightened on forward bending, suggestive of a non-structural scoliosis. Challenge revealed a category two right pelvic-spinal MAP. Additionally, his left sacroiliac joint had a grade two sprain, and the pelvis was shifted underneath the lumbar spine (category three) with compressed intervertebral discs from L3 to L5. The left facet joints L3 to L5 were imbricated. Both psoas muscles were hypertonic, and moderate foot pronation was noted bilaterally. The tarsal tunnel MAPs were bilaterally present. His left anterior tibialis was 0/5 and his left posterior tibialis was 3-/5.

The patient had a positive magnesium stretch test and a right-left-left cranial stress MAP. The thyroid and adrenal muscles were inhibited bilaterally, which together with inhibited systemic ligaments, is indicative of a dampening of the patient's neuro-endocrine axis.

Bilateral inhibition was present for stomach, pancreas, liver, gallbladder and small intestine related muscles. This indicated the need to up-regulate this patient's digestive and absorptive capabilities. Positive reflexes suggestive of a small intestine mold overgrowth and a leaky gut were present as well.

"There is only one issue in this country—campaign finance reform."
Cenk Uygu
Former MSNBC commentator

On his first visit, the cranial stress MAP was reduced, as well as the category two, three pelvic-spinal stress MAPs. Psoas muscle spasm was bilaterally reduced and foot/ankle and low back/pelvic muscles were balanced. The patient was instructed in the use of a sacroiliac belt and moist cold to promote healing of the chronic left grade two sacroiliac ligament stretch/tear, as well as proper body biomechanics. Both tarsal tunnel complex sprains were corrected, along with de-imbrications of the left L3-5 facets. Origin/insertion, golgi tendon and neuro-muscular spindle cell work had an immediate profound impact. Muscle testing now revealed his left anterior tibialis 2/5, left posterior tibialis 3+/5.

He started with betaine hydrochloride, two per meal; 15 mgs zinc, three times a day; 1 mg copper per day; magnesium glycinate, 200 mgs, two times a day; and Sea Klenz to debride accumulated debris. We also instructed the patient in how to utilize products proven to help blood sugar levels, lipoic acid, and a product called Meta-Glycemix.

The second visit one week later found the patient with some mild low back pain, which started after a session of deep muscle therapy. Posturally, his alignment was perfect. We corrected the Category 0 pelvic-spinal MAP, and used a Frequency Specific Microcurrent® treatment protocol to increase the healing energy along his left sciatic area, from his low back to his left foot. He was tested for foods and molds. All molds were positive, negated by olive leaf extract. He was sensitive to corn, millet, oat, wheat, cheddar cheese, Monterey jack cheese, green pepper, string beans, walnuts, turkey and cherry. He was advised to avoid these foods, was put on a low sugar diet, and advised to take two olive leaf capsules two times a day, on an empty stomach.

Three weeks later, all molds were clear. Food sensitivities were reduced as follows: cottage cheese, green olives, green peas and coffee. Olive leaf was reduced to three, three times a week on an empty stomach. Just two lumbar vertebrae were rotated L4-L, L3-R, and no lumbar intervertebral disc weakness was found. We casted him for orthotics. His left anterior and posterior tibialis muscles were both 3-/5 and 4/5 respectively. His entire left leg and foot were percussed. The patient was given exercises to strengthen his plantar flexors bilaterally. Frequency Specific Microcurrent® was utilized as on the previous visit.

One month later he presented with increased low back pain of two days duration, aggravated by trans-Atlantic travel. His overall energy was better, and the patient noted post-treatment, that he felt much better each time. He was treated with Frequency Specific Microcurrant® as on the two previous visits.

'Until it gets fixed, governance will remain stalled. The challenge is to get America to see and then act."

Lawrence Lessig, JD
Director Edmond J Safra Center for Ethics
Harvard University

On his fifth visit the left posterior tibialis was 5/5 and his left anterior tibialis was 3+/5. He was given orthotics, and no longer needed to wear the foot brace.

The patient was seen six weeks later. He complained of low back sensitivity of two days duration, in certain positions. We found and corrected a Category 0 right pelvic-spinal MAP and de-imbricated the last three left lumbar facets.

The seventh visit, one month later, revealed his left anterior tibialis at 4/5! Patient noted that he was able to fully function without his brace, and had very little residual symptoms. His foot drop was gone.

"That the thing that we were once most proud of—this, our republic—is the one thing that we have all learned to ignore. Government is an embarrassment. It has lost the capacity to make the most essential decisions. And slowly it begins to dawn upon us: a ship that can't be steered is a ship that will sink.

We inherited an extraordinary estate.
On our watch we have let it fall to ruin."

L. Lessig

43. Irritable Bowel Syndrome (IBS), Abdominal Pain, Cervical Dysplasia, Vulvodynia

A 45-year-old female presented with a three-year history of severe (8/10) abdominal pain which was stabbing and intermittent in quality. It was present 50% of the time. She noted the pain was "all over." She had been hospitalized about one month earlier, where they performed an endoscopy, a colonoscopy and an abdominal CAT scan with contrast. All of these tests were normal. The resultant diagnosis was irritable bowel syndrome. She noted that she moved her bowels all day long, and two days out of the week experienced severe diarrhea. She noted she bloated less than one hour after eating, and that her abdominal pain was much worse after sweets and carbohydrates. The pain in her left lower rib areas was "really painful."

Additionally, she had a ten-year history of sinus and upper respiratory congestion (6/10) that was constant in the winter. It would also become a problem at the change of seasons (3-4 times per year) with copious sinus drainage, a sore throat and increased urination all day long. She noted these symptoms also appeared to be aggravated by wool, mold, animals, and certain chemicals.

She noted recurrent colds after frequent contact with sick young children over the past few years in her job as a paraprofessional aid to disabled and special needs children. Her energy level was fair, her ears rang continuously, and in the past year, she noticed a decreased sense of smell and taste. For the last four years, she had also experienced vulvodynia (7/10) which she described as an intermittent sharp ache, relieved with an ice pack.

For the previous two months, she had severe insomnia (9/10). This is was intermittently causing problems three to four nights of the week. On the nights that this occurred, she would doze off and then jolt awake every 20 minutes for the first few hours. She noted that her skin and rectum itched at these times as well. She was tested for parasites, and they were negative.

She had two children, aged 21 and 18, that were normal vaginal deliveries. At age 35, she had jaw surgery involving the fracture and resetting of both her maxillae and mandible. She noted that an ultrasound of several years ago showed gallstones. Eight years previously, she had mononucleosis that turned into chronic fatigue syndrome. She received treatment at the Country Clinic in Las Vegas, Nevada which included hyperbaric oxygen, EDTA chelation and protein-electrophoresis. She responded well to this treatment. She had used armor thyroid, 120 mg per day for thirty years. She used .5mg of Lorazepam for the past year, but noted that it was no longer helping her. She also used quite a few nutritional supplements. Her MSQ (Medical Symptoms Questionnaire) score was 70, which is quite high.

Physical examination revealed an alert, but distraught 45-year-old, 5'5", 135-pound female. Posturally, her left iliac crest and left shoulder were both elevated by one inch. Her head was level. A mild "S" scoliosis was present; right lumbar, left thoracic that straightened on forward bending suggestive of a functional scoliosis. Challenge revealed a right major cranial stress MAP, a category two right pelvic-spinal stress MAP with a grade two left sacroiliac sprain (externally-rotated sacroiliac joint), and a bilateral tarsal tunnel complex stress MAP.

Extra pelvic-spinal complex and spinal dysarthrias were present as follows: T1-8 right with ribs right; T9-12 anterior left with ribs left. The psoas muscles were hypertonic bilaterally and a strained diaphragm was present.

The muscles relating to the following organs were bilaterally inhibited: stomach, liver, gall-bladder and small intestine. Murphy's test caused moderate pain, suggesting biliary stasis. The magnesium stretch test was positive. Repetitive muscle testing created muscle inhibition, which indicated a need to increase her essential fatty acid intake or to improve their assimilation. Reflexes were positive suggestive of both a leaky gut, and ongoing food and mold sensitivities. The patient's thyroid and adrenal muscles were bilaterally inhibited, which together with a marked systemic ligamentous laxity, is suggestive of a dampening of the neuro-endocrine axis.

On her first visit, we reduced her right major cranial stress MAP, the category two right pelvic-spinal stress MAP, the extra pelvic-spinal and rib lesions, as well as the bilateral tarsal tunnel complex stress MAPs. Muscle inhibitions were facilitated and balanced. We instructed the patient in the use of moist cold, a sacroiliac (SI) belt, and pelvic diaphragm exercise to stabilize her SI joint complex. She was tested and found to be sensitive to her multivitamins and B-complex formulas.

We instructed her to use the following nutritional protocol: betaine hydrochloride, two per meal; magnesium glycinate, 400 mgs per day; zinc, 20 mg per meal; copper 1 mg per day, and also was instructed to begin an inflammatory-modulating medical food in powdered drink form, to replace one meal per day. She was advised to miss no meals, and to use beets and beet greens on a regular basis to help thin her bile. A product to debride the small intestine of undigested food and mucus was started.

> "We are, to steal from Thoreau, the "thousand[s] hacking at the branches of evil" with "[n]one striking at the root."
>
> The root, the thing that feeds the other ills, and the thing that we must kill first. The cure that would be generative—the single, if impossibly difficult, intervention that would give us the chance to repair the rest."
>
> L. Lessig

On her second visit, everything was a little better: the abdominal pain was reduced (5/10) ; vulvadynia (6/10); insomnia (5/10) and congestion, post-nasal drip (5/10). She noted that for the past month, the use of a banana before bed had helped to decrease her irregular heart beat and muscle symptoms. A recent Ob-Gyn visit had revealed a mild to moderate squamous dysplasia with marked HPV effect. She was given two choices: 1) do nothing, and recheck in six months or 2) cryosurgery.

On her next visit two weeks later, her posture was improved, with a level head and pelvis. The left shoulder was slightly elevated by one half inch. We found and corrected a category one pelvic-spinal MAP and bilateral post tarsal tunnel MAPs. Neuro-musculoskeletal testing revealed sensitivity to all 12 molds and the following foods: oat, wheat, American cheese, cow's milk, white potato, soy, tuna, bananas, grapes, chocolate and MSG. We instructed the patient in the use of olive leaf (two, twice per day on an empty stomach), the avoidance of the offending foods and a low sugar diet. We also started the patient on magnesium/potassium aspartate, two a day and reduced the magnesium glycinate to 200 mgs per day. We started her on a better multivitamin and mineral, two per meal; B12 folate, three capsules per meal for one week (then two per meal for one week, then one per meal); vitamin E, two a day; and vitamin A protocol starting at 200,000 IU a day for two weeks; (followed by a tapering), Vitamin E - 200 IU/100 gammatocopherol, 100-alpha.

Five weeks later, we rechecked the food and mold sensitivities. All molds were negative and turkey was the only reactive food. We reduced the olive leaf extract to three, two to three times a week on an empty stomach. The patient had been pushed, and had fallen on her right shoulder, which was now quite painful (8/10). The following day, she became sick with marked sinus congestion. Posturally, her pelvis was level, her left shoulder was elevated by one half inch, and her right occiput was high on the right by one half inch. Challenge revealed T1-5 right with ribs right and multiple cervical spinal dysarthrias (C1, 2, 3 RLR; C5, 6, 7 RLR) with a right lateral clavicle, occiput and holographic TMJ. The right acromioclavicular ligament was sprained.

Lab work revealed normal white and red cells and negative viral titers for CMV, herpes I and II, and mono. The infraspinatus muscles (thymus related) were facilitated with Vitamin D, olive leaf and a combination anti-viral product. She was instructed to use vitamin D3, 2000 IU a day, olive leaf, one tablet, two-three times a week on an empty stomach, and the antiviral combination, six a day for three days, then three a day until symptoms subsided.

> *"Our planet spins furiously to a radically changed climate, certain to impose catastrophic costs on a huge portion of the world's population. We ignore this, too. Everything our government touches—from healthcare to Social Security to the monopoly rights we call patents and copy right,—it poisons.*
> *Yet our leaders seem oblivious to the thought that there's anything that needs fixing."*
>
> L. Lessig

The patient was seen one month later, noting an aggravation of her insomnia, fatigue, dull supra-orbital headaches and mild joint pain. Her tinnitus was constant (6/10). Posturally, her head, shoulders and hips were level. Challenge revealed Category 0 pelvic-spinal MAP, with T1-5 right with ribs right; C5, 6, 7 R-L-R, right lateral T3-5 anterior with ribs bilaterally lateral, occiput and clavicle.

Treatment consisted of the reduction of the category 0 pelvic-spinal MAP, and extra pelvic-spinal complex spinal dysarthrias. Strain counter-strain were performed on the medial pterygoid muscles bilaterally. We instructed the patient in the use of ginko biloba; Vitamin D3, 2000 IUs, and to increase B12 folate.

A follow-up pap smear revealed rare atypical squamous cells of undetermined significance. This indicated a marked improvement over the first one, six months earlier, and no need for culposcopy.

Patient presented one month later with neck discomfort, increased sensitivity in her mouth and tongue. She described her taste buds as being oversensitive. After having a stressful conversation recently, her hair had started falling out in clumps. Structurally, challenge revealed a pure right cranial MAP, category two right pelvic-spinal MAP, and bilateral tarsal tunnel MAPs. Extra pelvic spinal listings included C5, 6, 7 R-L-R; T1-6 right with ribs right and T3-6 anterior with ribs bilaterally lateral. These areas were corrected and related muscles were facilitated and balanced. The stomach related muscles were bilaterally inhibited. Hydrochloric acid and zinc facilitated these muscles, so we advised her how to use them.

At this point, the patient noted that her vulvodynia had recently been more on than off, at a fairly steady 6-7/10. We therefore utilized the Frequency Specific Microcurrent protocol to his area.

Three months later the patient presented feeling much better overall. Her energy was way up. Her abdominal symptoms were gone. She noted that the one frequency specific microcurrent treatment given to her on the previous visit had completely cleared up her vulvodynia, with no residuals. This was huge for her, since it had been a four year problem. The last five weeks she felt moderately achy "all over." Recent lab work revealed an elevated anti-nuclear antibody test. Examination and correction involved on this visit included: a category one right pelvic-spinal MAP and bilateral tarsal tunnel complex stress MAPs. Both carpal tunnels were sprained. A leaky gut reflex was positive, so we started her on an antifungal and instructed her in a low sugar diet.

A follow-up pap smear was normal. This, together with the correction of her irritable bowel syndrome and chronic vulvodynia, made for one extremely happy patient.

> *"Ben Franklin would weep. The republic that he helped birth is lost. The 89% of Americans who have no confidence in Congress (as reported by the latest Gallup poll) are not idiots. We were here at least once before...70% of America had said 'This democracy is corrupted, we demand it fixed.' The year was 1912."*
>
> L. Lessig

44. Thirty Years of Pre-menstrual Migraines, Fibromyalgia, Chronic Fatigue Syndrome (CFS), Irritable Bowel Syndrome (IBS)

A 43-year-old female presented with a laundry list of complaints, including severe indigestion, diarrhea, fatigue, foggy thinking, headaches, and emotional ups and downs. For the prior six years she had experienced three to four sub-occipital to frontal headaches a week. She noted that they began after a car accident six years earlier. They were brought on by stress and began in sleep, as she frequently awoke with them. Additionally she experienced severe two-day migraine headaches, one and one half weeks premenstrually. These had been ongoing since age 13, when her periods began: thirty years of premenstrual migraines!

Six months earlier, she developed severe indigestion after having two bouts of bronchitis, back to back. This was treated medically with Zithromax. Since then she had noticed that if she ate anything with wheat, she would get severe abdominal pain (8/10) and diarrhea, and she had become exhausted. She was now having six bouts of diarrhea daily. She usually slept from 10:00 p.m. or 11:00 p.m. until 5:30 am and had recently been waking up at 4:00 a.m. For the last month her knees hurt going up and down stairs. She also had right shoulder pain, which she had injured pulling a heavy suitcase one month earlier. Several medical people she had seen gave her the following diagnoses: fibromyalgia, chronic fatigue syndrome and irritable bowel syndrome. She was self-employed as an interior designer, with moderate job stress.

Physical examination revealed an alert 43-year-old female, 5' 7.5" weighing 140 pounds. Posturally she had an elevated right occiput by one half inch, left shoulder by two inches, and left hip by one inch. Her spine demonstrated a mild "S" scoliosis; left lumbar, right thoracic that straightened on forward bending, suggestive of a less severe functional scoliosis. Both feet were mildly supinated.

Challenge revealed the following: a pure right cranial stress MAP, a category two right pelvic-spinal stress MAP and bilateral tarsal tunnel complex stress MAPs. Extra category pelvic-spinal disarthrias included: C5, 6, 7 RLR, T1-6 right with ribs right, and T3-5 anterior with ribs laterally lateral. Approximation of the right acromio-clavicular joint facilitated the right mid-deltoid muscle indicating a sprain of the acromio-clavicular ligament. The opponens pollicis and digiti minimi muscles were bilaterally inhibited, and became facilitated with the patient bending her head to the opposite side. This suggested compression of the nerve roots, where they exit the spine, as part of the cause of the hand muscle weakness (i.e., a double crush injury). Challenge was positive to the cervical 4-6 inter-vertebral discs (non-weight bearing) as well as to the atlas (first cervical vertebrae) being anteriorly displaced.

"The great threat to our republic today is the economy of influence now transparent to all, which has normalized a process that draws our democracy away form the will of the people. For the single most

salient feature of the government that we have evolved is not that it discriminates in favor of one side and against another. The single most salient feature is that it discriminates against all sides to favor itself. We have created an engine of influence that seeks simply to make those the most connected rich."
L. Lessig

Her Medical Symptoms Questionnaire was scored at 70. Anything greater than 50 is indicative of multiple systems dysfunction and toxicity. Both the magnesium stretch test and the repeat muscle test inhibition (suggesting a need for essential fatty acids) were positive. Paired muscle inhibition was noted for muscles related to digestion indicative of mal-absorption of nutrients. Reflexes were positive suggesting a small intestine mold overgrowth, leaky gut, and ongoing food and mold sensitivities. Thyroid and adrenal muscles were inhibited, due to dampening of her neuro-endocrine axis.

On her first visit we reduced the major complex stress MAPs: cranial, pelvic-spinal and tarsal tunnel. We corrected the extra pelvic-spinal vertebral subluxation complexes, and tractioned her C4-6 inter-vertebral discs. We taught her the correct use of moist cold for her areas of chronic pain—occiput/C1, lower cervical, right acromio-clavicular joint. We treated these areas with interferential to reduce pain, swelling and promote healing. She was instructed to use the Sea Klenz protocol, magnesium glycinate (200 mgs twice a day), and lipogen (one with each meal) [a lipotrophic agent to mobilize bile and improve assimilation of fats].

Two weeks later on her second visit, she noted that her energy level was much better. Her neck was still tight and her headaches were "still there but less intense." Posturally her head and pelvis were level, and her left shoulder was elevated by one half inch. We found and corrected a category one right, pelvic-spinal complex with C5, 6, 7 right and T4 anterior. The C4-6 inter-vertebral discs were sixty percent reduced (a torque pattern)—these were once again manually tractioned, along with her right acromio-clavicular joint. Interferential current was also applied to the area. Neuro-musculoskeletal testing revealed multiple molds positive, sensitive to olive leaf extract. The following foods were positive: corn, string beans, rice, wheat, peanuts, walnuts, salmon, chicken, mozzarella cheese, Monterey jack cheese, cow's milk, tomatoes, tuna, chic peas, cabbage, cucumbers, lettuce, grapes, strawberries, oranges, vodka and chocolate. She was advised to avoid the offending foods, stay on a low sugar diet and use olive leaf extract (two, twice per day on an empty stomach). We reviewed cervical disc exercises, lumbar disc exercises and pelvic diaphragm exercises.

204

On her third visit, one month later, her energy had continued to improve, and her neck pain was gone. She noted mid-stomach pain which was worse at night, for the past one and one half weeks, as well as a couple of mild headaches over the past few days. She had mild nausea and diarrhea recently from eating strawberries. Posturally, her hips were level, her left shoulder was elevated by one inch, and her right occiput was elevated by one half inch. Challenge revealed bilateral tarsal tunnel MAPs, and a category one right, pelvic-spinal MAP. Thoracic vertebral segments ten through twelve were anterior, with ribs bilaterally lateral. Her diaphragm was strained, and both psoas muscles were hypertonic.

Treatment consisted of the correction of the category one right, pelvic-spinal MAP, the bilateral tarsal tunnel MAPs, and the T10-12 anterior thoracics and bilaterally lateral ribs. The hiatal hernia was reduced and psoas muscle spindles turned down. Neuro-musculoskeletal re-testing was performed and revealed one mold and several foods including: wheat, yogurt, onions, almonds and blueberries. The patient was advised to stay on the olive leaf extract, two/twice a day. We had her use a product containing glutamine to help heal her leaky gut, since that reflex persisted; along with an acidophilus strain to re-inoculate her intestinal tract. The patient was treated once every six to eight weeks, with various areas recurrently strained due to travel on airplanes, especially her upper cervical spine and thoraco-lumbar junction. We suggested 10 sessions in a far infrared sauna, both to detoxify her, and diminish her chronic pain. After her third session, she began to sweat, and as time went by, she felt better and better.

After completing the detox program, we began a program of first line therapy. We used the bio-impedance analysis (BIA) to measure her body composition. This machine was created by NASA to monitor astronaut's body composition in space, and had input into its research and development from many state universities making it, presently, one of the most researched and accurate tools to measure and monitor the human body's response to nutrient and lifestyle interventions.

The major information gleaned consists of the phase angle, total water (intra and extra-cellular), fat and lean muscle as percentages. The phase angle gives an indirect measure of the cellular redox potential (think of cellular bioenergetics), and thus, is useful in assessing the trajectory of general health of an individual. The higher the phase angle, the more robust a person's cell membranes and overall fitness. The phase angle range is from 2.1 (lower is death) to robust health (8.9 and greater). It is both age and sex adjusted, with the norms gradually declining from age 20 to age 80 as follows: men 7.9 to 5.1; and women 7.3 to 4.5. The normal range for total body water is 55% to 65%. Healthy values for body cell mass or lean muscle mass are above 40%. Healthy fat ranges are 15%-20% for men, and 20% to 25% for women.

"The second element is lost trust: When a democracy seems a charade, we lose faith in it's process."

L. Lessig

On her first test, her phase angle was 4.5. The normal reading is 6.7, so her cell membrane health was less than optimal. Her total body water was 44 (normal 55-65) so she was dehydrated. Her lean muscle mass was 26 (normal is greater than 40); and her fat was 42 (normal range is 20-25).

We started her on a medical food intervention program that consisted of one meal replacement a day with Ultra Clear Plus. We had her use a whole food diet supplemented with a multi-vitamin/mineral formula (2/meal), digestive enzymes (2/meal), magnesium potassium aspartate (4/day for a total of 200 mgs magnesium aspartate and 320 mgs potassium aspartate). We re-inoculated her gut with lactobacillus acidophilus NCFM strain, and advised her to use 2 grams of buffered vitamin C per day.

As she felt more energy and less pain, she increased her physical activity to include several aerobic exercise and pilates classes per week. Within three months time, the BIA test results improved dramatically. Her phase angle increased to 7.9 (normal 6.7). Her total body water went up to 55 (normal 55-65). Her lean muscle mass rose from 26 to 37, and her fat decreased from 42 to 28. Overall her Medical Symptom Questionnaire dropped from 70 to 8. Her thinking was now clear, her mood was steady, instead of up and down, but best of all, her fatigue and body pain had resolved. The 30 year premenstrual migraines were gone. Her gastrointestinal tract was also functioning without a symptom. She continues to get checked on a periodic basis (quarterly) to maintain her improved state of health.

> *"If we want to protect the environment, design a better healthcare system or improve our energy policy, we need a political system that encourages law makers to listen more to voters than to oil and gas companies, pharmaceutical giants and other industries. The Fair Elections Now Act (S 2023 and HR 1404) is a bold solution to the problem of special interest money in politics."*
>
> Craig Holman, Gov't affairs lobbyist
> Public Citizen's Congress Watch Division

> *The prognosis is not good. The disease we face is not one that nations cure, or, at least, cure easily. But we should understand the options. For few who work to understand what has gone wrong will be willing to accept defeat—without a fight.*
>
> L. Lessig

45. Exhaustion, Severe Depression, Chronic Cervico-Thoracic Pain

A woman in her late forties presented for treatment of severe depression, constant moderate neck and upper back pain, as well as extremely low energy level. She noted that these symptoms had been present for three years. She had been treated by her primary care physician with medications. At this time she was using 4-8 ibuprofen pills a day. She took Premarin for hormone replacement, Prozac for depression and an antihistamine for a hot and cold sensitivity that caused rashes.

The patient noted she heard one of my lectures at a seminar, and decided to give my methods a try. She had never been to a chiropractor previously, and felt as though it would be unlikely that chiropractic would help her, except for some possible short term results.

Physical examination revealed a five foot, four inch tall, one hundred forty five pound, 48-year-old female. She appeared depressed and exhausted from dealing with constant neck and upper back pain. Posturally, her right occiput was elevated by one inch, right shoulder by two inches, and left hip by one and a half inches. Challenge revealed a pure right, cranial MAP.

A category two right, pelvic-spinal complex stress MAP was found. Extra pelvic-spinal complex lesions included the following: thoracic one through seven right with ribs right; C5, 6, 7 RLR; thoracic three through five anterior with ribs bilaterally lateral. Bilateral tarsal tunnel MAPs were also present.

Bilateral muscle inhibition was noted for the following digestive organs: stomach, small intestine and liver. The thyroid and adrenal-related muscles were also inhibited as a downstream result of her cranial stress MAP. The magnesium stretch test was positive. Repetitive muscle testing created inhibition, suggesting a need to up-regulate her essential fatty acid metabolism. Reflexes tested positive for ongoing food and mold sensitivities, small intestine mold overgrowth and a leaky gut.

On her first visit we reduced the cranial, pelvic-spinal and tarsal tunnel complex stress MAPs.

The extra category cervical, thoracic and rib luxations were also reduced. Her right neck flexors and several right shoulder muscles were facilitated.

"We need to reframe and change tax structures so they have more meaning.

This is due to the fact that the current economies system has a major flaw due to lack of feedback."

Paul Guilding
The Great Disruption

All of the right cervical facet joints were de-imbricated. The right acromio-clavicular joint was treated with interferential therapy to promote healing. Both psoas muscles were inhibited, and a hiatal hernia was reduced.

The patient was instructed in correct spinal posture to prevent restrain of her thoracic and cervical areas. She was given full spine stretching exercises, and was instructed in the use of moist cold for her cervical, thoracic and right acromio-clavicular areas to reduce inflammation and promote healing.

She was advised to use two betaine hydrochloride tablets with each meal to improve her stomach's digestive function. Sea-klenz was given to be used one half hour prior to two meals a day to debride the small intestine of undigested food and mucous. Additionally, she was instructed to use a multi-vitamin/mineral, fish oil, and an extra 400 mgs of magnesium citrate daily. were unexpectedly reduced. She noted that her energy level had gotten a little bit better as well. Posturally her pelvis, shoulders and head were level. Challenge revealed a bilateral post-tarsal tunnel complex stress MAP, a category one right, pelvic-spinal complex stress MAP with extra complex T2-3 anterior with ribs bilaterally lateral, and C5, 6, 7 RLR. We performed the cervical ligament stress technique and taught her cervical inter-vertebral disc and thoraco-lumbar spine stretching exercises.

At this point we tested her for food and mold sensitivities. We found a number of molds tested positive. We recommended a low sugar diet, and the use of olive leaf extract as an anti-fungal. Foods that created a sensitivity reaction included: wheat, corn, cow's milk, potatoes, peas.

Three weeks later, she reported that her neck and upper back pain were no long present (she had been able to reduce, and then discontinue her use of ibuprofen). She had gone on a step down program, under the guidance of her physician, to eliminate her anti-depressant medication. She was really happy about the fact that her mood was quite improved. On this visit we found and corrected a category zero right pelvic-spinal complex stress map. Neuro-musculoskeletal sensitivity retesting revealed just one mold and two foods: soy and citrus. We had her continue the low sugar diet, and reduced the use of olive leaf to 2-3 times per week on an empty stomach.

Two months later, on the patient's next visit she noted that her energy level was back to normal. The hot and cold sensitivity that created skin rashes had diminished, and then vanished. She was ecstatic that her mood was stable and that she had been able to discontinue her use of, not only anti-depressants, but also anti-inflammatory medications and antihistamines. Her outlook was very bright, being both pain and drug free.

As we learn more about the Web of Wellness in which we live, it is becoming more apparent that when cells talk to each other with inflammatory language (pro-inflammatory cytokines) the distinction between pain and depression pathways vanishes. Go ask Alice.

"We need to think about what the future capitalist model will look like and plan to achieve it. We need to learn to live in a finite world. The current system exceeds earth recharge by 150% and if left unchanged will, by 2050, with an increased population of 30-percent, we'll exceed by 3 to 400%. This, of course, will push the system until it collapses.

Paul Guilding

46. Shingles, and Spine and Shoulder Pain

A 57-year-old male presented for treatment of severe pain in the right side of his neck, upper back, chest wall and shoulder. He stated that about one week earlier he had physically overworked himself cutting, splitting and then stacking cord wood. A couple of days later, he developed a rash of small vesicles on his right upper back, chest wall and neck. They were extremely painful, so he went to his primary care physician who diagnosed shingles, and prescribed Zovirox. The medication was not touching his severe pain.

Physical examination revealed an alert but distraught 5'10" one hundred eighty five pound male. Posturally his right occiput, shoulder and left hip were all elevated by one inch. Challenge revealed a pure right cranial stress MAP, a category two right, pelvic-spinal MAP and bilateral tarsal tunnel MAPs. Extra pelvic-spinal complex lesions included: C5, 6, 7 RLR; T1-7 right with ribs right; and T3-5 anterior with ribs bilaterally lateral. Visually he had a dozen small vesicular lesions located in his right upper back and anterior chest wall in the right T3 nerve root distribution.

The paired muscles relating to his thymus gland were inhibited. The anti-viral formula Total VirX facilitated these muscles, so we advised that he use six per day. The magnesium stretch test was positive, so we suggested he us 200 mgs of magnesium glycinate, twice a day.

We reduced the cranial, pelvic-spinal, and tarsal tunnel complex stress MAPs, along with the extra pelvic-spinal lesions. We then applied the Frequency Specific Microcurrent to the shingles affected area for 30 minutes.

The next day he was feeling considerably better. The herpetic lesions had started to dry up and shrink. We identified and reduced a category one right, pelvic-spinal complex stress MAP and bilateral post tarsal tunnel MAPs. The third thoracic was anterior with the third rib still right lateral: these were gently reduced. We performed another 30 minutes of Frequency Specific Microcurrent to the infected area.

The patient made a remarkably complete and quick recovery. In fact, the vesicles dried up and were gone two days after the second treatment. His herpetic pain was 100% gone the day following the second visit.

Discussion:

It has been both the author's experience with five separate cases, as well as the experience of the Frequency Specific Microcurrent manufacturer, that this response to shingles is reproducible. Given the fact that we spend $1.1B a year for anti-viral medications that don't work as well as this method, this should be a best practice.

"Sometimes you gotta create what you want to be part of."
Geri Weitzman

47. Empty Nest Syndrome and Sciatica

A 44-year-old female presented for the treatment of low back pain and a right grade III (meaning the pain went all the way from her leg into her calf and foot) sciatic neuralgia of three weeks duration. She noted that she was a massage therapist, and had strained her back lifting a heavy client. Initially the pain was mild but gradually worsened to the point where she could no longer work. Tears were continuously rolling down both of her cheeks, so I asked her if she was crying due to her back and leg pain. At this point I was rather shocked by her answer to my query. She stated that her back and leg pain were 9/10 but the tears were due to "empty nest syndrome." This had started one year earlier when her younger daughter moved out of her house to go away to college. I had never heard of this before, so I asked her if she had ever stopped crying in the past year, and to my amazement, she replied, "no."

Physical examination revealed a 5'3" 160-pound female. Postural examination revealed an elevated right occiput by one half inch, an elevated right shoulder by two inches, and an elevated left iliac crest by two inches. Challenge revealed a pure right cranial MAP, a category two, three right external pelvic-spinal MAP, and bilateral tarsal tunnel MAPs. Extra pelvic-spinal complex lesions included: C5, 6, 7 RLR, T1-5 right with ribs right, a bilateral carpal tunnel syndrome, and non-weight bearing discs from L3-L5. Raising her right leg off the table with her lying on her back, caused back and leg pain at 20 degrees. This is called a positive straight leg raise test and means the sciatic nerve is inflamed.

Treatment on her first visit consisted of the reduction of the cranial, category two/three right, external pelvic-spinal, and bilateral tarsal tunnel MAPs. All of the extra pelvic-spinal complex lesions were also corrected. We inhibited (muscle spindle/golgi tendon approach) both psoas muscles and de-imbricated the right L3-5 facet joints. Interferential was placed from her thoraco-lumbar junction to the base of her right calf. She was instructed in the use of moist cold, pelvic diaphragm exercises, and a sacroiliac belt.

I saw her the next day, and to my amazement, she was no longer crying. In fact, she stated the empty nest feelings had vanished within one hour of leaving our office the previous day! Her low back and leg pain were 50% better (5/10).

We found and corrected a category one right, external pelvic-spinal complex stress MAP, and bilateral post tarsal tunnel MAPs. The lumbar discs challenged positive in a torque or gait mode, so we used lumbar inter-segmental traction and interferential. We also had her begin a program of lumbar inter-vertebral disc exercises. She was seen a week later for her third visit, much improved, and happy to be able to work without pain. The only remaining symptoms were low back stiffness in the mornings.

Discussion:

This case was really interesting to me because it was the first time I clearly experienced what a huge effect cranial adjusting has on mental well being. It was after this case that I really focused attention to the systemic endocrine response in the reduction of cranial stress complex, which led me to some of my present ideas and understanding.

"Your brain is all about attachment, until the heart shines through. The heart is the geographic center of your universe - Thinking about what the heart loves is the ultimate freedom."
Zoe Marae, PhD

48. Incontinence

A 58-year-old female presented for the treatment of mild low back pain and bilateral foot and knee pain. These symptoms were constant and mild. Her medical history was positive for mental instability (bipolar disorder), and she used a number of psychotropic medications to remain functional. For several years, she had experienced a profound lack of bladder control. Typically she would get to the front door of her apartment, realize the urge to urinate, and then before she could make it to the bathroom, would lose control and have an accident. She had to, therefore, wear protective panties, and she attributed this to a side effect of her medications.

Physical examination revealed a pleasant 5'5" 160-pound female. Posturally, her occiput was elevated on the left by one half inch, her right shoulder by one inch, and her left iliac crest by two inches. Challenge revealed a pure left cranial complex MAP, a category two right pelvic-spinal MAP, and bilateral tarsal tunnel MAPs. Superimposed on these findings was a gross shift of her pelvis underneath her lumbar spine. Thus, it formed a category three pelvic-spinal category. This creates a lateral shear effect on the lumbar spine, compressing and wedging the lower lumbar inter-vertebral discs. The L3-5 lumbar inter-vertebral discs were found positive in a non-weight bearing position.

Paired muscle inhibition was positive for the stomach-related muscles, suggesting a need to increase this organ's function. The magnesium stretch test was positive.

> *"Chronic pelvic pain, the most commonly encountered and single most prevalent symptom of the mechanically induced pelvic pain organ dysfunction (PPOD) syndrome, continues to be one of the true enigmas of medical practice today."*
>
> James E Browning, DC

We reduced the cranial, pelvic-spinal and tarsal tunnel MAPs. We suggested the use of two betaine hydrochloride tablets with each meal, and 200 mg of magnesium glycinate twice a day. She was instructed in the components of a good shoe.

She was followed up one week later and she was feeling much better overall. Her low back, knee and foot pain were gone. She noted that her incontinence had also cleared up.

Discussion:

Over the years, a number of patients—mostly female—with incontinence, have reported marked improvements in their bladder control secondary to treatment of pelvic-spinal stress maps. Recently, Dr. Scott Cuthbert and Dr. Anthony Rosner published a retrospective case series[1] that showed improvement in urinary incontinence symptoms over time.

In the United States alone, "many millions of men and women suffer from the far reaching and devastating effects of this disorder"[2] (mechanically induced PPOD syndrome). Affecting people of all ages, it is often intertwined with disturbances of bowel, bladder, gynecologic and sexual function. It is "devastating because the relentless and intractable nature of the condition has caused untold physical, emotional, psychological and financial ruin."[3]

> *"I learned about the (Mother Standard) - a model of care practiced at the CTCA (Cancer Treatment Centers Of America) where every patient and caregiver is treated like one would treat a member of their own family."*
>
> Jeff Sklar, DC

49. Severe Abdominal Pain

A 60-year-old female presented for the treatment of severe left lower abdominal pain. It was located about two inches to the left of her umbilicus and would come and go without rhyme or reason. At times it would become so intense that she could not move and could hardly breathe. During these intense episodes, the area of pain would expand to include her entire left abdomen, hip and low back. The episodes would occur anywhere from one to ten times a day and would last anywhere from a few minutes to one hour. Pain medications had no effect at all.

She had undergone extensive medical testing. This had included an Ob-Gyn bi manual examination and abdominal ultrasound. Next, she had an abdominal CAT Scan and a barium enema to evaluate her colon. Everything, including blood chemistries, came back normal. The problem had been ongoing for two years, and had escalated in frequency, intensity and duration in the previous three months.

Physical examination revealed an alert, but highly distressed 5'8" 160-pound female. Posturally her head and shoulders were level, but her right iliac crest was elevated by two inches. Challenge revealed a right major cranial MAP, a category two left external pelvic-spinal MAP, and bilateral tarsal tunnel MAPs. The left psoas was in marked spasm, and the ileo-colic reflex was positive, suggestive of spasm of the muscles in the sigmoid flexure of the large intestine. The magnesium stretch test was positive and inhibition was present in the paired muscles related to the following organs: stomach, liver, small and large intestine.

On her first visit, we reduced the cranial, pelvic-spinal and tarsal tunnel MAPs. We percussed and balanced the related muscles. Interferential therapy was used from her thoraco-lumbar junction to the bottom of her buttocks. We instructed her in the use of moist cold, corrective exercises, and a sacroiliac belt. Nutritionally, we advised the use of two betaine hydrochloride with each meal, 200 mg of magnesium glycinate twice a day, and the Sea Klenz protocol to debride the small intestine of undigested food and mucous.

She presented one week later for her second visit feeling somewhat better. She noted that her pain episodes had diminished in frequency, duration and intensity. We found and fixed a category one left external pelvic-spinal complex stress map, and a bilateral post tarsal tunnel complex stress map.

Upon examination of her acupuncture pulse points, the lung/large intestine pulse point therapy localized. This led me to check the alarm points for these two meridians, and the alarm point for the large intestine was positive. From the work of Dr. John Diamond, I understood that there is a relationship between our emotions and a meridian's function. The healing affirmation for this meridian is: "I am worthy of my mother's love."

*"You make a living by what you get. You make a life
by what you give. "*

Winston Churchill

*"It's time for everyone to step forward and make a life for themselves,
their family, their community, their country and our world."*

Dave Janda, MD
Davejanda.com

Naturally, the next question that I asked her is what her relationship with her mother was like. I was flabbergasted when she responded to me that her mother hated her. I then asked what her mother's attitude was towards her other siblings, and she told me that she had one sister and that her mother hated her as well. I told her that I thought it was highly unusual that a mother would hate her only two children, and deduced that she (the mother) was probably mentally impaired. We had her repeat the affirmation: "I am worthy of my mother's love" several times a day.

About five weeks later, we saw her for the third visit and she gratefully informed us that her chief complaint had entirely resolved. She was pain free.

Discussion:

We have two to three hundred neurotransmitters and neuropeptides that flow through our cerebrospinal and other body fluids. According to Dr. Candace Pert, who discovered the receptor for beta-endorphin (one of the first neurotransmitters to be discovered), these molecules are how we experience emotion. Her book, *The Molecules of Emotion* is a great read! Evidently these neurotransmitters carry or store the emotions in our bodies, which serves to explain, in part, our bodily emotional experience. (e.g., a heart-felt sympathy or a gut-wrenching experience).

The ability to tie the emotions to the acupuncture system, and make this connection into a profoundly effective emotional treatment modality "is pure genius" which is exactly what Dr. George Goodheart had to say about Dr. John Diamond. I agree, as this work has proven time and time again to expedite the resolution of a patient's condition. This energetic engagement mirrors the socio-genomic concept of community affecting behavior put forward by Dr. Mark Hyman (see Appendix: *The Meridians and their Emotions*).

> *It is really important for us to know that our elected officials don't write the laws of the land anymore. They are all written by corporate lobbyists who run them through elected officials that they own. It is also non-denominational.*
>
> John Perkins

50. Severe Epicondylitis and Two Torn Rotator Cuffs

A 48-year-old male presented for treatment of a right lateral epicondylitis ("tennis elbow"). It had started ten months earlier. He had an MRI, which showed some fraying of the forearm extensor tendon at its origin, with fluid surrounding the area, for which surgery had been recommended. They were going to place a titanium claw into his humerus, and then anchor the tendon of his extensor muscle to this. He wanted to avoid this if at all possible.

The pain he had was moderate to severe. It was made worse by flexing his forearm and squeezing with his hand. It was relieved only with non-use, and this was a major bummer for him, as he loved tennis.

His medical history was positive for a surgical repair of an L4/L5 disc 20 years earlier, as a result of a football injury. He had a tracheotomy secondary to an infectious process in his throat. He had been involved in a few motor vehicle "fender benders" with no obvious (to him) injuries sustained. Overall he was quite healthy and extremely physically active, enjoying a number of aerobic activities including cycling, tennis (until he injured his elbow), swimming, water aerobics, running and snow skiing.

Chronically, he had two torn rotator cuffs and he had been unable to do pushups for the last four years. He noted his shoulders were aggravated doing dips. He needed to use good support shoes because he had a tendency for inversion ankle strains.

Physical examination revealed an alert 48-year-old male, 6', 173 lbs.

Posturally, his head was level, right shoulder elevated by 2" and left hip iliac crest elevated by 1". Both feet were moderate to severely pronated (inner arch dropped). He exhibited global musculoskeletal compromise. Multiple cranial structural dysrelationships were present, which along with weakening of the muscles relating to his thyroid and adrenals, was indicative of a dampening of his neurendocrine axis. Multiple muscles weakened after a quick stretch, suggestive of insufficient magnesium. Repetitive muscle testing caused weakness, suggestive of an essential fatty acid imbalance.

An orthopedic test to check for a torn forearm extensor tendon (Cozen's test) was positive on his right side. The right hand muscles that bring together the thumb and the little finger were weak when tested. They became strong when he bent his neck to the left, suggesting a double crush injury.[1]

Testing of his arm abductors (arm side raising–deltoid muscles) showed marked weakness on both sides. This weakness went away when we approximated the joint where the top of the shoulder blade (acromion process) meets the end of the clavicle (acromioclavicular joint). This means that both shoulders had a sprain of the acromioclavicular ligament. This is commonly referred to as a "separated shoulder". This injury often leads to rotator cuff problems.

"Action is eloquence."
William Shakespeare

"One person can make a difference and everyone must try. This is a call to arms to keep the republic."

John Perkins, author of *Confessions of a Economic Hit Man* and *Hoodwinked* - (JohnPerkins.org)

The muscles relating to his stomach, liver, gallbladder and small intestines were weak. Reflexes were also present suggestive of a mold overgrowth in the small intestine, leading to inflammation and leaking of the gut, with related food and mold sensitivities.

We jump started his normal stomach acid production with a product containing betaine hydrochloride. We cleared the small intestine of built up mucus and undigested foods to promote nutrient absorption and healing the inflammation of his gut wall. We utilized natural antifungal and anti-inflammatory compounds with turmeric, ginger and boswellia. He was instructed in the use of moist cold. His first visit was at the end of September, and he had three visits in October, one in November and one in December. By this time he could do 50 push ups at one time.

He was seen once again in April for a low back flair-up. He was completely healed in six visits, with no drugs and no surgery. Needless to say, he was very pleased with what had been accomplished.

Footnote:

In our forearms, we have two major muscle groups that start above the elbow (on the humerus) and extend into our hands. Imagine yourself standing with your hands at your sides, with your palms facing forward—the anatomical position. The forearm flexors start on the inside (medial) of your elbow and raise your palms up towards the sky. The extensor muscles start on the outside (lateral) of the elbow and raise the backs of your hands towards the sky. All of our muscles, as a functional organ, have a variety of working parts, including a beginning and ending (origin and insertion). In the middle is the belly, with contractile nerve fibers called neuromuscular spindles. On either side of the spindles are built in safety releases, called golgi tendons, which release and lengthen, to avoid rupture of the belly, if the total muscle load is too heavy. The origin and insertion, have Sharpey's fibers, which are like plant rootlets that anchor the muscle tendon into the outer shell of the bone (periosteum). With overuse, these are torn out, away from the periosteum causing exquisite pain, called epicondylitis. The outside/lateral epicondylitis is called tennis elbow, and inside/medial is called golfer's elbow. These are obviously named for the sports that most commonly create the repetitive injury.

The evidence-based literature supports a multi-modal treatment approach for shoulder sprains.[1] This represents a huge expense with 13.7 million rotator cuff surgeries done per year at 12.4 thousand dollars per case (162 billion dollars per year).[2] Shoulder injuries include rotator cuff injuries, shoulder complaints, dysfunction disorders or pain and adhesive capsulitis (frozen shoulder). The evidence is clear that the First Line of Therapy is manual muscle testing combined with MAP reduction, soft tissue treatment and exercise therapy.

Deep Politics

"Looking beneath public formation of policy issues to the bureaucratic, economic and ultimately covert criminal activities that underlie them."

Peter Dale Scott

51. Post Coronary Artery Bypass Graft (CABG), With Singultis (Hiccups)

I received a phone call one day from a patient whose husband had just received a quadruple coronary artery bypass graft (CABG). When he awoke from the general anesthesia, he had a severe case of hiccups which was not responding to medications. This situation was creating high anxiety, as the fear of breaking the sutures on the newly sewn grafts took its toll on this couple.

He had just gotten home from the hospital when I arrived and assessed the situation. I used his wife's arm, and utilized surrogate testing, as the poor man was beside himself, unable to sleep a wink due to the non-stop hiccups. I couldn't imagine a more uncomfortable, fear-provoking situation. They informed me that the medications he was given had diminished the frequency of hiccups by 50% (from once a second to once every two seconds).

Challenge revealed a pure right cranial complex stress MAP and a category two right pelvic- spinal complex stress MAP. Extra pelvic-spinal complex lesions included: C5, 6, 7 RLR and C3 anterior. The thoracics were also locked up, but given the circumstances I wasn't going to go there. Besides, I found what I was looking for right off the bat. It has been my experience that when the C3 vertebra subluxes anteriorly, it creates stress in the medulla oblongata, which is the part of the midbrain where the respiratory control center resides. Within minutes of the reduction of the aforementioned complexes and extra complex lesions, his hiccups stopped.

> *"It isn't the mountain ahead that wears you out; it's the grain of sand in your shoe."*
> Robert Service

52. A Twenty-Year Cluster Headache

I think that deviation from the regular format will add some color to this wonderful story. My patient tells the following story in his own words:

"Since 1973, without reason, I suffered from cluster headaches, usually 2 or 3 times daily, and twice at night. Cluster headaches are so severe that banging your head on the floor or the wall is frequent, and committing suicide is never out of the question. After consulting with several (many) neurologists over the years, I was referred to Dr. Maykel. I remembered I smiled and said, renown neurologists say there is no hope, what is a chiropractor going to do? Dr. Maykel and his staff did many things, too numerous to mention. But most importantly, he cured me. Not a trace of a cluster headache in almost a year. Don't stare at me, if you see me kiss him on the cheek. I just love him."

A 62-year-old male presented with a 20 year history of classic cluster headaches. The headaches typically occurred either a half-hour after lunch or 1-2 hours after falling asleep. They had a duration of one half to four hours. The headache was daily in frequency, constant in intensity, and worse with increased stress levels. The patient also felt they were possibly related to allergy (MSG, alcohol, wheat, chocolate).

The pain was severe and located over the entire left side of the face, and was accompanied by belching, facial pallor, conjunctival injection, nasal stuffiness and rhinorrhea, bradycardia and lacrimation. He used Fibrinol to relieve the pain and although he thoroughly medicated, the severity was such that often he would lie on his back on the floor in his office during lunch hour, pounding the back of his head on the floor for relief.

He had a history of multiple fractures and trauma from an extensive history of participation in sports, although there was no trauma directly antecedent to the onset of the chronic headaches. He was under the care of an orthodontist for a temporomandibular joint problem, and had seen numerous neurologists.

At the initial physical examination, cervical ranges of motion were within normal limits. The masseter, temporalis and pterygoid muscles were bilaterally hypertonic. Challenge revealed a pure left major cranial MAP, a category two left bilateral external pelvic-spinal MAP, and bilateral tarsal tunnel MAPs. Extra pelvic-spinal category lesions included: C5, 6, 7 LRL, T1-5 left with ribs left. The left acromio-clavicular joint was sprained, and all the left cervical facet joints were imbricated.

The cervical 4-6 inter-vertebral discs challenged in a non-weight position, suggestive of severe compressive trauma to these soft tissues. The biceps and Achilles deep tendon reflexes were diminished at plus one bilaterally.

"When plundering becomes a way of life for a group of men living together in society, they create for themselves, in the course of time, a legal system that authorizes it and a moral code that glorifies it."
Frederick Bestrat

Cervical spine films revealed a hypolordosis of the cervical spine, with no reversal. Moderately-decreased discs were noted at C2/3, 4/5; and severe loss of disc height was noted at C5/6 and 6/7. Moderate to severe lateral canal stenosis was noted from C3/4 to C7/T1 bilaterally. Moderate to severe osteoarthritic degenerative changes were seen throughout his cervical spine, representing phase two spinal degenerative changes. The C3 and C5 articular pillars were hypertrophied, as well as the Von Luschka joints at C4-6.

Testing revealed bilaterally-inhibited muscles related to the stomach, pancreas, liver and small intestine. The diaphragm was strained. Comprehensive stool and digestive analysis revealed mildly elevated undigested meat fibers and moderately elevated vegetable oils and fibers, with an elevated urobilinogen of 12 mg/cc (normal is less than 1 mg/cc). Reflexes were positive for a small intestine mold overgrowth, ongoing food and mold sensitivities, and a leaky gut.

Treatment consisted of the reduction of the cranial, pelvic-spinal and tarsal tunnel MAPs. The chronic cervical inter-vertebral disc syndromes were tractioned, interferentialled and exercised. The use of betaine hydrochloride, sea klenz and neuromuscular food and mold sensitivity identification and elimination were incorporated. Medical foods to up-regulate liver function were utilized. He was treated 30 times in a five-month period, with gradual diminution, and then complete cessation of his headaches!

Discussion:

We routinely see patients whose lives have been incapacitated by chronic pain and within a short time are able to have them dramatically reduce or discontinue their medications and make them feel and move "better than ever".

Cluster headaches represent one of the severest forms of headaches. With no known cure, the severity of these headaches is documented to have caused sufferers to commit suicide. I believe this is the first documented cure[1] for this horrible condition. I hope this information spreads so that many more may enjoy the life this patient enjoyed with 10 years of freedom from headaches, before his death.

"To be persuasive we must be believable, to be believable we must be credible, to be credible we must be truthful."

Edward R Murrow

What follows is a sequence of thought underlying this case from an anatomical patho-physiological point of view: The distribution of pain in cluster headache is in the trigeminal system, and neuronal discharge is thought to be a primary factor in the patho-physiology of cluster headache, rather than vascular discharge.[2] A particular type of neuron, the "Substance P" (SP) neurons, have unique characteristics, including the ability to excite ganglion cells and activate mast cells through their motor components, as well as sensory nerves, etc.[3] SP neurons are found in the ophthalmic and maxillary divisions of the trigeminal nerve, and are connected to the spheno-palatine ganglion and internal carotid perivascular sympathetic plexus. Blocking or inhibiting these neurons reduces both intensity and duration of cluster headache attacks.[4]

Many circadian rhythms are disrupted in cluster headache, returning to normal in the headache-free interval.[5] The circadian pacemaker is thought to be in the suprachiasmatic nuclei (SCN).[6] The SCN is responsive to serotonin, and is linked to various structures in the central nervous system, including the nuclei of the trigeminal nerve. There is much evidence to support a hypothesis that the activation of the substance P fibers in the trigeminal nerve comes from disturbances in the circadian pacemaker in the SCN.[7] Neuro-anatomy can then link, through the trigeminal system and the circadian pacemaker, the timing, autonomic features, and pain distribution in cluster headache.[8]

Sumatriptan was developed more than 20 years ago as a 5 HT1B/1D receptor agonist. This was the first drug in a new class of specific anti-migraine drugs, the triptans. Recent expert opinion is that oral sumatriptan is effective[9], but not in a convincing majority (60%) of patients in clinical trials. It has failed to show superiority over more standard and cheaper treatment such as aspirin. Thus there is still an unmet need to develop new non-triptan, anti-migraine drugs which act as effective treatment for those who suffer migraines.[10]

As discussed above, vascular changes are probably secondary in cluster headaches, with neuronal factors primary, as it has been found that vascular changes occur after the onset of pain.[11,12] The possible role of the pineal gland in cluster headache has been described and summarized by Sandyk. He proposed that "the pathogenesis of cluster headache is associated with alterations in pineal melatonin

222

functions," and went on to state that "the occurrence of cluster headache, with its distinctive circadian and clockwise regularity, and the prophylactic effects of lithium are highly suggestive of a causal relationship."

There are reports linking cluster headache with trauma to the head and facial area.[14, 15] Mathews and colleagues have observed patients with cluster-like headaches following head and facial trauma, but with atypical features in the clinical profile (relative unresponsiveness to prophylactic and abortive drug treatment).[16]

This patient's headaches were an example of the "chronic cluster headache, unremitting from onset" as noted in the International Headache Society (Classification I), having been daily from the onset.

"Given the overwhelming burden of pain in human lives, dollars and social consequence, relieving pain should be a national priority."
Relieving Pain in America—Institutes of Medicine 2011

The traditional treatment of the cluster headache is palliative, there being no known cure. Various drugs have been used including oxygen, ergotamines, local anesthetics, and most recently sumatriptin (Imitrex™).

Prevention through lifestyle alterations and prophylactic drug therapy using steroids, lithium (because of the frequent manic-like hyperactivity) calcium channel blockers, anti-inflammatory drugs, etc. is also stressed. Surgery is an option in severe cases.

In the patient reported here, the trigeminal nerve was subject to abnormal mechanical stress from multiple cranial structural dis-relationships and temporomandibular joint imbalance.

The anatomy and bio-chemistry described above provide linkages which support a possible connection between the altered structural anatomy, and the clinical problem of cluster headache in this patient.

The sequence of events in the pathogenesis of this condition is conceived of as follows:

1. Structural abnormalities leading to direct pressure on the trigeminal nerve, resulting in abnormal nerve function and/or disturbed afferent stimuli to brainstem structures, leading to disturbed visceral and somatic responses (e.g., pain).

2. Structural abnormalities leading to changes in tension on dural structures (which are innervated supratentorially by the trigeminal nerve), leading to disturbed

afferent stimuli to brainstem structures, leading to disturbed visceral and somatic responses (e.g., pain).

3. Impaired digestive function leading to multiple food sensitivities and subsequent increase in pro-inflammatory immune complexes, adding to the overall inflammatory load on the dural membranes and trigeminal nerve.

Treatment was aimed at correcting all the skeletal positional abnormalities, so as to reduce the afferent barrage of noxious stimuli from soft-tissue mechanoreceptors. This was done, specifically, in the stomatognathic system and entire skeletal system simultaneously, thus affecting both local and whole-body kinematic chains. He was also given nutritional support for his digestive system.

This clinical response, while not presented as proof of the hypothesized pathogenesis of cluster headache, is at least consistent with the hypothesis. A prospective, controlled trial of chiropractic management in this condition is warranted, especially considering the absence of otherwise suitable therapy.

"The cost of chronic illness is depleting healthcare resources. But there is now significant clinical research demonstrating that therapeutic lifestyle change programs combined with a medical food are more effective in preventing and treating certain chronic illnesses."

Jeff Katke

53. Chronic Testicular Pain (Orchitis)

A 65-year-old male presented for treatment of a chronic, low to moderate grade, pain in his testicles. He noted a gradual onset several years earlier. Urological work-ups turned up empty handed as to a probable cause, so he had "learned to live with it." The patient's wife had previously responded extremely well to our care, so he thought he would give us a try.

Physical examination revealed an alert, 6'1" 220-pound male. Visually, he had an elevated right occiput by one inch, right shoulder by one and one half inches, and an elevated left hip by two inches. Challenge revealed a pure right cranial MAP, a category two right bilateral external pelvic spinal MAP and bilateral tarsal tunnel MAPs map. Extra pelvic-spinal complex lesions included T9-12 anterior with ribs bilaterally lateral, and L1/2 anterior. Both of his psoas muscles were markedly hypertonic. Oddly enough, this patient's spine demonstrated a marked dishing in the lower thoracic spine, usually only seen in the upper thoracic spine.

His previous medical history was unremarkable, except for the fact that he had a history of prolonged sitting on a daily basis, as CEO of a large corporation. This will predispose a person to develop very tight psoas muscles. It's kind of a chicken-egg question with respect to tight hamstrings. With prolonged sitting, those huge muscle groups shorten and tighten and, of course, this happens with children sitting in school for years on end!

Treatment consisted of the reduction of the cranial, pelvic-spinal and tarsal tunnel complex MAPs. The psoas muscles were inhibited prior to the correction of the four anterior lower thoracics and the upper two lumbars, since the lumbar vertebrae provide the origin for this massive muscle. We percussed and balanced his core muscles, abdominals and back extensors, and applied interferential current to his spine from T8 to the base of his buttocks. The patient was instructed in the use of moist cold, correct posture, corrective exercises, and the use of a sacroiliac belt.

At his follow-up visit a couple of days later, he described a very profound change, his testicular pain of several years duration had vanished! We found and corrected a category one right external pelvic-spinal MAP, and bilateral post tarsal tunnel MAPs, along with T12, L1 anterior vertebrae. We taught him the rock and roll, arch and sway, and child pose stretches.

Follow-up phone conversation months later revealed an ongoing testicular pain-free patient.

"In a study of community-living persons aged 50 and older, 24% of participants had significant pain (moderate to severe intensity). Participants with pain had much higher rates of functional limitations than subjects without pain. Participants with pain were similar in terms of their degree of functional limitation to participants two to three decades older."

Kenneth E Covinsky, MD, et al
"Pain, Functional Limitations and Aging" J Am Geriatric Soc. 57: 1556-1561, 2009

Discussion:

Dr. Goodheart told the following story of how a man presented with a similar case of testicular pain: After doing everything he could find, this man's chief complaint remained unchanged.

Dr. Goodheart, wasn't giving up. There was a computerized goniometer (range of motion machine) he was fond of using at this point in his career, called the Metrocom. He remarked that with his use of this machine, he detected abnormal motion at this patient's thoraco-lumbar junction. So he had the patient forcefully extend his spine (bend backwards, pushing his belly forward) and he found that L1 was anterior. After carefully adjusting this hidden structural glitch, the pain was immediately gone.

Evidently this is another example of an organ not functioning correctly due to a strained lumbosacral nerve plexus.

> *"The number one problem is that the greatest minds in the country don't recognize the number one problem."*
>
> Norman Cousins

54. Erectile Dysfunction

A 62-year-old man presented with a chief complaint of erectile dysfunction (ED). He had noticed that bouts of low back pain would exacerbate his ability to achieve an erection. This condition had been ongoing for several years, but it really flared up over the past few months.

Physical examination revealed a well-nourished 5'9" 190-pound male. Posturally, his left occiput was elevated by one half inch, his left shoulder by one inch, and his left iliac crest by two and one half inches. Challenge revealed a right-left-left cranial complex stress MAP, a category two/three right pelvic-spinal complex stress map, and a bilateral tarsal tunnel complex stress MAP. Extra pelvic-spinal complex lesions included the following: T1-4 left with ribs left, C5, 6, 7 LRL, T10-12 anterior with ribs bilaterally lateral.

The magnesium stretch test was positive. Repetitive muscle testing provoked inhibition, indicating a need to up-regulate his essential fatty acid metabolism. The shock absorber test was positive, indicating a need for a good multivitamin, with trace minerals, to provide the necessary nutrients for strong ligaments. The stomach-related muscles were inhibited bilaterally, indicative of a need to use hydrochloric acid to improve protein digestion and mineral absorption. The adrenal-related muscles were bilaterally inhibited and responded to a product with several adaptogenic herbs in it.

On his first visit, we reduced the cranial, pelvic-spinal, extra pelvic-spinal, and tarsal tunnel complex stress maps. We percussed and balanced his core and pelvic diaphragm musculature. We used interferential current from his thoracolumbar spine to the base of his buttocks. We taught him how to use moist cold, corrective exercises, and a sacroiliac belt. He was advised to eat a clean, well-balanced diet, with the addition of betaine hydrochloride, magnesium, a multivitamin and mineral, EPA/DHA, and the adrenal support adaptogens—including rhodiola, ginseng and cordyceps.

Within the first two treatments his problem abated, and then vanished. Over the years, he noticed marked improvement in all areas of his life.

ED or erectile dysfunction is essentially synonymous with endothelial dysfunction. The one celled thick layer of our 62,000 miles of blood vessels is the tissue, which when damaged may respond as all cells do, with one of three options: the processes of inflammation, oxidation and immune dysregulation. I highly recommend Dr Houston's book, *What Your Doctor May Not Tell You About Heart Disease*. As a cardiologist with a degree in nutrition, he exemplifies the functional approach to heart disease. You may have the health of your endothelium checked with the Endopat test and see if your endothelium is healthy 10 years before you have a problem with a stroke or heart attack.

"Logic will get you from A to B. Imagination will take you everywhere."
Albert Einstein

55. Vocal Cord Paralysis—Spasmodic Dysphonia

A 67-year-old retired school teacher presented for treatment of chronic low back pain, rheumatoid arthritis and spasmodic dysphonia. She was referred to our office by another team member, Dr. Judith Swack.[1] She had a 43-year history of intermittent low back pain that was relieved by chiropractic and physical therapy exercises. One month earlier, she had a laminectomy of L4/5 which relieved her sciatic, but she still had a "slapping step" on the right. This had persisted for the last three months. Her present complaints involved a mild ache (3/10) and stiffness in the midline of her lumbar spine.

She had been diagnosed two years earlier with rheumatoid arthritis. Her symptoms were: chronic ache (3/10) of all fingers and both wrists, as well as both knees and anterior shoulders. These symptoms were constant, and were improved with the medications Arava (leflunomide 20 mg) and Prednisone (5mg).

"A quality of life issue" for her was a condition that had started eight years earlier with the death of her father, called spasmodic dysphonia. This condition (5/10) was intermittent, but frequent, and definitely worse with stress. The condition would cause her voice to "quaver." She had been prescribed 300 mgs of Neurontin to help with this condition.

Her medical history was also remarkable for a severe (8/10) tinnitus of 14 years duration, relieved slightly with a traditional chinese herb formula (Zhi Bai Di Huang Wan). She experienced a chronic catch in her left knee (4/10) for the previous 14 months, lasting a few seconds each time. She had quite a string of previous traumas: two fractured ankles (two years earlier from a sledding accident), and three concussions, at ages 17, 23, and 31 from falls on ice and skiing. She was extremely active gardening, biking, golfing and kayaking. She also had a history of heartburn and high blood pressure, for which she used Prilosec and HCTZ (25 ms). She used a C-Pap machine for sleep apnea.

Physical examination revealed a pleasant 5'6" 169-pound female. Her occiput was slightly elevated on the left, her left shoulder and left hip were both elevated by one inch. Challenge revealed a right, right left cranial MAP, a category two/three right external pelvic-spinal MAP, and bilateral tarsal tunnel MAPs. The left tarsal tunnel complex sprain was the atypical medial talus, internal tibia type. The cervical 4-6 and lumbar 3-5 inter-vertebral discs challenged positive in a weight-bearing position. Extra pelvic-spinal complex lesions included: T1-6 left with ribs left; C5, 6, 7 LRL; T3-5 and T10-12 anterior with ribs bilaterally lateral. The left acromio-clavicular ligament was sprained and her diaphragm was sprained with a hiatal hernia.

Paired muscle inhibition was present relating to the following organs: stomach, pancreas, liver, gallbladder, small intestine, thyroid and adrenals. The magnesium stretch test was positive and repetitive muscle test inhibition, and shock absorber tests were positive.

"Every day, think as you wake up, today I am fortunate to have woken up. I am alive, I have a precious human life, I am going to use all my energies to develop myself. To expand my heart out to others, to achieve enlightenment for the benefit of all beings, I am going to have kind thoughts towards others, I am not going to get angry or think badly about others. I am going to benefit others as much as I can."

HH the XIVth— Dalai Lama

On her first visit, we fixed everything we found. We tested all of her medications and supplements. She was sensitive to several of them including the HCTZ, Prilosec, Simvastatin, calcium, magnesium and omega 3, 6, 9. We suggested a different form of magnesium (glycinate instead of oxide, as it is more readily absorbed), and suggested she try to not use the Prilosec. We also recommended Sea Klenz.

All of her neck flexors were inhibited bilaterally, so we facilitated them. We tractioned the compressed cervical and lumbar inter-vertebral discs. We reviewed correct posture, corrective exercises and moist cold. We followed up with interferential therapy to upper and lower back/pelvis.

One month later, on her second visit, she presented with aggravated low back pain (8/10) from shoveling snow, and some left-sided cervico-thoracic pain (8/10), with numbness in her left hand when she held the phone. She noted her "acid" reflux was definitely better after the first treatment. Her posture was improved, with level hips and shoulders, and just a slight elevated left occiput by one half inch.

We found and corrected the following: a category one right pelvic-spinal MAP, bilateral post tarsal tunnel MAPs; C5, 6, 7 LRL; T1-5 left with ribs left. The right psoas was inhibited and the hiatal hernia reduced.

Her voice was really "quavering" (5/10), so I rechecked her neck flexors and they were all 5/5. I challenged her hyoid bone and found that it was positive in a straight downward direction. I balanced her intrinsic hyoid musculature by facilitating the upward hyoid muscles (anterior and posterior digastrics, geniohyoid, mylohyoids) and inhibiting the downward pulling hyoid muscles (sterno and thyrohyoideus).

Immediately after I balanced the hyoid muscles, she began to speak, and to both our amazement, the words flowed out of her throat perfectly! She was beginning to say "I can't do this," when in fact, she did! We both wept with joy.

On a subsequent follow-up visit, her musculoskeletal complaints were all (2/10) and her vocal cords were "90% better."

Discussion:

Fine tuning and maintaining balance in the muscles of the throat and neck should be the first line of approach for spasmodic dysphonia.

> *"After thirty, a body has a mind of its own."*
> Bette Midler

56. Lumbar Disc Herniation, Bulging Degenerative Discs with Severe Leg Pain

A 76-year-old gentleman presented to our office with a severely degenerated lumbar spine. He experienced severe left leg pain (9/10), and chronic low back pain (8/10). This had been an ongoing problem for 10 years or so, gradually worsening until it became a crippling condition. He had seen many different top orthopedic surgeons at his home in Manila, and they all wanted to perform a complete lumbar spinal fusion. Lumbar MRIs had shown advanced spinal degenerative changes, with bulging discs at all lumbar levels, and two small herniations at L4/5 and L5/S1.

Physical examination revealed a pleasant 5'5" 150-pound male. Posturally, his left occiput was elevated by one half inch, his left shoulder and hip were both elevated by one and a half inches. Challenge revealed a right-left-left cranial MAP; a category two, three right pelvic spinal MAP; and bilateral tarsal tunnel MAPs. Challenge to all of his lumbar inter-vertebral discs was found positive in non-weight bearing.

The magnesium stretch test was positive. The shock absorber and repetitive muscle inhibition tests were also positive. The paired muscles were inhibited for the following organs: thyroid, adrenals, stomach, small intestine and liver.

We worked with this gentleman daily, Monday through Friday, for three weeks. Our treatment consisted initially of the reduction of his cranial, pelvic-spinal and tarsal tunnel complex stress MAPs. We taught him the concepts of a whole foods balanced diet, including instruction on the glycemic index of carbohydrates and the use of key nutritional supplements as indicated (multivitamin and mineral, EPA/DHA, betaine hydrochloride, magnesium). We cleared a leaky gut and eliminated food sensitivities.

We vigorously tractioned his lumbar spine, and had him build core strength. We used foot leveler orthotics to support his arches and our corrections.

He left three weeks later, pain free, and returned one year later for a check-up. He was healed—without surgery!

Discussion:

Our national bill for chronic pain is estimated to be between $535 to $650 billion dollars per year, which is more than heart disease and stroke at $445B/year. This is a category we can steadily drive to zero, with healthcare teams of physical and functional medicine doctors, first-line therapists, massage therapists and acupuncturists. Decreased morbidities, related to mental health (depression), cardiovascular diseases, stroke, diabetes and obesity (diabesity) can be realized. Decreased pharmaceutical drug use, and advanced health, nutrition and detoxification knowledge will lead to massive cost savings.

> *"There is a 2.6 fold increased risk of heart disease with wheezing, and a 40% higher risk with rhinoconjunctivitis (stuffy nose blocking the fluid drainage of the eyes) compared to no allergies. The results from this study suggest that common allergic symptoms raise the risk of coronary heart disease, particularly in women younger than 50 years."*
>
> J Kim, et al.
> "Relation Between Common Allergic Symptoms and Coronary Heart Disease Among NHANES III Participants."
> Am. J Cardiology, Oct 2011.

57. Severe 10-year Leg Itching, Recurrent Bronchitis and Allergies

A 75-year-old male presented for treatment for a severe (9/10) bilateral intermittent leg itch, which typically lasted three to nine days per month. This condition had been ongoing for 10 years. He noted that there was a slight rash associated with the itch, which occurred around his ankles. The patient also noted that his veins became more pronounced and slightly swollen, associated with increased bowel stress and a tendency towards constipation.

This man also noted a 15-year history of frequent urination. He felt the need to get up to urinate twice a night. This problem was intermittent, and definitely worse in the spring. He had a 20-year history of spring allergies, with a large amount of post-nasal drip, and a fading of his energy in the late afternoons. This "seasonal allergy" had recently increased in prevalence, expanding to the winter as well. He was non-responsive to Benadryl. One other nagging condition was bronchitis, which flared up once a year for 30 years. It usually created a severe, two-week cough, and twice had progressed to pneumonia.

Physical examination revealed an alert, pleasant 6' tall, 180-pound male. Posturally, he had level hips, shoulders and head. His spine was straight. Challenge revealed a pure right cranial MAP, a category two right pelvic-spinal MAP and bilateral tarsal tunnel MAPs. The extra complex spinal dysarthsias were C5, 6, 7 RLR.

Bilateral muscle inhibition was noted for the following related digestive organs: stomach, liver and small intestine. Reflexes were positive for a leaky gut and neuro-musculoskeletal sensitivities (food/mold sensitivities). The magnesium stretch test was positive. Systemic ligamentous instability was present, which together with inhibited adrenal and thyroid-related muscles, is indicative of a dampened neuro-endocrine axis. The muscles energetically related to his prostate were bilaterally inhibited as well.

We corrected the cranial, pelvic-spinal and bilateral tarsal tunnel MAPs. We facilitated and balanced his major muscle groups and instructed him in corrective exercises, posture and dietary know-how. We recommended related nutritional supplementation as follows: two betaine hydrochloride tablets per meal; 200 mgs, magnesium glycinate twice a day with meals. Additionally, we advised the patient to use Advaclear, which is a liver detoxification support product, and another product to cleanse his small intestine.

On his second visit, one and a half weeks later, the patient noted an increased range of motion in his feet, but the itch was still a 9/10. He complained of difficulty breathing at night, due to tightness in the axillary (armpit) areas. We structurally corrected a category one pelvic-spinal MAP, and bilateral post tarsal tunnel MAPs. We found and corrected three anteriorly-displaced upper thoracic vertebrae (T2-4) and their related bilaterally-displaced ribs. This distortion complex would create decreased upper rib cage motion, and thereby cause a pressure in his axillary areas.

Neuro-musculoskeletal testing revealed a positive sensitivity to all molds and the following foods: oats, rice, wheat, cow's milk, salmon and chocolate. Based on these findings he was instructed in the use of a natural anti-fungal, (citrus-based extract) and a low sugar diet.

Three weeks later, on his third visit, the itch was now a 4/10. His breathing was fine. Structural listings were found and corrected for pelvic-spinal category zero MAP. As I like to say, he was playing par chiropractic golf. In other words, his sequential healing was excellent. Re-neuro-musculoskeletal stress testing revealed zero mold sensitivities, with only food sensitivities to soy and string beans. We also started the patient on an anti-inflammatory medical food in an effort to speed up the itch resolution.

The patient was next seen three and a half months later. At this point, the leg itch was 0-1/10, and in his words, "90% better." His feet were stiff and sore, and his calves had been heavy and cramping. He also noted moderate bilateral knee pain (a recent flare-up of his knee arthritis). He presented with a bilateral tarsal tunnel complex stress MAP and a category two pelvic-spinal MAP. The patient was quite ecstatic regarding the itch resolution. We reduced the anti-fungal to a small amount, three times per week.

The patient was next seen six months later, with no lung infection and no itch.

58. Incapacitating Foot Pain

A 72-year-old woman presented at this office for treatment of left foot pain. She graded the pain at 5/10, worse with walking and relieved by staying off of it.

She had experienced the pain for two years and had been told that she had posterior tibial tendonitis. She had undergone a series of physical therapy treatments with no real change. The pain was somewhat relieved with the use of a therapeutic boot. She had been using Nabumetone (Relafen), an anti-inflammatory 500 mgs/3 times per day. This was in addition to aspirin, high blood pressure medication and a number of supplements (omega 3, multi, vitamin C, zinc, calcium citrate). She also had neck pain and stiffness which had been ongoing for years. Her energy level had been low for several months. She was very anxious to relieve her foot pain, not only because it hurt, but also because it was cramping her lifestyle. She wanted to travel abroad, and had booked an upcoming trip to Europe, which she feared she would be unable to physically manage.

Physical examination revealed an alert, but distraught 72-year-old female. Posturally, her left hip was elevated by one inch, her left shoulder was elevated by one half inch, and her head was level. Both of her feet were severely pronated. Challenge revealed bilateral tarsal tunnel MAPs with a right lateral talus, and externally-rotated tibia, a left medially-displaced talus and internally-rotated tibia. She had a category two right pelvic-spinal complex stress MAP with a grade two right sacroiliac ligament sprain. A right cranial complex MAP was present.

The magnesium stretch test was positive, suggestive of a need to increase her magnesium. Multiple facilitated muscles became inhibited with repetitive testing, suggesting a need to increase her essential fatty acid intake. Inhibition of muscles relating to the patient's thyroid and adrenals, plus a marked systemic ligamentous laxity was present, suggesting a dampening of the patient's neuro-endocrine axis. Muscles related to the patient's stomach, liver and small intestine were bilaterally inhibited, suggestive of poor digestion, food mal-absorption and impaired detoxification.

On her first visit we reduced the cranial, pelvic-spinal and bilateral tarsal tunnel MAPs. The related muscles were facilitated and balanced. The left anterior and posterior tibialis muscles were percussed, to break up fibrous adhesions and improve strength. We recommended nutritional supplementation as follows: betaine hydrochloride, two per meal; magnesium glycinate 200 mgs, twice per day; two grams of fish oil and Sea Klenz to clear the small intestine lining.

One week later on her second visit, her left foot was much improved. We found and corrected bilateral post-tarsal tunnel MAPs and category one right pelvic-spinal MAP.

Neuro-musculoskeletal testing revealed four mold sensitivities, and food sensitivities as follows: mushrooms, rice, almonds, cow's milk, haddock, tuna, white potato, baking powder and msg. She was advised to avoid the offending foods, take olive leaf extract, (two, twice per day between meals) and follow a low sugar diet.

Three weeks later, the pain in her left first metatarsal was now mild and her walking was more normal. Structurally, we found and corrected the following: category zero right pelvic-spinal MAP, a dropped left first metatarsal and left anterior tibialis muscles 3/5. We casted a foot levelers orthotic, to promote lasting stability to our corrections. All mold and food sensitivities were gone.

One month later, the patient had completely improved, and was able to travel in Europe on a trip that involved extensive walking.

59. High Blood Pressure, Blocked Nasal Lacrimal Duct, Vertigo

A 77-year-old female presented with complaints of her right eye "not draining properly." Tears would continuously roll from her right lower lid onto her cheek. This had been going on for several months. She also had some mild vertigo, which she attributed to a stiff neck from a "bad pillow." Her blood pressure had also recently increased, and was reading at 150/100.

Physical examination revealed an alert 5' 4" 140-pound 77-year-old female. Posturally her head was elevated on the right by one half inch, and her left shoulder was elevated by one inch. Challenge revealed the following: a pure right cranial

MAP; a category two right pelvic-spinal MAP with extra complex lesions, a C1-anterior, C5, 6, 7 RLR; T1-5 right with ribs right; and bilateral tarsal tunnel MAPs. Blood pressure in her right arm supine was 150/78, and dropped to 140/90 standing, suggestive of both high blood pressure and decreased adrenal gland function.

Treatment consisted of the reduction of the cranial, category two right pelvic-spinal, and bilateral tarsal tunnel MAPs. The extra pelvic-spinal sequences were also reduced along with the de-imbrication of the C4-C7 cervical facets bilaterally, followed by percussion to the cervical thoracic spine. Interferential current was used through the occipit-C7 to reduce inflammation and improve blood flow. [Frequency Specific Microcurrent was used from the right forehead to the right cheek (channel A- 50, 40, 284, 970, 18, 30, 81 49), (channel B- 62, 13, 103).] Post adjustment her right arm, blood pressure readings were 134/78 supine and 122/80 standing, showing a good reduction in blood pressure, but still demonstrating diminished adrenal gland function.

N-acetyl cysteine, 500 mgs, taken twice per day, and quercetin ascobate, 500 mgs, taken three times per day, were recommended to help reduce inflammation in the right eye, and naso-lacrimal canal, as well as support adrenal gland function. Four hundred mgs of magnesium citrate was also recommended, as the magnesium stretch test was positive. The patient was instructed in the use of the lion exercise to diminish temporo-mandibular muscle tightness.

A few weeks later the right eye had a 60% to 70% reduction in both redness and tearing. The patient was thrilled, and had cancelled the upcoming surgery to open her right tear duct. Posturally, her head, shoulders and pelvis were level. Challenge revealed a category one right, pelvic-spinal MAP, and bilateral post tarsal tunnel MAP. The cranial complex was within normal limits. Blood pressure in her right arm supine was 118/78 and rose to 126/80 standing, suggestive of both improved blood pressure and adrenal gland function. The category one right, pelvic-spinal MAP was reduced along with the post tarsal tunnel MAPs. On subsequent visits, the eye function remained completely cleared up, and her blood pressure remained normal.

"Neglect starts out as an infection then becomes a disease."
Jim Rohn

60. Global Body Pain

An 85-year-old female presented for treatment of whole-body pain that began after raking leaves. She had a marked inability to move her hands, and to move around in general, due to severe back and arm pain. Initially, she was taken to her medical doctor who examined her, put her on pain medication, and sent her home. As the weeks passed she had no improvement and she tried one pain medication after another, with no relief. She developed a severe rash from the medication and was hospitalized for one week. By this time, she was so incapacitated that she was not able to eat or drink by herself. She sought osteopathic care, but was denied because of her age.

Physical examination revealed a 5'5" 130-pound female. Prior medical history was unremarkable. Posturally, her left occiput was elevated by one half inch, her left shoulder was elevated by two inches, and her left hip was elevated by one and one half inches. Challenge revealed a pure left cranial MAP, a category two right pelvic-spinal MAP, and bilateral tarsal tunnel MAPs. Extra pelvic-spinal complex lesions included T1-7 left with ribs left; C5, 6, 7 LRL; T3-5 and T9-12 anterior with ribs bilaterally lateral. Muscle testing revealed a marked inhibition of opponens pollicis and digiti minimi bilaterally, indicative of a bilateral carpal tunnel sprain. Those muscles were facilitated when the patient bent and rolled away from the side being tested. The maneuver indicated the presence of a double crush injury. The cervical 4-6 inter-vertebral discs challenged positive in non-weight bearing, suggesting severe compression of these shock absorbers. She self-rated her neck, bilateral arm/hand and low back pain at a 9/10 scale.

The magnesium stretch test was positive. Repetitive muscle test inhibition was positive, suggesting a need to increase her essential fatty acid status. Paired muscle inhibition was present relating to the following organs: stomach, liver and small intestine. The reflexes for ongoing food and mold sensitivities, a small intestine mold overgrowth, and a leaky gut, were all positive.

Initial treatment consisted of the reduction of the cranial, pelvic-spinal and tarsal tunnel complex stress MAPs. The extra pelvic-spinal lesions were also reduced. All of her cervical facet joints were de-imbricated bilaterally. The cervical inter-vertebral discs were manually tractioned and treated with interferential. The carpal tunnel sprains were reduced. Both pronator quadratus and pronator teres were facilitated bilaterally. Correct posture, the use of moist cold and corrective spinal exercises were reviewed with the patient. She was advised to use: 2 betaine hydrochloride tablets with each meal, 200 mgs magnesium glycinate twice per day,

1 gm of EPA-DHA and the Sea Klenz protocol.

One week later, on her return visit, her previous pain ratings were all down to a 4/10. We found and corrected a category one right pelvic-spinal complex stress MAP, and a bilateral post tarsal tunnel complex stress MAP. The cervical 4-6 intervertebral discs challenged in torque position, which indicated a 50%-60% improvement. They were again manually tractioned and interferential current was applied.

"The tragedy of old age is not that one is old,
but that one is young."

Oscar Wilde

Neuromuscular sensitivity testing was performed. All molds tested positive. Their sensitivity was negated with olive leaf, so she was advised to use this antifungal (two between meals, twice a day). She was instructed to follow a low sugar diet and avoid the few foods to which she tested sensitive, including: wheat, corn, eggs, and chocolate.

She was seen a few weeks later for a follow-up visit. At this time, all of her neuro-musculoskeletal pain had gone (0/10). Her energy level was much improved, as was her overall state of mind. We found and corrected a category 0 pelvic-spinal complex.

Discussion:

Stress MAPs may be readily identified and corrected. Substantial monies (and many uncomfortable patient hours) can be saved by avoiding unnecessary diagnostic tests, hospitalizations and pain medications. The Hippocratic Order of Treatment—least invasive first—utilizing these gentle, highly effective technologies, clearly represents best practices. (H O T ™ Medicine!)

Gentle respiratory adjusting is a true gem, and allows treatment to not only the frail elderly and newborns, but also those with metastatic bone cancers who find themselves with sciatica or other severe pain syndromes. Its widespread use will be a true blessing for mankind.

Thank you Dr. Goodheart for PAK and thank you Dr. Bland for FM!

"The Body is intricately simple and simply intricate."
George Goodheart, DC
Inventor of PAK

THE ONE SYSTEM TENSEGRITY BODY

This term denotes that the body's geometry is so highly interconnected that if you simply alter one tension the entire structure rearranges. In the big picture, it is body geometry that gets us and keeps us well. Unfortunately, until now, this has been an extremely under appreciated fact. Good body geometry builds adaptive fitness. This means that body alignment allows for the dissipation of stress and shock. This improves body communication. Geometry up-regulates all body systems and thus has a "systemic effect".

We know that the extra-cellular matrix or ECM has its own memory. This means that the connective tissues of our body is its own reservoir of information. The entire body, right down to most individual cells, is connected by receptors that are pressure and position sensitive. Single cells are spot welded by receptors called integrins to the ECM. It is the push/pull here, or mechanotransduction, that creates proteins that tell our genes what to do next. Mechanical stimuli appear to activate the same signaling pathways that are activated by hormones, growth factors and inflammatory mediators. It is hypothesized that the synergy between these mediators may be altered during aging and repair processes. Activation of the phosphor relay system by physical forces mitogen-activated-protein-kinases (MAPKs) are part of a phosphor relay system, which are activated through cell membrane and cytoskeletal stretching. Cell mitosis, gene expression and protein synthesis occur by generation of secondary messengers that activate a number of kinase pathways.

We live in a body that is controlled and coordinated by a receptor dependent nervous system. As Dr. James Oschman, author of the book *Energy Medicine* states, "The more flexible and balanced the network, the more readily it absorbs shock and converts them to information rather than damage."

YOUR HEALTH MEANS BALANCE - ARE YOU ANABOLIC OR CATABOLIC?

Our autonomic nervous system is made up of two basic components—the parasympathetic and sympathetic nervous systems. The sympathetic part comes out of the spine in the neck and chest regions. The parasympathetic part, as its name implies, comes out on either side of the sympathetics in the head and pelvis. When a person becomes stressed or traumatized, they become sympathetic dominant. Structurally speaking, their cranial and pelvic bones are misaligned. These distortions in their geometry make their body catabolic. This creates an inability to repair and enhances the destructive mode. At idle or rest, the body consumes vast amounts of energy which accelerates loss of function and promotes degeneration and aging. An unstable body is in a state of compression. Fields created by this type of strain create magnetic fields that lay down, "bone like concrete and muscles like leather," says Jeffrey Spencer, DC. The body becomes a shock transmitter.

With correct function of the cranium and pelvis the person may experience a parasympathetic dominant state. This makes the body anabolic, which is the rest and repair mode. This up-regulates protein synthesis, strengthens the immune system and the body's cellular energetics. Adenosine triphosphate (ATP) is the name of the high energy molecule formed by our consumption of food. You can think of it as cellular money. With increased ATP production, the reversal of all disease is supported as it aids every single important physiological job.

Improved blood flow (vaso-dilation) is promoted. Parasympathetic dominance takes place. Subsequently, increased levels of key body antioxidants like catalase and glutathione peroxidase are produced.

Increased protein synthesis takes place, helping to reactivate the body's major anti-oxidant systems. This improves immune function and supports tissue regeneration. Good body geometry means that energy consumption is neutral at idle which is anti-aging.

What follows is a brief review of the body's four key complexes: the cranium, pelvic-spinal and upper and lower extremities. Normal function is described, as well as the specific ways that stress and trauma cause them to maladapt. I refer to these changes as stress maladaptation patterns or MAPs.

Taking full responsibility for your body's health may be likened to car ownership. Your body is your vehicle to get you through space. In much the same way that you should pay attention to a warning light on your dashboard or take your car in for an annual inspection, so should you with your body. Pain is caused by tissue being physically strained or crushed somewhere in your body. This is analogous to a red light lighting up on the dashboard of your car, warning you to take a specific immediate action. The way in which you choose to deal with this is your choice. You could cover up the light with a post-it. This would be like taking a pain medication to cover up the pain. You could try to find and eliminate the actual cause (Stress MAP reduction).

Adequately protecting your vehicular investment goes well beyond acute emergencies and involves your ongoing maintenance such as oil changes, engine tuning, and tire balancing and rotation. In much the same way, your body requires specific attention to maintain optimal functioning of its four key complexes. Making sure you are parasympathetic dominant is readily accomplished by getting a Tune-Up by a skilled PAK™ provider. It is important to maintain the balance in your autonomic nervous system because increased heart rate variability lowers all causes of mortality. Keep in mind that better body geometry upgrades all systems. Reductions in body geometry often don't result in pain, but do diminish function which may be incorrectly interpreted as normal aging. It is wise to incorporate regular body care, with an occasional full body PAK™ tune-up. Regular chiropractic adjustments, massages and acupuncture visits should be a part of your lifestyle.

It is my vision that by the elucidation of stress MAPs, people will be able to recognize their presence and respond by getting the treatment they need to be and stay in balance. This type of proactive ongoing care will help everyone to realize better function and improved performance with less disease and more longevity. Getting and staying tuned-up changes everyone's life for the better. I totally agree with Dr. Joel Fuhrman, who states in his book *The End of Dieting*, "The most effective healthcare is self care." This will result in a huge positive economic impact.

Professional Applied Kinesiology - Functional Neurological Tools

The nervous, digestive, immune and endocrine systems may be approached diagnostically by the use of several tools. What follows is a brief explanation and examples of their use.

I. **Challenge**—The challenge is the manual application of a vector of force into a physiological area while simultaneously testing an intact muscle to see if a change in the muscle strength occurs, resulting in an inhibition of the muscle to fire. This is an excellent, quick, non-invasive tool to assess joint malfunction. For example, it may be used to determine cranial suture jamming, vertebral biomechanical lesions, rib luxations, etc. Basically any joint can be challenged to assess its biomechanical status.. Stress MAP assessment is facilitated. If altered they can be adjusted and immediately re-challenged to assess the outcome. Intervertebral discs may be challenged to not only assess their degree of compression, but also monitor their healing (see Appendix: Using PAK™ Challenge to Diagnose IVD Problems, p.264).

Specific key components of the gastro-intestinal tract may be challenged, such as the stomach-esophagus-diaphragm relationship, and the illeo-cecal valve (see Appendix: Key Gastrointestinal and Immune Function Areas, p.281).

II.   **Therapy Localization**—A positive therapy localization is the term used to describe the change in a muscle's state when a person simultaneously touches an area of their body. Areas of dysfunction are found which may correlate to a number of different causes (e.g., lymphatic blockage, visceral reflex point, acupuncture point, aberrant skin receptor, etc).
A few of the major reflex points include the lymphatic reflex areas for the endocrine, digestive and immune organs.
One other area that has been developed is the therapy localization of acupuncture points. Key points known as alarm points act as windows into these flows of electromagnetic energy. When these flows are blocked, they may arise from subconscious emotional blockage (see Appendix: Dr. John Diamond's chart, p. 282). It is very important to keep in mind that health is all about generating and promoting intelligent energy fields.

III.   **Manual Muscle Test (MMT)**—The isolation and testing of muscles to directly examine a person's nervous system function either locally or systemically. For example, specific, single muscle may be isolated, tested, and its proprioceptive components assessed and corrected. Paired bilateral muscle inhibitions guide the care to the related organ or glandular system for appropriate treatment.

IV.   **Functional Tests For Key Nutrient Processing/Presence**—These are a few key functional nutrient assessments: Proteins, Fats, Water/Hydration, Trace Minerals, Magnesium, Iron

UNDERSTANDING THE CRANIAL COMPLEX

Our brains are divided into three compartments by a hammock of ligaments called the tough mother or the dura mater. The tough mother then proceeds to line the inside of our cranium and extends down the spine, forming a tube that the spinal cord sits in. These dural membranes are known as meninges; they are both cranial and spinal. Another name for the meninges is the reciprocal tension membrane which describes the great balancing act this tissue accomplishes. Our heads are made up of 22 cranial bones. They move throughout our entire life and interconnect to one another by a series of tiny boney interdigitations called sutures. Although they only move a few hundreths of a millimeter, this motion is crucial to the production and flow of cerebrospinal fluid and the normal function of the brain at the highest point where we deal with stress. This brain area is called the neurendocrine axis. This is literally where the nervous system becomes the endocrine system. Small motion here allows for the production and flow of hundreds of informational substances called neurotransmitters, neuropeptides and hormones that control the body's physiological functions.

There are twelve pair of nerves that come directly out of the cranium that have various functions. One of these nerves is called the vagus nerve. This nerve is thought to be responsible for the majority (75%) of the parasympathetic nervous system. This is not just a nerve, but is actually a complex of nerve centers. Derived from the Latin name for "wanderer", the vagus nerve controls the function of the digestive tract from the mouth right down to the first half of the large intestine. Not only does it create our ability to eat, digest, assimilate and detoxify, but also excrete and slow down the heart's rate known as the vagal brake, this slows the heartbeat which typically speeds up with inspiration. The stronger the vagal outflow, the greater the heart rate variability is. The greater the person's overall health is. Because of its vast functional repertoire it is often used, albeit incorrectly, as a synonymous term for the entire parasympathetic nervous system.

NORMAL CRANIAL COMPLEX MOTION

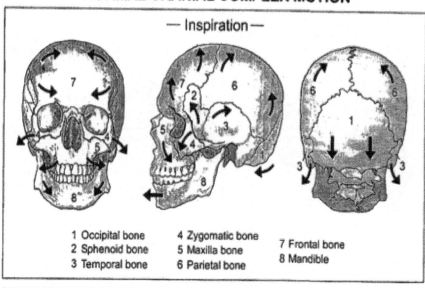

— Inspiration —

1 Occipital bone   4 Zygomatic bone
2 Sphenoid bone   5 Maxilla bone   7 Frontal bone
3 Temporal bone   6 Parietal bone   8 Mandible

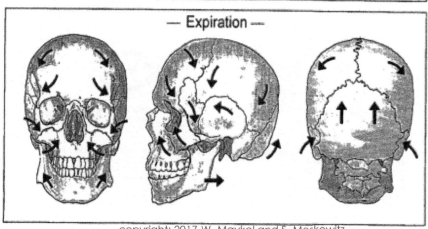

— Expiration —

The meninges have three layers that line the inside of the skull, and then extend down the entire spinal column as a series of 3 tubes within tubes.

Spinal cord

Spinal nerve

Spinal meninges
- Pia mater (inner)
- Arachnoid (middle)
- Dura mater (outer)

The spinal cord and its meninges

Motor unit

Position of spinal cord

Anterior motor unit

Posterior motor unit

(Cross-section)

CSF flow

Dorsal Dura root   Arachnoid

Ventral root

Posterior motor unit

Anterior motor unit

Vertebral body with disc

The inner layer is the pia, the middle layer is the arachnoid, and the outer layer is the dura. These help expedite motion while protecting the delicate spinal cord. Research done back in the 1960's at the University of Colorado, School of Aerospace Engineering showed that as little as 2 grams of pressure on the exiting spinal nerve decreased axoplasmic flow, carrying nutrients and informational substances to the organs and glands by 60%. Dissection studies have shown a direct correlation between spinal distortion and diseased organs of all types. Likewise, it just takes a little bit of stretch or compressive concentration to create the experience of exquisite pain from these pain sensitive tissues.

UNDERSTANDING THE PELVIC—SPINAL COMPLEX

The spinal column consists of 24 vertebrae stacked one upon the other connected by ligaments called intervertebral discs. The spine sits upon the pelvis, which is really a downward continuation of the spine and why I refer to the whole structure as the pelvic spinal complex. A healthy spine has three curves; two forward (lordotic) in the neck and low back and one backward (kyphotic) in between. Those three curves give the spine as an organ 20 times more strength and resiliency.

The pelvis is a composite of three bones. In the center is the sacrum which is a fusion of five bone growth centers. The top of the sacrum is called the sacral base because it provides the physical base for the spine above it. At its lower end sits the coccyx or tail bone. On either side of the sacrum are the ilia. Each of these iliac or innominant bones are so called because no one could figure out what they looked like. Thus they're called the innominant or "unnamed" bones. The ligaments that attach the sacrum to the two ilia are the sacro-iliac ligaments. These joints are beveled at a 45° angle from back to front and have a little "boot" in them that allows the sacrum to move back and forth (flex and extend) between them with respiration. Since they support the entire torso, the sacroiliac joints only move a very small amount, about 2° in a type of figure eight motion with ambulation.

Everything moves together in a dynamic fluid manner with motion. With a right step forward, the sacral base lowers on the right side. This unleveling causes the last three lumbar vertebral bodies to rotate right-left-right. For ease of reference, you can think of right as clockwise when viewed from above.

"The ability to walk and to maintain posture depends on a complex integration of many intrinsic and extrinsic factors. The basic walking rhythm is generated by a neuronal network which is located within the spinal cord."

J. M. Ramirez

ADAPTIVE PROPERTIES OF MOTOR BEHAVIOR

Simultaneously, the top three cervical vertebrae rotate right-left-right to keep your eyes level with the horizon. This helps maintain your balance in motion. This vertebral rotation and counter rotation takes place at the same time that the spinal curves decrease and increase in dimension coincident with inspiration and expiration. As you move through space there is an instantaneous action of motion throughout the entire pelvic-spine, cranium and tarsal tunnel complexes. Visually, healthy human motion appears to function like fluid dynamics.

All of this motion is fundamentally generated by internal pattern generators in the brain and spinal cord which are adapted to the specific internal and external conditions by proprioceptors. For example, with walking the regulation of phase transitions (re: heel strike, mid-stance, toe-off) are precisely timed by input from muscles spindles and golgi tendon organs. These proprioceptors are ideal for this

246

role as they synthesize information regarding body movement with that of the state of the environments.

NORMAL PELVIC-SPINAL COMPLEX MOTION

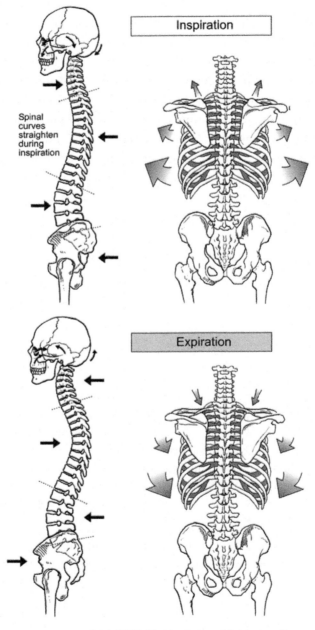

THE FLUID DYNAMICS OF HUMAN MOTION

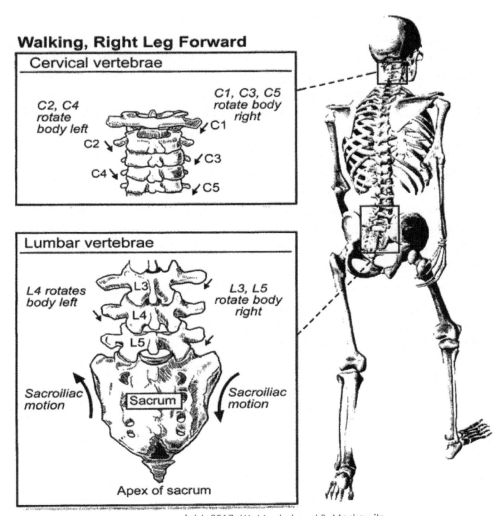

Walking, Right Leg Forward

Cervical vertebrae

C2, C4 rotate body left

C1, C3, C5 rotate body right

C1
C2
C3
C4
C5

Lumbar vertebrae

L4 rotates body left

L3, L5 rotate body right

L3
L4
L5

Sacroiliac motion

Sacroiliac motion

Sacrum

Apex of sacrum

Just being in a body and being sentient is a cause for celebration and joy.

Rumi

THE NORMAL VERTEBRAL COMPLEX

For ease of analyzing the individual spinal components, the term motor unit is used as its basis. Each motor unit consists of two vertebrae joined by an intervertebral disc. The motor unit is divided into anterior and posterior sections. As the drawing shows, the anterior section consists of the bodies of the two vertebrae (1) and the intervertebral disc (2) between them. Each intervertebral disc is made up of two components. The central ball bearing is called the nucleus pulposus (2A). This allows for flexion, extension, lateral bending and rotation. Due to this ball bearing-like function it is under a tremendous amount of pressure and is therefore held in place by 15 to 20 rings of ligaments called the annulus fibrosis (2B). Each of these rings has bands that run at opposing $30°$ angles to ensure strength.

The posterior motor units allow space for the neural elements of the spinal cord and the spinal nerve roots. Two sets of gliding joints, called facet joints, create the ability for flexion and extension as well as lateral bending and rotation. Between the facet joints, especially in the neck, are small pain sensitive cartilaginous menisci.

There is a fluid dynamism here that works in exquisite synchronicity with the normal vertebral complex motion. This allows for the circulation of cerebral spinal fluid (CSF) throughout the body while at the same time providing core structural support and allowing conscious complex motion. It's empowering to understand that all of this function is simultaneously taking place at every moment.

THE NORMAL VERTEBRAL COMPLEX

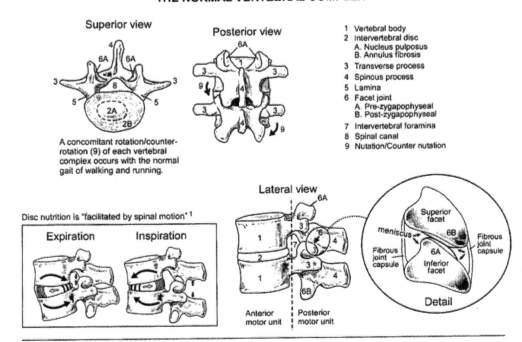

Superior view

A concomitant rotation/counter-rotation (9) of each vertebral complex occurs with the normal gait of walking and running.

Posterior view

1 Vertebral body
2 Intervertebral disc
  A. Nucleus pulposus
  B. Annulus fibrosis
3 Transverse process
4 Spinous process
5 Lamina
6 Facet joint
  A. Pre-zygapophyseal
  B. Post-zygapophyseal
7 Intervertebral foramina
8 Spinal canal
9 Nutation/Counter nutation

Disc nutrition is "facilitated by spinal motion"[1]

Expiration   Inspiration

Lateral view

meniscus

Superior facet

Fibrous joint capsule

Fibrous joint capsule

Inferior facet

Fibrous joint capsule

Detail

Anterior motor unit   Posterior motor unit

DURA-ARACHNOID SLEEVE

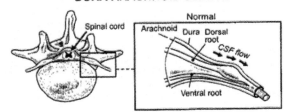

Spinal cord

Normal

Arachnoid Dura Dorsal root

CSF flow

Ventral root

The small amount of inherent motion in the vertebral complex consisting of flexion and extension together with nutation and counter-nutation act as local hydraulic pumps. This maintains the health of the disc and the facet joints by providing nutrients and facilitating the flow of cerebral spinal fluid (CSF) throughout the entire nervous system. Normal motion promotes bodymind balance by the unimpeded flow of informational substances.

1 Martin, Michael et al., Pathophysiology of lumbar disc degeneration: a review of the literature. Neurosurg. Focus 13(2):August 2002

UNDERSTANDING THE TARSAL TUNNEL COMPLEX

Each foot has 26 bones that make up three arches referred to as the plantar vault as noted on the next page. Good geometry here allows for the neutral transmission of forces allowing stable, fluid knee and hip motion. The posterior tibial nerve provides strength to the four layers of plantar flexors, which together with the anterior and posterior tibialis muscles keep the vault intact for a smooth ride. The three phases of gait are quite a symphony as this complex sets the tone from the bottom up.

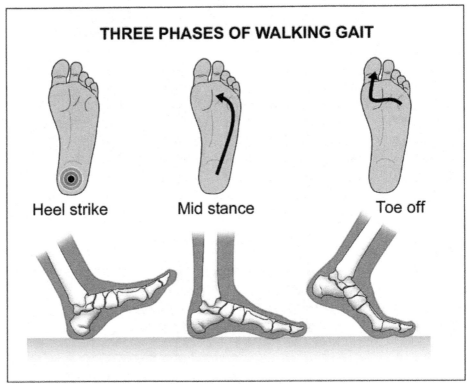

THREE PHASES OF WALKING GAIT

Heel strike   Mid stance   Toe off

Note: The natural motion during barefoot running is to land mid-foot or even somewhat fore-foot

THE TARSAL TUNNEL COMPLEX

Every foot has three arches that interconnect to form the extremely strong, supportive plantar vault, which allows movement, flexibility and strength.

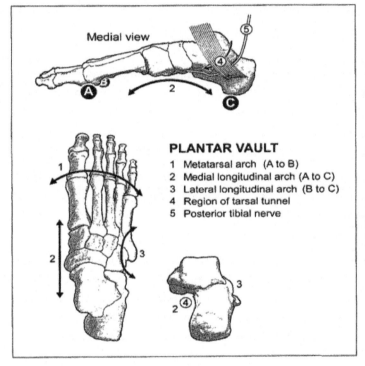

PLANTAR VAULT

1 Metatarsal arch (A to B)
2 Medial longitudinal arch (A to C)
3 Lateral longitudinal arch (B to C)
4 Region of tarsal tunnel
5 Posterior tibial nerve

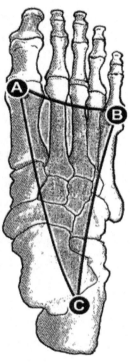

"An understanding of the magnitudes and rates of force application to the lower extremity, combined with a knowledge of the normal responses of joints and muscles to these forces, are important in the prevention, treatment, and rehabilitation of musculoskeletal injury."

Joseph M. Czernicki, MD. Foot and Ankle Biomechanics in Walking and Running - a Review; Am J of Phys Med and Rehab. 1988

"The injury of the intra-cranial and sub-cranial structures is thus the rule, not the exception. The ability of most newborns to overcome and repair these lesions shows the enormous capacity of the not yet fully developed brain to cope with trauma at this stage."

H. Biedermann, MD - Manual Therapy in Children

Cranial Complex Stress MAPs

Normal cranial complex motion is in and of itself complex. There are seven basic causes of cranial stress MAPs in this area. The first three involve trauma:

1. The birthing process—whether vaginal or caesarian delivery. A direct blow to the head, such as walking into a pole or a beam, slipping, falling and hitting your head.

2. Missing molar teeth, a malocclusion or misaligned bite, as well as grinding one's teeth at night or clenching during the day, all may cause or contribute to these MAPs. Invasive dental procedures like orthodontics, root canals, tooth extractions, implants, crown/bridge work or multiple fillings, are probable causes. A heavy handed hygienist may possibly create one as well.

3. A motor vehicle accident—even at 3 to 5 miles per hour with no physical car damage. Research has proven that the soft tissues in the occupant's head, neck and upper back are exposed to an exponential magnification of the forces of the two colliding vehicles' momentum.

4. Inadequate magnesium levels. Remember, your red blood cell magnesium level needs to be in the optimal range of 6.0-6.5mg/dl. You can order your own by going on the web to RequestATest.com or Directlabs.com and typing in "magnesium RBC." Plasma magnesium tests are useless. Low levels of this mineral cause your jaw muscles to over-contract when chewing food and over time, jams the cranial sutures .

5. Inadequate amounts of hydrochloric acid produced by the stomach leads to not only protein maldigestion, but also a failure to cleave the bonds in nutritional supplements (like magnesium), so that they are not absorbed. A sympathetic dominant state - which the majority of people are - precludes adequate production of this important digestive enzyme.

6. When a person has an acute immune system challenge like a flu or infection somewhere (e.g., bladder, kidney, sinus) or perhaps a severe cold with violent sneezing and coughing, this will often create a stress MAP. The neuromusculoskeletal system takes a back seat to immune function. After all, if your immune system fails you are not going anywhere.

7.   Last but not least is exposure to abnormal electromagnetic fields (EMFs). We have found that prolonged cell or cordless phone use, wifi areas, electric blankets, heating pads and car seat heaters also create cranial stress MAPs. The pineal gland is your GPS and it is very EMF sensitive.

The underlying reason for this is that we are electromagnetic creatures. The brain itself and the surrounding dural membranes are directly affected by EMFs due to the fact that every gram of brain tissue contains 5 million magnetite crystals; the strongest magnets known to man. Every gram of dural tissue has twenty times that amount or 100 million magnetite crystals per gram. The central nervous system has been described as the antenna to the universe.

In an effort to describe and easily understand how this complex system goes awry, I think that the analogy of a simple one story house fits the bill. You have three levels; the basement, the first floor and the roof. With a basic left or right asymmetry, the three levels offer 3^2 or nine possible permutations.

The basement or foundation—just like in a house—sets in motion predictable changes when a shift occurs.   The related cranial structures are the occiput and mandible (TMJ), along with their anchor, the clavicle.

The first floor consists of the sphenobasilar joint, which is the connection between the occiput and the sphenoid (like the stairway from the basement to the first floor). The lateral wings of the sphenoid, palatine and zygomatic bones are also parts of this floor.

The roof consists of the temporal, parietal and frontal bones.

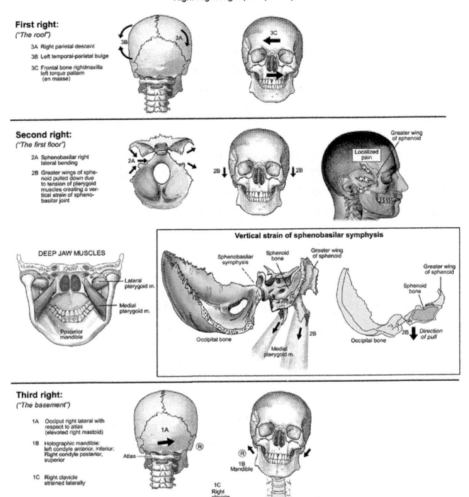

A CRANIAL STRESS MALADAPTATION PATTERN
Right-Right-Right (RRR) example

First right:
("The roof")

3A Right parietal descent
3B Left temporal-parietal bulge
3C Frontal bone right/maxilla
    left torque pattern
    (en masse)

Second right:
("The first floor")

2A Sphenobasilar right
   lateral bending
2B Greater wings of sphe-
   noid pulled down due
   to tension of pterygoid
   muscles creating a vertical strain of spheno-
   basilar joint

Localized pain

Vertical strain of sphenobasilar symphysis

DEEP JAW MUSCLES

Lateral pterygoid m.
Medial pterygoid m.
Posterior mandible

Sphenobasilar symphysis
Sphenoid bone
Greater wing of sphenoid
Occipital bone
Medial pterygoid m.

Greater wing of sphenoid
Sphenoid bone
Occipital bone
Direction of pull

Third right:
("The basement")

1A Occiput right lateral with
   respect to atlas
   (elevated right mastoid)
1B Holographic mandible:
   left condyle anterior, inferior;
   Right condyle posterior,
   superior
1C Right clavicle
   strained laterally

Atlas
1B Mandible
1C Right clavicle

Pelvic-Spinal Complex MAPs

MAPs here involve functional shifts in the pelvis and their subsequent effects up and downstream from there. Like all other parts of the Web of Wellness, structural balance has a multi-factorial input. Motor vehicle accidents, falls, sports injuries and repetitive trauma, including poor seating posture, all have a direct physical impact to the sacroiliac joints where it's not difficult to understand the stress MAP origin. The destabilization of the key soft tissues, the sacroiliac ligaments, resulting in pelvic-spinal MAPs may occur from a number of different sources.

What follows is a list of the most common contributors: cranial stress MAPs resulting in systemically diminished ligamentous tone, nutritional insufficiencies (especially trace minerals that maintain strong ligaments, like zinc, copper and manganese), diminished adrenal gland function, decreased stomach acid secretion, metabolic endotoxemia (leaky gut), hepato-biliary dysfunction and tarsal tunnel MAPs.

The sacroiliac joint is somewhat "sketchy", in terms of it's overall stability. This is no better stated than in the following fact. Low back pain is the number one disability in the world today. This is due to the fact that it has duel functions at odds with one another. These joints must both hold the majority of the weight of the body while at the same time allowing the sacrum to flex and extend a few degrees to facilitate CSF flow. The joints are large, beveled from back to front at a 45 angle, and have a boot built into their center to allow the rocking flexion and extension.

The stress MAPs that follow are simple common ones. The bilateral sacro-iliac sprain (category 2 MAP) with one sacroiliac joint rotated back and the opposite forward is one of the most frequently found pelvic-spinal stress MAPs. Nine vertebral biomechanical lesions usually accompany each of these three MAPs.

Other pelvic-spinal MAPs creating more extreme forms of low back pain and disability leading to intervertebral disc lesions are possible, but are beyond the scope of this text. For those inclined to learn more, you may look at my upcoming book *Body Stress MAPs.*

Utilizing the challenge technique in PAK™, a provider may assess not only the individual components of the cranium, pelvic-spine, upper and lower extremities, but also their related soft tissues. The concept that balance in the upper neck has more to do than the inner ear is presented by Dr. Barry Wyke. This sits on a huge branch of the tree of logic as we now experience an estimated 4 trillion dollar annual loss in gross domestic product (GDP) as a result of death from unintentional falls. The application of these truths will exponentially leverage our health system forward.

The ability to challenge each intervertebral disc to assess its functional health is presented. When utilized sequentially, as illustrated, it provides an elegant tool to monitor patient improvement or lack thereof.

Next, the most common tarsal tunnel MAP is presented with its specific bony misalignments and their associated upstream muscle inhibitions. The relationship to paired muscle functions related to gait imbalances is included to show another degree of the complexity of the web of the extracellular matrix with its acupuncture meridian component.

PELVIC SPINAL COMPLEX STRESS MALADAPTATION PATTERNS
(All examples are right-sided)

Other MAP presence	Category 0 (No stress - Mild)	Category 1 (Mild - Moderate)	Category 2 (Moderate- Severe)
CRANIAL COMPLEX:	No	Usually No	Usually Yes

Vertebral rotational patterns common to all:

C1, C2, C3 (R, L, R)

T10, T11, T12 (R, L, R)

L3, L4, L5 (R, L, R)

Sacrum drops right

TARSAL TUNNEL:	No	Yes; Post MAP	Yes; Bilateral MAPs
Right-sided example:	No pelvic involvement	Low sacral base right	Bilateral sacro-iliac spine right posterior, left anterior

Nota: Vertebral rotations present throughout the drawings. They would be the opposite for a left-sided case.

"It seems to be the implication of the data reviewed here that in the course of evolution of the erect from the quadruped posture that there has been a shift in the relative perceptual and reflexogenic significance of the mechanoreceptors in the labyrinth of the internal ear and those located in the cervical spinal joints in favor of the latter."

Barry Wyke, MD

Intrinsic Spinal Muscles
A Prescient Point of View on Balance

By Dr. Barry Wyke

It may also be relevant to note that the cervical articular mechanoreceptors become functionally active in the developing human fetus long before the vestibular mechanoreceptors.

It should be pointed out that the symptoms and physical signs occasioned by such impairment of cervical articular mechanoreceptor function (which often include vertigo, nystagmus, disordered jaw movement, arm dyspraxia and ataxia) may closely resemble that produced by inadequate blood flow in the vertebrobasilar arterial system.

Loss of the normal afferent input from the Type I cervical articular mechanoreceptors (small corpuscles in the fibrous capsule of the joint with reflexogenic effects on eye, jaw, neck and limb muscles, pain suppression, postural and kinesthetic sensation) for any reason gives rise to clinically significant disturbances of postural sensation (often involving vertigo) and of kinaestheisis (upon which precise control of voluntary movements, including walking, depends), even in the presence of a normally functioning vestibular system.

"Since increasing age is inevitably associated with progressive degenerative loss of mechanoreceptor afferent systems related to all parts of the body, it seems probable that involvement of the cervical spinal articular mechano receptor systems in this process contributes significantly to the impairment of postural and kinaesthetic sensation from which the majority of elderly people suffer to varying degrees. Furthermore, it will be clear the acceleration of this natural senile degenerative loss of mechanoreceptor afferent activity by in involvement of the cervical spine joints in inflammatory and degenerative diseases, or in trauma of the neck, will serve to intensify these perceptual disorders."

Barry Wyke, MD
Cervical Articular Contributions to Posture and Gait: Their Relation to Senile Disequilibrium British Geriatric's Society's Conference on the Aging Brain, Portugal, Dec 1978

"About 90% of all patients with LBP have non-specific LBP, which is, in essence, a diagnosis by exclusion. At present no reliable and valid classification system exists for most cases of nonspecific LBP."

BW Koes, PhD
Diagnosis and treatment of Low Back Pain– BMJ 2006;332:1430-34

The Intervertebral Disc (IVD) and PAK™ Challenge Diagnostics Understanding the Composition of Intervertebral Discs - A Tipping Point for Action

It is my hope that by understanding the following information it will empower you to take daily action and if already injured, provide you with new metrics to gauge your recovery.

- The intervertebral disc (IVD) is the shock absorber between two vertebrae that consists of a central ball bearing called the nucleus pulposis. This is held in place by 15-20 rings of ligaments called the annulus fibrosis. Each of these rings orients in a $30°$ opposing direction to provide stability.

- The healthy center of the IVD—the nucleus pulposis—acts like a ball bearing between the vertebrae because it provides the basis for flexion, extension, lateral bending and rotation. It is continuously under a large amount of compressive pressure and is greatest when sitting.

259

- The intervertebral discs are highly avascular, which means that they do not have much of a blood supply. After age 20, the IVDs get their nutrition by passive imbibition or diffusion of water through the end plates of the vertebrae above and below the disc. The vascular and lymphatics to the annulus are not present after this time.

    The supply of nutrients to the cells within the disc has been described as "barely adequate" for normal requirements. The nucleus pulposis can withstand low oxygen, but they die if the extracellular concentration of glucose falls below a certain level for a period of several days.

- The integrity of a disc is dependent on its proteoglycan content because proleoglycans draw water. Also known as glycosaminoglycans, they include such structures as glucose, chondroitin and collagen. Disc collagen suffers from oxidative stress with aging increasing degenerative disease.
- Disc nutrition is facilitated by spinal motion. A lack of motion due to mechanical stress (faulty biomechanics) leads to disc degeneration.[1]
- The IVD is richly innervated and degenerative discs have more nerve innervation than normal discs.

Diagnosing a Functional IVD problem with the PAK Challenge:

    The PAK™ challenge may be utilized to quickly and non-invasively diagnose disc problems as follows: When the disc is extremely compressed it will show with the person lying down. This is termed non-weight bearing (NW). As the disc imbibes more fluids it will then show in a weight bearing position (W) with the person sitting or standing. At this point, the clinician can advise the patient of a 25% improvement. As more fluid enters the IVD it may now be found in a torque position (T) with the person in a gait pose or twisting. At this point the clinician may advise the patient that their disc is 50% better. Typically the next diagnostic finding is with the patient flexing (FL). At this point the patient's disc is about 75% decompressed. The last phase of IVD challenge is with the patient's spine flexed and rotated (FL-T). At this point, the person is now at 90% improved. The process of utilizing the PAK™ challenge becomes rewarding for both the patient and the doctor as the functional healing phases of the injured intervertebral disc are predictable.

Strategies to maintain healthy discs throughout your life:

- Yoga–Stretch your discs daily to prevent and lessen degenerative changes. Perform the IVD exercises slowly with long deep breathing daily to maintain their nutrition (see Appendices: Cervical and Lumbar IVD Exercises, p. 271-273). Perform these as part of your daily routine and especially before resistance exercise as it will strengthen your muscles.

- Take antioxidants on a regular basis, especially vitamin C for adequate collagen formation. The current advice of leading nutritionally aware physicians is one gram (1,000mg) taken between meals three times per day. This is taken away from meals to prevent the increased absorption of iron that may be detrimental to the vascular tree.

- Use moist cold if acutely injured (whiplash, hit on head, lifting something too heavy, fall on butt, etc.). This is described in detail in Appendix: Correct Use of Moist Cold, page 278.

- Maintain good posture and support your posture with well designed chairs, sofa and beds (see Appendix: Mattress Matters, p.274).

- Remember, maintaining your height as you age promotes longevity. You truly are only as young as your spine is flexible. Your posture is a direct reflection of your brain.

- Get adjusted on a regular basis. The dental field should be looked up to for their model of preventative maintenance. Your spine is no different than your teeth and should be offered the same type of ongoing professional and daily personal care. Feed your discs with specific daily stretches.

Treatment Options:

- Most of the time (99.5/100) the correction of the body's major joint functions by adjustments allows the discs to become asymptomatic.

- As stress MAPs are reduced, inter-segmental traction, interferential, frequency specific micro-current, moist cold, and gentle stretching exercises will yield good results.

- The presence of a torque between the abdomen and pelvis, when viewed as two separate physiological compartments is the true underlying cause of al lumbar disc disease. This is due to the fact that all of the muscles attaching the lower rib cage to the pelvis are taught, thus putting the IVDs from T12/L4 to L5/S1 in a NW pattern. The simple correction of this torque pattern (called Category III) instantly restores normal function to these IVDs. There may be more work to do (traction and e-stim) to one or more of these IVDs but for the most part, that is usually all that is needed (given the resolution of the other MAPs).

- Surgery for disc problems is not indicated unless there is an extrusion or a sequestered fragment either impinging on the cord or spinal nerve root. A minimally invasive approach to remove the offending extrusion or sequestered fragment is reasonable. Herniation itself is not an indication, as studies have shown asymptomatic people with herniated discs at two or more levels.

THE INTERVERTEBRAL DISC - STRUCTURAL FACTS, PRO-ACTIVE THOUGHTS, DEGENERATIVE CHANGES AND RELATED TERMINOLOGY

The intervertebral discs are the complex structures positioned between the vertebral bodies whose primary function is to evenly transfer compressive forces from one vertebral body to the next while allowing small intervertebral movements (i.e. flexion, extension, lateral bending and rotation). The disc is composed of a soft proteoglycan-rich center called the nucleus pulposus (1). Due to its high water content and loose collagen network, it resembles a fluid, and in fact its behavior has been described as a tethered fluid.

This is surrounded by 15 to 25 concentric lamellae or rings of collagenous fiber bundles called the annulus (2). Each annular ring contains alternating fiber angles of about 30° to add strength. Due to nuclear fluid inhibition there is a diurnal cycle of nocturnal swelling - increasing human stature by 2 cm overnight - and daytime height loss.

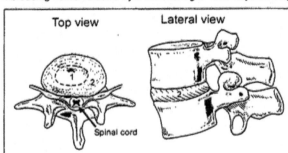

Top view | Lateral view

Spinal cord

Outer lamellae function as a strong ligament resisting excessive bending and twisting. Middle lamellae are sufficiently deformable acting like fluid in a young healthy disc and as a fibrous solid by age 35. The innermost lamellae act like a pressurized fluid.

The water content of the nucleus depends on a number of factors including age, loading history (trauma), and it has a profound effect on internal mechanics of the disc. Any increase in water content reduces disc bulging, increases disc height and strength.

"LIKE PUMPING AIR INTO A TIRE"
- Better function of the spine and nervous system
- Do your disc exercises daily
- Consume plenty of the anti-oxidant network daily
- Get/ stay tuned up and massaged regularly

STAGES OF DISC TRAUMA

1) Micro-trauma from repetitive stress creates injury to the inner rings of the annulus.

2) Over time, this creates a bulge which is a symmetrical extension of the disc beyond the end plates.

3) A protrusion is a focal area of extension still attached to the disc. If this breaks off and is no longer connected to the disc, it is then known as an extruded fragment.

4) A sequestered fragment is contained within the posterior longitudinal ligament (between the disc and the spinal cord).

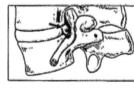
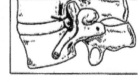

USING PAK CHALLENGE TO DIAGNOSE IVD PROBLEMS

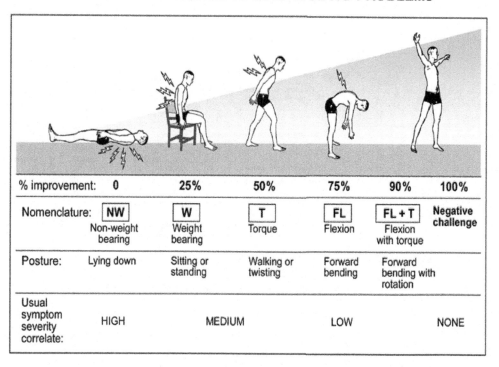

% improvement:	0	25%	50%	75%	90%	100%
Nomenclature:	**NW** Non-weight bearing	**W** Weight bearing	**T** Torque	**FL** Flexion	**FL + T** Flexion with torque	Negative challenge
Posture:	Lying down	Sitting or standing	Walking or twisting	Forward bending	Forward bending with rotation	
Usual symptom severity correlate:	HIGH	MEDIUM		LOW		NONE

The utilization of the PAK "challenge" test is a quick, non-invasive test that may be utilized to determine the location and severity of spinal intervertebral disc compression. As the discs become more healthy and less compressed the nucleus absorbs more water. This chart represents the stages by which discs normally heal and may be utilized as a guideline by your PAK doctor to evaluate your progress and compliance with your posture, stretching and nutrition related to your healing.

THE TARSAL TUNNEL COMPLEX
Its Most Common Stress Maladaptation Pattern

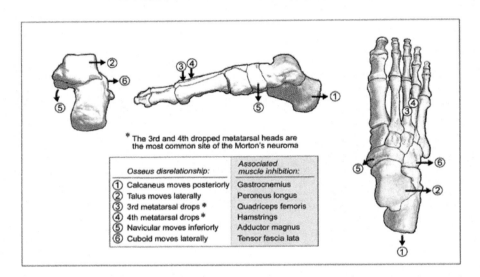

* The 3rd and 4th dropped metatarsal heads are the most common site of the Morton's neuroma

Osseus disrelationship:	Associated muscle inhibition:
① Calcaneus moves posteriorly	Gastrocnemius
② Talus moves laterally	Peroneus longus
③ 3rd metatarsal drops *	Quadriceps femoris
④ 4th metatarsal drops *	Hamstrings
⑤ Navicular moves inferiorly	Adductor magnus
⑥ Cuboid moves laterally	Tensor fascia lata

Gait Function - Paired Muscle Function Related to Foot Acupuncture Points

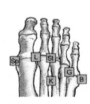

Acupuncture Meridian Point	Location	Related muscles	
		Same side	Opposite side
K Kidney 1	Plantar surface between 2nd and 3rd metatarsal	Psoas	Pectoralis major sternal
Sp Spleen 3	Medial side 1st metatarsal - phalangeal	Gluteus maximus	Triceps
L Liver 2	1st and 2nd metatarsal - phalangeal	Quadriceps	Biceps
St Stomach 44	Between 2nd and 3rd metatarsal - phalangeal	Tensor fascia lata	Deltoid
G Gallbladder 42	Between 4th and 5th metatarsal - phalangeal	Gluteus medius	Abdominal oblique
B Bladder 65	Lateral side 5th metatarsal - phalangeal	Adductor magnus	Latissimus dorsi

PAK has demonstrated this information system may become disrupted with MAPs here.

"Alignment is key since mechanics or lack thereof form the molecular basis of a wide range of diseases included within virtually all fields of medicine and surgery. The common feature they share is that their etiology or clinical presentation results from abnormal mechanotransduction. Mechanotransduction is the process by which cells sense and respond to mechanical signals. It is mediated by extracellular matrix, trans membrane integrin receptors, cytoskeletal structures and associated signaling molecules."

Donald Z Ingber, MD, PhD

Children's Hospital and Harvard Medical School

Stay Well Adjusted

Stay Tuned Up—What's The Evidence?

Recent findings:

- Chiropractic adjustments may enhance creativity and divergent thinking.[1]
- Chiropractic adjustments improved movement time by 9.2%. These improvements in function may result in improved balance, work productivity and athletic ability.[2]
- Chiropractic care enhances heart rate variability[3], indicating a better balance in the autonomic nervous system. This means that chiropractic adjustments turn back the effects of stress that amplify the sympathetic nervous system and prevent healing. This is a predictor of less mortality from all causes.[4]
- Chiropractic adjustments are five times more effective than Celebrex or Vioxx in treating chronic spinal pain.[5,6]
- A recent report of chiropractic effect on Medicare patients was submitted to Congress.[7] The two most frequent complaints cited were: musculoskeletal pain and difficulty walking. The results? Sixty percent reported substantial or complete relief from their symptoms under chiropractic care. This compares to 11% reporting this level of relief when treated with pain pills, injections, surgery and other non-chiropractic interventions.
- As far as neck pain goes, a systematic review of the literature concludes that the "best evidence synthesis suggests that therapies involving manual therapy and exercise are more effective than alternative strategies for patients with neck pain, this was also true of therapies which include educational interventions addressing self-efficacy."[8]

"While pain relief is an impressive benefit, the importance of walking should not be overlooked."
Charles Masarsky, DC

- As you increase the sympathetic nervous system, it decreases the body's temperature and this is associated with decreased immunity. Chiropractic care balances the two hands of the nervous system.
- Chiropractic management can have a highly significant, positive impact on gastro-esophageal reflux disorder symptoms, with the majority of patients reporting decreased frequency and severity of symptoms and many being able to reduce or eliminate their requirement for medication. [9]

"Imagine that your head is an apple, one half inch in front of and above your neck." The key postural takeaway of the Alexander postural positioning technique.

Dr. George Goodheart

Good Posture Promotes Good Health

Good posture promotes good health and longevity. By understanding a few basics you can prevent a world of trouble. Remember posture may be interpreted as the orientation of adjacent vertebrae. As you now know, mechanical loading of the spine does not have to be severe to cause pain. Small forces to the right areas of tissue can result in exquisite pain. The way you sit, stand and sleep affects your alignment. Good posture is a constant process involving awareness. As you may recall, the spinal column is an organ composed of 24 vertebrae that make up three curves. The preservation of those curves is the key to good posture. There are two forward or lordotic curves, one in the low back and one in the neck. The one in the neck is composed of seven vertebrae and the one in the low back is composed of five vertebrae. Sitting in the middle of these two is the backward facing or kyphotic curve of the thoracic spine. This is from the base of the neck to the top of the low back. Each of these 12 vertebrae articulates (or is connected) to a rib. This curve can be injured by a variety of ways but poor posture is right up there at the top.

These three curves make the spine a spring loaded organ and the maintenance of these curves is preventive medicine since they contribute twenty times more resiliency to the spine. All of the spine's motions behave a little differently due to these curves. Forward bending (flexion) and backward bending (extension) take place in a straight forward manner. It is with rotation and lateral bending that a "twist" occurs. Due to the combination of the shape of the facet joints and the spinal curves, "coupled motion" occurs. For example, when you turn your neck to the right to back up your car, your spine also laterally bends to the left. Thus us function blurs the anatomical distinctions of the three spinal curves, blending them together in series to create the complexity known as a full range of motion. If you flatten the middle and upper thoracic curve it decreases neck range of motion and function. If you can't couple, you will hurt. So it is important to understand the following do's and don'ts for good spine function.

DO:

- Sit up straight so that you have a small forward curve in your low back. There is a neutral sweet spot that you want to find and maintain. This keeps your weight on the ischial bones (the ones at the base of your buttocks) and allows free motion of your sacrum.
- Use a lumbar support if you need to, but don't let this be your excuse not to get up and move around frequently.
- Sit on a good, firm surface.
- Sleep on a moderately firm surface
- Go to bed when you are tired. Falling asleep sitting up is actually very dangerous as it may negatively affect the brain stem; coordinator of your balance, blood pressure, etc.
- Turn to face directly anything you intend to pick up. Keep your shoulders, hips and knees parallel to avoid flexing and twisting at the same time.
- Stand with a slight bend in your knees to prevent too much stress in the lower back

DON'T:
- Sit in a slouched position as this flattens the thoracic kyphosis and causes biomechanical distortions of this area
- Put your feet up on a desk or chair while seated as this leverages vertebra in a misaligned position
- Sleep or nap on a soft couch
- Sleep on your stomach as it reverses the neck and thoracic curves
- Twist to reach
- Read in bed unless you are properly supported (sitting up straight with a back cushion support)

Good posture helps maintain normal vertebral alignment and lessens the chance of developing high concentrations of stress in the intervertebral discs, ligaments and zygapophyseal (facet) joints. Besides good posture there are two other mechanisms that can prevent functional pathology in the spine. One is that of sustained 'creep' loading. This applies to the fact that sustained loading of the intervertebral disc causes them to lose height gradually. Most of disc creep is due to the expulsion of water with 25% of it due to viscoelastic deformation of the outer disc or annulus. The third factor that can place abnormal stress on the spine is asymmetrical muscle activity. The creep and asymmetrical muscle activity may be minimized with daily stretching exercises.

On the following pages are your lifestyle directions to maintain a healthy, pain free spine. Properly performed on a daily basis these exercise will help to provide you with a solid foundation in the structural aspect of your Web of Wellness. The return on investment is exponential. Like a smile on your face, a healthy spine with good posture signals a healthy body mind. Failure to take appropriate care of your spine will cause spinal decay as shown on the following page.

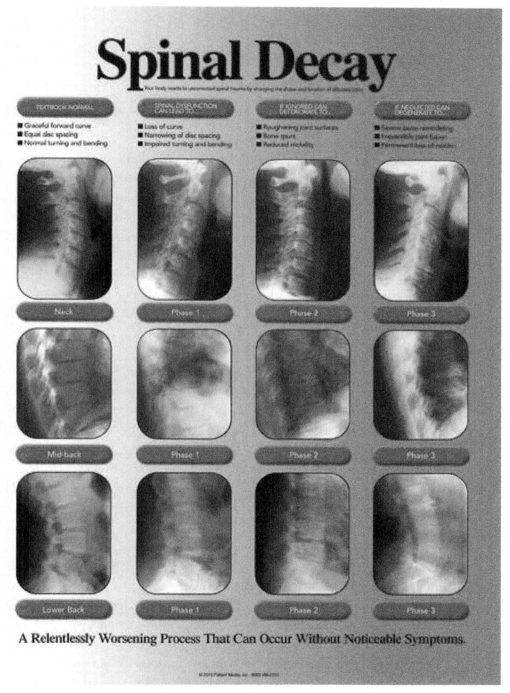

Pay attention to "the largest avascular structures in the body" your intervertebral discs.
Michael Adams, et al.
The Biomechanics of Back Pain

Cervical Intervertebral Disc Exercises

In order to promote the health and healing of the soft tissues in your neck (mainly your intervertebral discs, ligaments and facet menisci) you need to stretch your neck through full ranges of motion, slowly with synchronized breathing. This encourages nutritional fluids to get into tissues from the body of the vertebra above and below the discs. These motions encourage normal vertebral alignment, which promotes a wider range of pain free motion. This is true for the facet joints as well as the discs. This passive influx of fluids providing nutrition is very important to get these tissues to heal and keep them healthy since they do not have a good blood supply. Performed on a daily basis, these will slow down, stop and reverse to some degree degenerative changes, like osteoarthritis, in your neck and upper back.

In order to achieve good results do the following exercises twice a day:

If possible perform two repetitions (reps) in the morning and two reps in the evening. It is very important that you stand with your feet shoulder width apart and breathe deeply for each of these exercises. Do not attempt these while driving a vehicle.

1. **Flexion**–Stand nice and straight, take a deep breath in and bring your chin towards your chest as you inhale. Inhale as deeply as possible and bring your head as far forward as you can. Then slowly exhale and come back up to the neutral position.
2. **Extension**–Inhale deeply and tilt your head backwards as far as you can comfortably while you are inhaling as deeply as possible. Then slowly exhale and bring your head back to the full upright position.
3. **Series of Four**–The next four steps will bring your head through an X range of motion. Imagine yourself looking at the top of your head from above and the figure you will create is an X shape.
   • The first range of motion will have you stretch the muscles in the back left side of your neck by having you inhale and bend your head forward and to the right at a 45° angle. Inhale while you go through the range of motion to the full extent and then exhale as you go back to neutral.

271

- Inhale and extend your head back and to the left at a 45° angle feeling the right anterior neck muscles stretch. Exhale to neutral.
- Inhale and bend your head forward and left at a 45° angle, coming back to neutral as you exhale.
- Inhale and bend backwards and right at a 45° angle, exhaling to neutral.

4. **Lateral Bending** - Inhale and tilt your right ear towards your right shoulder as far as you can and exhale returning to neutral. Then inhale and tilt your left ear towards your left shoulder, then exhale fully coming back to neutral.
5. **Rotation** - Inhale and look as far as you can to your left over your left shoulder rotating your torso so that you turn and face 180% behind you. Exhale and come back to center. Then inhale and turn your head to the right as far as possible and exhale coming back to center.

This completes one full range of motion and works all of the joints in your neck to realign them and pump fluid into all the discs, ligaments and facet joints. Some crepitus or joint noise is completely normal when performing these exercises.

Repeat these exercises until you can go through all of these ranges of motion with absolutely no pain. If at any time you feel sharp pain, do not force that range of motion but rather do all the other ranges of motion. In general, concentrate on your long deep breaths with long slow stretches. Joint noise is normal—pain is not. If pain persists in any of these range of motion exercises, you need to get adjusted. Otherwise, make these a part of your daily routine. Properly executed on a regular basis they will make your spine resistant to degenerative joint changes and improve upper body strength, so a good time to do them is before you work out.

Thoracic Spine Stretches
Thoracic Intervertebral disc exercises

Stand with your feet shoulder width apart. Slightly bend your knees. Reach above your head with your right arm as high as you can comfortably. With your left arm reach for the floor. Laterally bend to the left until you feel a good stretch on your right side. Take a deep breath in as you stretch up, over and down. Exhale as you come up. Repeat this to the right side. To complete the step inhale and bend as far forward as you can as you inhale. Exhale as you come back up to the starting position. Do three repetitions, two times a day.

Remember that a little stretch is better than no stretch at all, so if time is a consideration, do at least two repetitions once a day. If you have thoracic challenges, do more reps. As your symptoms abate, maintain at least two repetitions a day as part of your lifetime wellness program.

Another good thing to do is to free hang from a chin bar with your hands as far apart as possible. Do this at the end of your day for 15 to 30 seconds. It is a great habit to develop, especially after sitting for prolonged periods of time. This action will also realign the bones in your forearms and wrists, stopping and reversing repetitive strain sprain injuries here, thus preventing carpal tunnel syndromes.

Thoracic Curve Stretches:
Rock and Roll Exercise

Sit on the floor with your knees bent and with a padded surface under you. Place your arms around your knees and as you exhale, roll backwards until your shoulders and the base of your skull touch the floor. Keep the motion going. As you inhale, rock forward, pulling your knees with your arms. Establish a rhythm and do 10-20 rock and rolls whenever you work out or stretch.

Arch and Sway (aka Cat/Cow)

Get on your hands and knees. Inhale deeply while you simultaneously tuck your chin to your chest, arching your back up and contracting your abs (pelvic tilt). Exhale, extending your head looking up to the ceiling, dropping your midback towards the floor. Repeat with long, deep breathing, 5-6 times, slowly increasing the amount of spinal flexion and extension coincidental with your breathing.

Another good stretch while on all fours is to inhale and look to the right as far as you can, exhaling back to neutral and then inhaling as you look all the way to your left. Do this a couple of times each way and you'll feel a lot of energy go into your shoulders and arms. Crepitus or joint noise is totally normal. Some of the noise is believed to be from fluids entering and moving around in the facet capsules.

Lumbar Disc Exercises

Stand with your feet shoulder width apart with your arms by your sides. Inhale while slowly bending as far to your left as you can without pain, sliding your left hand down the side of your leg (helps to keep you on plane). Exhale fully as you slowly come up. Repeat the exercise to your right side. Next, inhale as you slowly bend forward, sliding your hands down over your knees towards the floor. While bending forward, no pain should be felt. You should only feel a stretch in your hamstring muscles (in the back of your thighs). Exhale as you slowly come up.

Your breath is an integral part of the success of this stretch. It should be purposeful, relaxed and full. It helps to physiologically pump fluids into the spinal tissues by straightening out the curves and relaxing the spinal muscles with movement.

One lumbar disc exercise repetition includes a left-a right-a forward bend. This is one repetition (rep). Try to do two sets of five reps per day.

Mattress Matters

As a specialist in preventing and treating spinal injuries, I've paid very close attention to the support (or lack thereof) that various sleep surfaces provide. What follows is my opinion, based on decades of clinical practice; the good, the bad and the ugly. It's important to know that your spine resets itself while you sleep. What I mean by this is that the intervertebral discs which hold your vertebrae apart and allow for spinal curves, strength and range of motion, expand while you sleep by imbibing water. You are actually one inch taller in the morning than you are when you go to sleep at night. In order for you to do this, your spine needs a firm surface that offers support so that the weight of your body at your hips and shoulders does not sink in and make an uphill path for your spine to travel. That's not a good idea. Recent peer reviewed research has shown that patients with low back trouble do well on a moderately firm surface. Failure to reset your spinal length means you are losing your height as you age, which becomes a risk factor for an earlier death.

THE GOOD: The best mattress that I've found is the Stearns & Foster line. They have recently merged with Sealy, so any of those brands are good.

Some of the mattresses feel firm, but previous experience has taught me that this is not the only criteria for quality. If the top coiled spring is not firmly prevented from moving laterally, by appropriate internal construction connecting the coiled springs at the top to the bottom ones, there can be a "lateral sheer" created that leads to back problems. This frequently happens on air mattresses. The only way short of being muscle tested on the mattress is to ask about the construction from a knowledgeable sales person. Since the night's rest is so key to good health, if you are not sure talk to your PAK™ doctor about testing you on it before you buy it.

THE BAD: Foam mattresses, in general, do not provide enough upward support for all the discs to separate adequately. The misaligned spine tends to stay misaligned. The foam used in the NASA space shuttles was meant to mold to the astronaut's back to prevent injury on acceleration and is not firm enough to adequately support the human spine at night.

THE UGLY: Futons, water beds and other non-supportive surfaces are a recipe for disaster. Our research has shown that electric heaters (whether turned on or not) create electrical problems for the body so they don't heal. The same is true for electric blankets. Evidently the wire configuration aborts the body's electro-magnetic healing properties which leads to inflammation and, if prolonged, autoimmune disease.

SLEEP BREAKTHROUGH—Earthing refers to the process of connecting your body to the earth. Research has shown that electrons move from the earth to the body and vice-versa with the net effect giving the body the same negative-charge electrical potential as the earth. The grounding of the body shields it from electropollution. The effects are anti–inflammatory, pain relieving, stress reducing, blood pressure lowering and sleep promoting.[1]

The study of the shift of the body's nervous system into a parasympathetic state was published in the 2006 issue of the Journal of European Biology and Bioelectromagnetics. Read the book *Earthing: The most important discovery ever?* by Clint Ober, Stephen Sinatra, MD and Martin Zucker. Dr Sinatra, a world famous cardiologist, considers this to be the biggest breakthrough in healing in his 40 year career.

> *"Negative ions only exist in a clean environment. One cm3 of clean air contains 250-300 ions. Cells must balance positive and negative ions. If there is a lack of negative ions within the cells, effective nutrition absorption and waste excretion functions are declined. As you increase negative ions, you increase alkali levels in the blood which improve the body's waste clearance system."*
>
> Nebuhiro Yoshimizu, MD, PhD - *The Fourth Treatment for Medical Refugees*

There are several ways of grounding yourself such as bedcovers and workplace mats. Go to the earthing institute (www.earthinginstitute.net) or call (800) 228-1507.

I have seen positive results in my patients' joint pain, blood pressure, sleep patterns and overall well-being with the use of these products. The book lists a number of other conditions that have responded well, including no bedsores for an invalid, enhanced athletic recovery, resolution of osteopenia, decreased pre-menstrual symptoms, period regularity, decreased atrial fibrillation, chronic fatigue syndrome and fibromyalgia.

The research that I found most fascinating was the change in the zeta potential of the red blood cells. This relates to the degree of negative charge on the surface of the red blood cell. After being grounded in a reclining chair for two hours, 10 subjects showed an average 270% improvement. The results "suggest the discovery of a natural solution for blood thinning, an option of great interest not just for cardiologists like me, but also for any physician concerned about the relationship of blood viscosity and inflammation."[2]

Pillow Talk—Some Good News

As far as a good night's sleep goes, the next best thing to a great mattress is a great pillow. Given the fact that we should have a forward curve in our neck it is a great idea to support this when we lie on our backs. Lying on one's stomach is not a good idea as it reduces or reverses this curve. The average person rolls 80 to 100 times a night so a good amount of sleep time is spent on a person's side.

A company in Canada, Therapeutica, invented a pillow that is designed to not only support your neck curve while you are on your back, but also keeps your head from bending laterally while you're on your side. By measuring the distance from the angle of your lower neck and shoulder to the outer edge of your shoulder you may be sized for the correct pillow. I have found they make a huge difference and I highly recommend them as they are biomechanically sound. Ask your chiropractor to fit you with one. They even make a travel size.

This is truly one of the best inventions I've seen in practice. By preventing lateral cervical bending while sleeping on your side the cervical and upper thoracic facet joints are kept in an open position. To leverage this in combination with supporting a forward cervical curve while lying on your back is a physiological home run for your neck. They take a little while to acclimate to, but once you get used to them you will be sold. Their website is www.therapeuticainc.com

The Importance of Having A Body Therapy Team

One important concept that has emerged is the importance of every person having a team of healthcare providers to physically align, massage, needle and educate them. These promote a healthy plasticity in the nervous system.

From the "Big Picture" lens: It helps maintain allostasis.

Balance in the autonomic nervous system (ANS) is the key to healthy aging. Simply stated, the parasympathetic branch of the ANS promotes healing and repair and is thus anabolic. This represents a true anti-aging process. Attention to the cranial complex and lower pelvic-spine complex accomplish this, especially when one integrates deep muscle therapy with proven ability to lower inflammation and create new mitochondria.

On the other hand, unattended cranial and lower pelvic-spinal stress MAPs allow a sympathetic dominance of the ANS. This accelerates degenerative changes and is thus catabolic and accelerates aging. It puts you in an allostatic load state of wear and tear.

From the "Neurological Lens":

Neuro degeneration associated with aging is considered normal. It is common, but it is not normal. Plasticity offsets neuro degeneration which is progressive and accelerative.

Sensory input to stimulate the brain should be varied. Multiple adjustments drive and promote plasticity in the brain by mechanoreceptor stimulation of the muscle spindles and golgi tendons as well as the capsular joint receptors. The mechanoreceptor input to the spinal cord goes to the cerebellum which then sends signals to the mesencephelan (upper cervical area) which increases dopamine and serotonin. This also increases natural killer (NK) cell count. NK cells are the one's that kill cancer, viruses and mold. Thus EVERYONE should have adjustments, massage and acupuncture on a regular basis to maintain brain plasticity. A healthy cell, when properly stimulated, increases protein synthesis, increases mitochondrial function and maintains a normal resting membrane potential (electro-chemical gradient). Fire in the gut (imbalanced flora leading to inflammation and increased permeability) leads to fire in the brain and everywhere else. This promotes neurodegeneration.

The Correct Use of Moist Cold

The correct use of moist cold is an invaluable tool to stop pain and promote healing. It is useful for both acute and chronic situations.

Background Physiology: Mechanically, the nerve endings that allow us to sense pain (nociceptors) are activated by being stretched. Chemically, the sensation of pain is upregulated by pro-inflammatory chemicals produced in the area of acute injury or chronic overuse or imbalance. Cold works as a truly effective natural painkiller, with no side effects, by changing both the mechanical and chemical causes of pain, but only IF PROPERLY USED!

Steps to Proper Use:
1. Obtain a flexible gel pack. This will remain flexible when frozen, molding to fit the area of injury.
2. Place gel pack in freezer for one hour or longer.
3. Thoroughly soak a medium sized bath towel under ice cold water. Wring it out and wrap it around the gel pack. (Do not use a kitchen towel as it has no loft and could therefore cause the skin to freeze.) The importance of this step cannot be overemphasized because failure to put adequate moisture (wet, wet, very wet) around the ice pack will only result in failure. You need moisture to drive the effects of the cold deep into the tissue. Since our bodies are two-thirds water, water is the medium capable of transmitting the cold from the skin surface several centimeters deep into the underlying tissues.
4. You must leave the pack on the affected area for at least 20 minutes. After 60 seconds you will be numb. Failure to treat for 20 minutes will make the treatment ineffective for the following reason: In order to create a chemical change in the tissues, the blood supply must be increased to bring in healing nutrients, remove old tissue and inflammatory chemicals. The 20 minute treatment period allows enough time to not only act as an analgesic but also to flood the area with nutrients and pump the area lymphatically to remove the pro-inflammatory cytokines. This up-regulates the body's innate healing response.

Now that you understand why and how it works physiologically you can correctly make and use moist cold for any new (acute) injury. You can also apply them to old (chronic) injuries, especially after you have been adjusted. Share this knowledge with family and friends so that they too, can use this wonderful, often misused, natural method to stop pain and promote healing.

WHERE TO FIND FUNCTIONAL MEDICINE (FM) AND PROFESSIONAL APPLIED KINESIOLOGY (PAK™) PROVIDERS FOR YOUR HEALTH TEAM

You may find providers for these new medical specialties at the following web sites:

FM: www.functionalmedicine.org/practitioner

PAK: ICAKUSA.com

Your doctor may enhance his or her PAK™ expertise by taking the basic 100 hour PAK™ course online. For more information contact ... drcharlesonline/100hr

On the following pages are some guidelines used by these providers to individualize your treatment.

The Medical Symptoms questionnaire is a useful tool to evaluate your current state of health and when taken sequentially act as a yardstick for your improvement. A score of 50 or greater is considered high and calls for detoxification in conjunction with your FM provider.

The following page—Key Gastrointestinal and Immune Function Areas— is included to let you know how to go about unraveling your current state of health with your PAK™ provider.

Medical Symptoms Questionnaire

Initials _____ Number # _____ Visit # _____ Date _____

Rate each of the following symptoms based on the last 48 hours:

Point Scale		
0	Never or almost never have the symptom	
1	Occasionally have it, effect is not severe	3 Frequently have it, effect is not severe
2	Ocasionally have it, effect is severe	4 Frequently have it, effect is severe

HEAD
_____ Headaches
_____ Faintness
_____ Dizziness
_____ Insomnia
_____ TOTAL

EYES
_____ Watery or itchy eyes
_____ Swollen, red or sticky eyelids
_____ Bags or dark circles under eyes
_____ Blurred or tunnel vision (does not include near- or far-sightedness)
_____ TOTAL

EARS
_____ Itchy ears
_____ Earaches, ear infections
_____ Drainage from ear
_____ Ringing in ears, hearing loss
_____ TOTAL

NOSE
_____ Stuffy nose
_____ Sinus problems
_____ Hay fever
_____ Sneezing attacks
_____ Excessive mucus formation
_____ TOTAL

MOUTH/ THROAT
_____ Chronic coughing
_____ Gagging, need to clear throat
_____ Sore throat, hoarse, loss of voice
_____ Swollen or discolored tongue, gums or lips
_____ Canker sores
_____ TOTAL

SKIN
_____ Acne
_____ Hives, rashes, dry skin
_____ Hair loss
_____ Flushing, hot flashes
_____ Excessive sweating
_____ TOTAL

HEART
_____ Irregular or skipped heartbeat
_____ Rapid or pounding heartbeat
_____ Chest pain
_____ TOTAL

LUNGS
_____ Chest congestion
_____ Asthma, bronchitis
_____ Shortness of breath
_____ Difficulty breathing
_____ TOTAL

DIGESTIVE TRACT
_____ Nausea, vomiting
_____ Diarrhea
_____ Constipation
_____ Bloated feeling
_____ Belching, passing gas
_____ Heartburn
_____ Intestinal/stomach pain
_____ TOTAL

JOINTS/ MUSCLE
_____ Pain or aches in joints
_____ Arthritis
_____ Stiff or limitation of movement
_____ Pain or aches in muscles
_____ Feeling of weakness or tired
_____ TOTAL

WEIGHT
_____ Binge eating/drinking
_____ Craving certain foods
_____ Excessive weight
_____ Compulsive eating
_____ Water retention
_____ Underweight
_____ TOTAL

ENERGY/ ACTIVITY
_____ Fatigue, sluggishness
_____ Apathy, lethargy
_____ Hyperactivity
_____ Restlessness
_____ TOTAL

MIND
_____ Poor memory
_____ Confusion, poor comprehension
_____ Poor concentration
_____ Poor physical coordination
_____ Difficulty in making decisions
_____ Stuttering or stammering
_____ Slurred speech
_____ Learning disabilities
_____ TOTAL

EMOTIONS
_____ Mood swings
_____ Anxiety, fear, nervousness
_____ Anger, irritability, aggression
_____ Depression
_____ TOTAL

OTHER
_____ Frequent illness
_____ Frequent or urgent urination
_____ Genital itch or discharge
_____ TOTAL

GRAND TOTAL _____

KEY GASTROINTESTINAL AND IMMUNE FUNCTION AREAS

1 Cranial stress complex
may affect function of the vagus nerve which has control over the secretion of the digestive glands of the mouth, stomach and pancreas. It increases the peristalsis and tone of the gut and relaxes the sphincters

2 Infraspinatus
A bilateral inhibition is associated with a stressed thymus gland (2a), indicative of an activated immune response that may indicate need for antiviral or antibiotic treatment

3 Pectoralis Major - Clavicular division
A bilateral inhibition associated with hypochlorhydria or decreased stomach acid production may indicate a need to increase zinc

4 Triceps(4A) or latissimus dorsi(4B)
bilateral inhibition associated with poor pancreatic function and suggests a need for pancreatic enzymes or cofactors to help with insulin resistance

5 Neuromusculoskeletal sensitivity reflex point - associated with food and mold sensitivities

6 Bilateral inhibition of abdominal or quadraceps muscles -
associated with congestion of small intestine and probable malabsorption / dysbiosis

7 Ileocecal valve
the sphincter valve between the distal small intestine - may be stuck closed causing constipation or open creating general malaise - associated with L3 anterior

8 Pectoralis major sternal division -
bilateral inhibition is associated with liver malfunction and may signal a need for nutrients to upregulate detoxification

9 Hiatal Hernia
a strained diaphragm caused by bilateral psoas contracture usually secondary to pelvic-spinal stress maps; this causes the diaphragm to be pulled down, causing the stomach to ride up through the opening for the esophagus - this causes the lower esophageal sphincter to no longer be flush with the diaphragm: may lead to the signs and symptoms of gastro-esophageal reflex disease (GERD).

10 Umbilicus reflex positive therapy localization
here is indicative of a small intestine mold overgrowth; three inches superior and lateral is a secondary reflex associated with a breakdown of the integrity of the small intestinal mucosa with subsequent increase in permeability, aka "leaky gut."

11 Tensor fascia lata or hamstrings
a bilateral inhibition of these muscles is associated with dysfunction of the large intestine, signalling the need for increased fiber, probiotics or colon cleansing

12 Lower left quadrant -ileo-colic area
opposite the ileo-cecal valve is the ileocolic valve, not a true valve, but a thickening of the taenia coli - may become spastic-associated with L4 anterior, and / or a need to increase iron.

THE MERIDIANS AND THEIR EMOTIONS
By John Diamond, MD

Meridian	General	Negative Emotions	Positive Affirmation
Lung	Tolerance/ Intolerance	disdain, scorn, contempt, prejudice, haughtiness, false pride, intolerance	I am of the earth
Liver	Happiness/ Unhappiness	Unhappiness	My mother smiles on me
Gallbladder	Love/Rage	rage, fury, wrath	I reach out with love
Large Intestine	Self-worth/guilt	guilt	I am worthy of my mother's love
Kidney	sexual security/ sexual indecision	sexual indecision	My sex energies are balanced
Spleen	faith in the future/ anxiety about the future	realistic anxieties	My future is secure
Circulation Sex	renunciation of past generosity, relaxation/ regret, sexual tension, remorse, jealousy	regret and remorse	I freely surrender my love
Heart	Love, forgiveness/ anger	anger	My heart is filled
Stomach	contentment/ disappointment, disgust, greed	disgust, disappointment, bitterness, greed, emptiness, deprivation, nausea, hunger	I am content with my life
Thyroid	Lightness, buoyancy/ heaviness, depression	depression, despair, grief, hopelessness, despondency, loneliness, solitude	I am light and buoyant
Small Intestine	Joy/sorrow sadness	Saddness, sorrow	I am jumping with joy

Bladder	peace, harmony	restlessness, impatience	I am perfectly
	restlessness	frustration	peaceful
	impatience		
Thymus	I am love, faith	I have gratitude & courage	

"Nutrition is really the future of health in our generation."
Garth Nicholson, PhD

1972 Co-author with SJ Singer of the 'Fluid Mosaic Model of the Structure of Cell Membranes.' This was the most highly cited paper in all fields of science for nearly one decade. He has authored over 600 peer reviewed publications.

THE WONDERS OF MEDICAL FOOD

- Medical Foods are specially designed groups of nutrients to provide support or prevent areas of stress in the web of wellness.
- Your healthcare provider helps determine the best ones for you to use.
- Nutrients directly affect gene expression for health or disease.
- Nutrigenomics is the application of nutrition to create positive gene expression.
- Metagenics has created a suite of FDA-regulated medical foods and bars designed to create happy genes. They pack a wallop to get the job done.
- They are quick (2 scoops in a blender, 8 oz of water, with a few organic berries or just eat a bar.)
- They taste great and come in a variety of flavors.
- They are hypoallergenic and come in a variety of protein base, (i.e., whey, rice or soy) to accommodate everyone's biochemical individuality.
- UltraInFlamX–This formula is not to be taken just for inflammation, but may be considered a potent anti-aging formula as it contains 17,500 ORAC per serving. This is important as every cell gets over 100,000 free radical hits per day.

Product name	Conditions	Proteins	Flavors	Bars	Affects
Ultra Meal [R]	Metabolic Syndrome Cardio vascular	Rice	Chocolate Vanilla	Chocolate Fudge Vanilla Almond	supports healthy body comp Increases muscle
		Whey	Dutch Chocolate Vanilla		Decreases fat
		Soy	Vanilla Dutch Chocloate Strawberry Mocha Banana Blast Country Peach Raspberry Seasonal Flavora	Apple Cinnamon Lemon Zinger Chocolate banana Chocolate raspberry Chocolate fudge	
UltraMeal Plus R	Metabolic Syndrome	Soy	Vanilla, Mocha Dutch Chocolate Srawberry		Central Obesity Insulin Resistance Altered Body Cmposition
UltraMeal Plus 360[R]		Soy	Vanilla Strawberry Dutch Chocolate		Decreases both total and LDL Cholesterol & Triglycerides Increases HDL Decreases Homocysteine
Ultra GlycemX Plus 360[R]	Type 2 diabetes	Soy	Original Natural Chocolate		

Product name	Conditions	Proteins	Flavors	Bars	Affects
UltraClear Plus[R]	Chronic Fatigue Syndrome Liver Detox Support	Rice Banana Chai	Original Natural Berry Pineapple-		Increases Energy, Better focus Clears skin Reduces pain
UltraInflamX Plus360[R]	Irritable & Inflammatory Bowel Disease	Rice	Mango Pineapple-Banana Original Spice		
Estrium[R]	PMS	Rice	Mango		

"Alteration of autonomic nervous system pathways and cardiac centers regulating heart rate variability can be directly influenced by inflammation. The association of inflammation with heart disease is well established, with the measurement of the high sensitive c-reactive protein (hsCRP) often included in screenings."

Nicolas Hall, PhD

Diagnosing Cardiovascular Disease from the Perspective of the Brain and In lammation Alt. Ther. In *Health and Med; Heart Health* 2013, Vol. 199, suppl.1;p.8

TRICKS TO KEEP A POSTIVE MAGNESIUM STATUS

Who doesn't have stress? Stressors, such as exercise that makes you sweat, pollution, prescription and recreational drugs, alcohol, carbonated beverages, caffeinated beverages, sugar containing foods, calcium supplements and multivitamin/mineral supplements with a 2:1 calcium to magnesium ratio all deplete this mineral. Magnesium comes from the root word magneto, meaning magnet, and it pulls calcium into the bones.

Magnesium is the kingpin of the mineral world of the body. It controls the body's use of calcium, sodium and potassium. In the tissues of the body it acts as an antioxidant. It is anti-inflammatory. It prevents cardiovascular disease and performs every single function that cardiovascular medications are used for. For example, magnesium thins the blood (like Coumadin or Warfarin) and it lowers blood pressure. It is nature's calcium channel blocker (regulating calcium from entering cells) and it functions as an anti-arrhythmic (normalizing heart rate). Recent scientific evidence has also demonstrated that 85% of people are deficient in getting the RDA for magnesium.[1]

Magnesium directly correlated with phase angle, a BIA parameter and marker of cellular health and inversely correlated with hsCRP

(a sensitive cardiovascular marker) in peritoneal dialysis patients.
P. Fern, et al. (2010) Advances in Peritoneal Dialysis, 2: 112-5

- Magnesium is known as the stress mineral. As soon as you experience stress and the adrenal glands secrete adrenalin and cortisol, your magnesium becomes depleted because all of the enzymes necessary to metabolize these hormones are magnesium dependent.
Thus it is depleted by all types of stress. When you are low in it, it actually amplifies your response to stress of all types, since it is anti-inflammatory.
A positive magnesium status is important to maintain because of its profound effect on cell membrane integrity. It is difficult to maintain for the following reasons:
- The optimal concentration inside the cell is 42 times greater than in the fluids outside the cell.
- The enzyme that pumps magnesium into the cell is magnesium and potassium dependent.
- It is necessary for the formation of the tripeptide glutathione, which is important for phase two liver detoxification. It is the main reducing agent of all cells—it may be likened to the Fed-Ex of the cellular immune system, recharging key antioxidants and removing waste. It is a key nutrient for preventing cancers of all types.
- Failure to maintain liver detoxification results in a fatty liver (steatorrhea). Currently there is an epidemic of NASH (non-alcoholic steatorrhea).
- All the soils of the industrialized nations have been depleted of magnesium for the last 60 years.
- Seven hundred of the body's key enzymes are magnesium dependent. The conversion of food into energy and the stability of your genes so they make exact copies of each other (genomic stability) are two good examples of these.

"The expression of nitric oxide by endothelial nitric oxide synthase (eNOS) is known to be regulated in part by the interaction of vitamin C, vitamin D, biotin, taurine and polyphenols with low molecular weights, such as grape seed extracts. Other essential nutrients, such as vitamin B6 and magnesium, are know to regulate blood pressure through various mechanisms."

Marc Houston, MD, William Sparks, CN

"Combination Nutraceutical Supplement Lowers Blood Pressure in Hypertensive Individuals" Integrative Medicine Vol. 12. No.3, June 2013

Now the obvious questions are how do you get enough magnesium and what is enough magnesium? Because it is difficult to keep this mineral in our cells and everything washes it out, you should use several different forms on a regular basis to maintain adequate amounts without too much trouble. Tablet forms include magnesium glycinate and magnesium citrate. Avoid magnesium oxide because even though it has increased elemental magnesium, it is poorly absorbed by the body. Powdered magnesium citrate and magnesium ascorbate can be mixed with hot water. Liquid magnesium chloride is easily assimilated and can be added to any liquid.

A busy working male should be taking a baseline amount of 400-600mg per day and can increase that amount to 800–1000mg per day with increased exercise, stress or heat exposure. These same recommendations apply for busy working women, just at a level of 100-200mg less. We recommend using several different forms of magnesium to leverage cell membrane uptake to help maintain optimal levels. The only potential side effect of excessive magnesium intake is diarrhea or a loose stool. If this happens, several things can be done. First of all, change to the glycinate or chloride form as they are more easily assimilated. If this doesn't work consider using several grams of taurine and/or phosphatidyl choline to improve your cell membrane function.

Magnesium protects us from neurodegeneration. In healthy brain cells, magnesium functionally blocks the NMDA receptor. This receptor is involved in memory. This allows it to respond with a normal response to become activated. A lack of adequate magnesium causes the formation of dangerous free radicals which damage the mitochondria leading to DNA breaks and damage.

A recent study[2] found that a new form of magnesium was able to concentrate 5 times greater in the cerebrospinal fluid of test animals. This new, highly absorbable form of magnesium (called magnesium-L-threonate or MgT), rebuilds ruptured synapses and restores the degraded neuronal connections seen in Alzheimer's disease and other forms of memory loss. It has been shown to significantly enhance both short and long term memory by increasing synaptic density and plasticity. This is a huge breakthrough as a decrease in neural connectivity and adaptability (lack of plasticity) are the harbingers of neurodegenerative changes.

Adequate magnesium is the best insurance policy we as individuals and as a nation can have. Think about it: anti-inflammatory, neuroprotective, improves respiratory, vascular, insulin, immune and kidney function. Adequate amounts prevent the development of cranial stress MAPs by normalizing TMJ muscle function, thus preventing systemic pain. Talk about a great return on investment.

"The world is not dangerous because of those who do harm, but because of those who look at it without doing anything."
Albert Einstein

A SHORT LIST OF TECHNOLOGIES TO BE WARY OF:

1. Cell phones, cordless phones, wi-fi, "smart" meters and cell phone towers:

The non-ionizing radiation of these devices has definitely been shown by a growing number of scientists to promote cellular changes associated with cancer called micro-nuclei. In one of the biggest cover ups, and failures to protect American citizens, the FDA helped the cell phone (wireless technology) industry cover up the harm proven by their own chief scientist Dr. George Carlo. He was blacklisted by the industry after his research, which they funded, proved beyond a doubt exactly what they most feared. You can read the whole story in his book *Cell Phones, Invisible Hazards in the Wireless Age* (ISBN 0-7867-0960-X). Wireless communication devices pose extreme health hazards. The microwave radiation from cell phone antennas disrupts cardiac pacemakers, penetrates developing skulls of children, compromises the blood-brain barrier and inflicts genetic damage (micro-nuclei) that is a known diagnostic marker for cancer. Cell phone users have a 50% increase of risk in developing tumors of the auditory nerve. Carlo's book was written in 2001. Dr. Devra Davis, PhD, MPH, is the founding director of the Board on Environmental Studies and Toxicology of the United States National Research Council of the National Academy of Sciences. Her new book, *Disconnect*, brings forth updated research from around the world, which shows that cell phone radiation may be an epigenetic carcinogen due to its blocking repair of DNA. Go to her website www. ehtrust.org to learn more.

According to the documentary movie *Full Signal*, we now live in an ocean of one trillion times the normal radiation levels, which is a form of electromagnetic air pollution. The creators of this film note that the Swedish neurologist, Professor Leif Larson, states, "You are not safe anywhere," because the possible risks to this intense radiation are not yet fully understood. Dr. David Carpenter, director of the Institute for Health and Environment at the

University of Albany, NY states that 13 studies have shown both single and double DNA strand breaks which both lead to mutation. About 2 to 6% of the US population or 10 to 15 million people have sensitivity to electromagnetic frequencies (EMF) called electro-hypersensitivity. These people are the "canaries in the mine shafts" and suffer deteriorating health from allergies to various frequencies creating a functional impairment. The signs and symptoms consist of flu-like symptoms, burning unbearable pain, convulsions, black spots before their eyes, dizziness, abnormal menstrual cycles, inability to concentrate and sleep problems. The scientists consulted all agreed that we are part of a massive human experiment and that we need to be very cautious as this is a "very sensitive" public health issue.

These frequencies are identified by the World Health Organization as potential human carcinogens. The companies involved are not motivated to improve safety and in fact are pressing for everything to go wireless because this saves them a considerable amount of money. Dr. Louis Slessin, editor of *Microwave News* says the cell phone industry scammed the American Public and that no real research at State Universities, for example, is being done.

"Few people realize that cell phones have never been tested for safety."
Dr. Devra Davis

The really big concern is our children. It's the first time in human history that brain tumors in children are a leading cause of death ages 5 to 15 (www.cdc. gov/nchs/fastats/children.htm). The uniquely vulnerable group of kids less than 20 years of age have shown a fivefold increase in brain tumors. Twelve million dollars paid to senators and congressmen by phone company lobbyists from '94 to '98, with 7M in '96 bought and sold the ability to take control over our EMF exposure. In 1996 congress passed the Telecommunications Act of 1996, essentially pre-empting all state interference. This act said that regardless of peoples' health, the telecommunications companies could put cell towers anywhere to create a nationwide cell tower system. There has been an absolute failure of the FCC to set any standards for safety. The telecommunications companies have been very aggressive at oppressing any control of cell towers, which they hide in clocks and church steeples. Watch *Full Signal,* it is worth it.

Since there is currently no public policy in this area and studies are showing increased cancers associated with vicinity to cell towers, it is time to promote active urgent messages to your legislatures. This is one issue you really don't want to do leave unchecked; one million billion increase in radiation can't be good, even for stockholders.

2. Electric blankets, waterbed heaters and car seat heaters have been found to create cranial stress MAPs and other problems (autoimmune) for some people.

3. Microwaving food strains the human immune system and is thus, a risky technology to use. In my practice, I have found that foods that have been microwaved routinely inhibit previously strong muscles. Over the years people have brought in foods to be tested for sensitivity and on multiple occasions people have brought in the same food cooked both in conventional and microwave ovens. The foods cooked by microwave all created inhibition of strong muscles and there was zero bias as the people that brought in the foods had them labeled A or B and were blind to me. They all commented that it was interesting that the same food provided a totally different level of sensitivity with the microwaved one creating the sensitivity or muscle inhibition.

All foods are chains of carbon. Microwaving food causes these carbon chains to rotate over one billion times per second. This is what generates the heat to cook the food. The problem is that your immune system can't recognize the substance, so in effect it becomes a potential carcinogen. Since we are all already bathed in oceans of chemicals and radiation, why tip the scales of wellness further against yourself?

More information may be found at Dr. Mercola's website, www.mercola.com.

"The FDA classifies fructose as GRAS: Generally Regarded As Safe, which pretty much means nothing and is based on nothing."

Dr. Mercola

(www.mercola.com)

4. Genetically modified organisms (GMO) have been given to us by Monsanto. There is a plethora of information regarding their harm. The best source for

information is the website run by Geoffrey Smith called the Institute for Responsible Technology. You may read his book *Seeds of Deception* , but you absolutely must watch his movie *Genetic Roulette*. Your life and your family's lives depend on this! The potential scope of harm from this technology is truly unprecedented.

You are on your own here as the industry has purposely put its products under the radar avoiding labeling laws. The avoidance of processed foods is a good start since they are in the majority of these products, especially corn and soy. This area is quickly becoming a flashpoint as the latest research[1,2] is showing both shortened life spans and multi-organ system failure in test animals fed GMO food. Get involved with and financially support the Organic Consumers Association. Ron Cummings and his wife Rose are truly "fighting the fight". Their website (www.organicconsumers.org) has a report you can read called "GMO - Myths and Truths - An evidence-based examination of the claims made for the safety and efficacy of genetically modified crops."

"The average American consumes 50 grams of high fructose corn syrup per day. This contains the same level of mercury as getting two amalgam fillings per day."

Sherry Rogers, MD

5. High Fructose Corn Syrup: This is the number one calorie source consumed by the average American and is like consuming fat. A multi-billion dollar boon for the corn industry, high fructose corn syrup is made from genetically modified corn and may be tainted with mercury, arsenic, lead, chloride and heavy metals. Numerous studies have linked fructose, in any form, as a major contributor to insulin resistance and obesity, elevated blood pressure, blood lipids, depletion of vitamins and minerals, heart disease, liver disease, cancer, arthritis and gout. Increased risk of pancreatic cancer was found in a study done by Anthony P. Heaney and colleagues at the David Gaffen School of Medicine, University of California, Los Angeles. (Cancer Res:70(15);6368-76.) Visit Mercola.com to get an incredible picture of this challenge.

6. Ritalin and Adderall: Currently three million children take these drugs for problems in focusing. The consumption of these drugs to treat attention

deficit disorder has increased by twenty fold in the last 30 years. According to Dr. L. Alan Sroufe, a professor emeritus in psychology at the University of Minnesota's Institute of Child Development, it is the child's environment that predicts the development of ADD problems.

"We are medicating millions of children, but long term, the drugs don't work."

L. Alan Sroufe, PhD

"Sadly, few physicians and parents seem to be aware of what we have been learning about the lack of effectiveness of these drugs." The studies show that these drugs are only effective for four to eight weeks. These drugs can have serious side effects including stunting growth and sudden cardiac arrest.

It is an illusion that children's behavioral problems can be cured with drugs. This view prevents us as a society from seeking the more complex solutions that will be necessary. Dr. Sroufe says "Drugs get everyone; politicians, scientists, teachers and parents, off the hook. Everyone, except the children, that is."

With many of these children showing symptoms of anxiety and depression, as well as others showing family stressors, it's time to treat them as individuals. The technologies of PAK™ and FM are well suited to stem this epidemic.

7. Green Tea, White Tea: Be wary of all teas and plants grown in Southeast Asia. The environment there is so toxic that the plants are loaded with lead and mercury, even if they are labeled USDA organic. You ask, "how could this be?" The sad truth is that these wonderful plants may be grown without chemicals, but growing anything in that environment exposes it to heavy metals from the coal-fired plants. The air the tea plants need to survive and grow is poisoning the product from the plant. The air has been fouled and it's getting worse with two new non-scrubbing coal plants opening per day in China. I tracked my own elevated lead and mercury levels to the organic tea I was drinking from China. When the boxes or other containers were put in my energy field or any person's, they weakened the person's muscles at a distance of up to several feet.

"You might want to get your family off the junk drinks, as treating cancer is very expensive compared to preventing it."
Garry Gordon, MD,DO
President, Gordon Research Institute

"It is the environment that controls gene expression. Rather than endorsing the Primacy of DNA, we must acknowledge the Primacy of the Environment!"

FYI— RELATED BOOKS

Antioxidants

- *The Anti-oxidant Miracle—Rejuvenate Your Heart, Strengthen Your Immune System, Maximize Your Brain Power, Reverse the Aging Process*—Lester Packer, PhD
- *Curing the Incurable: Vitamin C, Infectious Diseases and Toxins*–Thomas E Levy, MD, JD
- *Primal Panacea*—Overwhelming documentation proves that in high enough doses this substance prevents and cures cancer, heart disease, infectious and degenerative diseases and even reverse damage from virtually all toxins, venoms, and radiation!—Thomas E Levy, MD, JD

Cardiovascular Disease

- *What Your Doctor May Not Tell You About Heart Disease* – The Revolutionary Book that Reveals the Truth Behind Coronary Illnesses and How You Can Fight Them? - Mark C. Houston, MD,MS
- *Is Your Cardiologist Killing You?* – Sherry A Rogers, MD
- *Dr Gundry's Diet Evolution* – Stephen R Gundry, MD, FACS, FACC
- *The Great Cholesterol Myth – Why Lowering Your Cholesterol Won't Prevent Heart Disease And the Statin-Free Plan That Will*—Johnny Bowden, PhD and Stephen Sinatra, MD.
- *Prevent and Reverse Heart Disease—The Revolutionary, Scientifically Proven Nutrition-Based Cure*—Caldwell B Esselstyn Jr, MD
- *The Nitric Oxide (NO) Solution—How to boost the miracle molecule to prevent and reverse chronic disease*—Nathan Bryan, PhD and Janet Zand, OMD

Cell Phones

- *Disconnect—The Truth About Cell Phone Radiation, What the Industry Has Done to Hide It, and How to Protect Your Family*—Devra Davis, PhD, MPH
- *Cell Phones—Invisible Hazards in the Wireless Age*—Dr. George Carlo and Martin Schram

Diabetes

- *The Blood Sugar Solution—The Ultra-healthy Program for Losing Weight, Preventing Disease and Feeling Great Now!*—Mark Hyman, MD
- *Dr. Neal Barnard's Program for Reversing Diabetes—the Scientifically Proven System for Reversing Diabetes without Drugs*—Neal D. Barnard, MD

Prevention

- *Generations At Risk—Reproductive Health and the Environment*—Ted Schletter, MD, Gina Solomon, MD, Maria Valenti and Annette Huddle
- *Healthy Child Healthy World—Creating a Cleaner, Greener Safer Home* — Christopher Gavigan

Chiropractic Neurology/Mental Health

- *Why Isn't My Brain Working?* - Datis Kharrazian, DHSc,DC,MS
- *Why You Get Sick and How Your Brain Can Fix It* - Richard Barwell, DC
- *What Do You Do When the Medications Don't Work? A Non-Drug Treatment of Dizziness, Migraine Headaches, Fibromyalgia and Other Chronic Conditions* —Michael Johnson, DC, DACNB
- *Pelvic Pain and Organic Dysfunction—The PPOD Syndrome*—James E Brauning, DC
- *Energize Your Brain ... Change Your Life*—Jeffrey Donatello, DC

New Technologies/Breakthroughs

• *Bombshell—Explosive Medical Secrets that Will Redefine Aging*—Suzanne Somers
• *Earthing—The Most Important Health Discovery Ever?* —Steve Sinatra
• *Frequency Specific Microcurrant in Pain Management*—Carolyn R McMakin, MA, DC

Weight Loss/Detoxify

• *Eat to Live—The Amazing Nutrient-Rich Program For Fast And Sustained Weight Loss*—Joel Fuhrman. MD
• *Clean Green and Lean – Get Rid of the Toxins That Make You Fat - Drop the Weight in 30 Days*—Walter Crinnion, ND
• *Detoxify or Die*—Sherry Rogers, MD
• *Eat Fat, Get Thin* - Mark Hyman, MD

Immunity/Energy

• *Super Immunity - The Essential Nutrition Guide for Boosting Your Body's Defenses to Live Longer, Stronger and Disease Free* - Joel Fuhrman, MD
• *Breast Cancer and Iodine*—David M. Dory, MD, PhD
• *Why Do I Still Have Thyroid Symptoms- When My Lab Tests Are Normal?* — Datis Kharrazian, DHSc., DC, MS

GMOs, Politics, Transparency, Health and Healing

• *Altered Genes, Twisted Truth* - Steven M. Drucker
• *A Return to Healing—Radical Health Care Reform and the Future of Medicine*—Len Suputo, MD with Byron Belitsos
• *Foodopoly—The Battle Over the Future of Food and Farming in America*—Wanonah Hauter

Epigenetics, Consciousness and Healing

• *One Mind—How our Individual Mind is Part of a Greater Consciousness and Why It Matters*—Larry Dossey, MD
• *The Genie in Your Genes—Epigenetic Medicine and the New Biology of Intention*— Dawson Church, PhD
• *Facets of a Diamond: Reflections of a Healer* - John Diamond, MD

SOME CDs OF INTEREST

1. www. The Beautiful Truth movie.com

This is a story about a young man whose mother died from breast cancer having used traditional medical therapy. What takes place is an enlightening investigation into alternative cancer therapies.

2. www.foodmatters.tv
A great review of the elephant in the waiting room of mainstream medicine-the fact that nutrition is the answer to a large part of our healthcare issues.

3. Brudzinski—The movie
Stanislau Brudzinski, MD, PhD, was the first in his class at medical school in Poland. He made the astonishing discovery that people with cancer are missing several hundred proteins in their blood. He manufactured the proteins and it increased the five year survival rate from 3% with traditional cancer treatments to 35%. Our National Cancer Institute's response was to steal his patents and give him 400 years of jail time. The Texas Medical Society's was to remove his MD license. Dr. Julian Whitaker helped raise him one million dollars to fight off these insane attacks. This is one you don't want to miss. Available from Whitaker Wellness for $20.00 (800 488-1500).

*4. Cancer, Nutrition and Healing—A Personal Odyssey—*Jerry Brunnetti
A movie about an aggressive form of lymphoma successfully treated with diet and nutrition. Available from www.acresusa.com—(800-355-5313)

5. Full Signal
An eye opening account of the unregulated field of non-ionizing radiation put out by the wireless telecommunications industry.

6. Blue Gold
A thought provoking movie about the world's water supplies. We have been pumping more groundwater than is being recharged for over 30 years. This is unsustainable practice will have to change for the good of our human family.

7. Oil Fracking and its Dangers—How it Affects You
A 27-minute documentary worth watching. Invented by Halliburton, in 2005 the Bush Administration exempted the industry from the Safe Drinking Water Act, allowing them to drill anywhere without a permit. The injection of 500+ toxic chemicals into the ground with 50% of the steel casing failing over the life of the well is a disaster. This is currently going on in 34 states! We already don't have enough water and people and animals are dying!

8. *Genetic Roulette*—This is a production of the Institute for Responsible Technology and Jeffrey M. Smith, author of the world's best selling book on GMOs—Seeds of Deception. This film exposes never-before-seen-evidence and points to genetically engineered foods as a major contributor to rising disease rates in the US population, especially among children. I was extremely disturbed to find out the fact that only GMO based baby formulas (Similac, Gerber, Enfamil Premium and Enfamil ProSobee) are the only ones, along with milk injected with Rbgh, that are approved for the WIC (food stamp) program. Gastrointestinal diseases, allergies, inflammatory diseases and infertility are just some of the problems implicated in humans, pets, livestock and lab animals that eat genetically modified soybeans and corn. The USDA is completely ignoring the roundup problem. Protect yourself and check out: www.nongmoshoppingguide.com.

9. *I AM* —is the story of a successful Hollywood director, Tom Shadyac, (Bruce Almighty, The Nutty Professor, Liar, Liar) who experienced a life threatening head injury and his ensuing journey to try and answer two very basic questions: What's wrong with our world? and What can we do about it? Dan Siegel of the Huffington Post states, "I AM is a true wake up call to the forces of good within each of us to write a new story for the world."

TED.COM

TED stands for Technology, Entertainment and Design. Starting back in the late '70s or early '80s, TED has provided a 15-minute platform per person twice per year—winters in California and summer in Edinburgh, Scotland–to allow people with creative insights a chance to express them to the world. These are all incredible. Below are a few to wet your appetite. What a gift! There are hundreds available to view on line.

1. Jill Bolte Tayler—*My Stroke of Insight*
   Dr. Tayler describes how her experience of a massive stroke involving her left cerebral hemisphere allowed her to experience the personalities of brain hemispherieity. Her insight is to consciously live in the peace of your right brain and only leave it when you have to.

2. Amy Cuddy—*Your Body Language Shapes Who You Are*
   "Tiny tweaks" in posture lead to "big changes". Her research shows that posture changes biochemistry as well as other people's perceptions. Power poses (e.g., standing with hands on hips, legs 45° apart or sitting legs on desk, arms over head) increases testosterone and lowers cortisol. "Don't fake it to make it, fake it till you become it."

3. Dan Barber—*The Fish I Fell in Love With*
   Chef Barber takes you on an insightful trip to the South West corner of Spain. Here the return of the natural estuary system from a failed cattle farm to it's natural state provides a vast cauldron of food from mother nature that is absolutely breathtaking.

Glossary

A.

Acupuncture

5,000 year old practice of promoting the flow of energy (chi) through 12 vessels or meridians. Every two hours the energy changes from one meridian to the next to nourish the related organs and tissues.

Adam's Test

A test used to determine a functional scoliosis from a structural one. If on forward bending, the scoliosis disappears without deformity of the rib cage, the scoliosis is said to be functional. This is noted as a positive Adam's Test. A failure of the ribs to normalize on forward flexion is indicative of a structural scoliosis, with potential for a greater negative impact throughout life.

Adaptogen

A term for natural, plant-derived substances (usually made by them in response to a stressor) that have the ability to increase the body's resistance to stress, trauma and fatigue

Adipocytes

Cells where body fat is stored—contrary to previous belief, body fat stored in the adipocyte is metabolically active, and a component of the neuro-endocrine immune system that produces inflammatory signaling agents (like cytokines IL-1 and TNF-alpha) that may contribute to the origin of heart disease, insulin resistance/Type 2 Diabetes and other chronic illnesses associated with obesity.

Adjustment

The term used to describe a specific thrust used to re-align an area of the body to normalize function. Usually applied to joints, it may also be used for soft tissues. These may be done with varying degrees of force and speed. (The two most common types are a high velocity adjustment [HVLA] or a low force respiratory adjustment.)

ADR

Adverse drug reaction. The Achilles heel of Western medicine, the third leading cause of death for the last 10 years in the U.S. are prescription drugs taken as prescribed. For every dollar used to purchase medication in nursing facilities another $1.33 is spent in healthcare resources to treat an ADR.

Adrenal Glands

Known as our "stress glands." Paired glands that sit atop the kidneys and participate in the production of three types of hormones: glucocorticoids that help regulate blood sugar, mineral corticoids to help balance bodily fluids, and corticosteroids to regulate inflammation and respond to stress. The paraventricular nucleus in the hypothalamus is the central center of these glands.

Aerobic Muscle Test

A term applied to weakening of a muscle upon slow repetitive testing (usually a slow twitch muscle) used to screen for iron insufficiency and or neuro-lymphatic congestion.

Alarm Points

A specific point on each acupuncture meridian that may be used to ascertain an imbalance in the related meridian.

Allostasis

The state of a balanced systemic stress response.

Allostatic Load

The imbalanced systemic stress response leading to wear and tear.

Anaerobic Muscle Test

A term applied to quick repetitive testing of the same muscle used (usually a fast twitch muscle) to screen for pantothenic acid insufficiency. Note: when multiple muscles weaken on both aerobic and anaerobic testing, this indicates an essential fatty acid insufficiency.

Antecedent

A term used to understand the origin of illness. These may be thought of as congenital; inherent like sex or genetics, acquired, or developmental (age). These relate to genomics.

Anterior Subluxation

The forward displacement of a vertebrae, which may occur at any spinal level (except C2). They may affect various physiological functions.

Antioxidants

Vitamins, minerals and phytochemicals that aid the body in removing or quenching free radicals and controlling free-radical production.

Annulus Fibrosus

The outer structure of the inter-vertebral disc that consists of 15 to 25 individual lamellae (or bands) that have alternating 30° fiber angles which hold the center of the disc or nucleus pulposus in place.

Applied Kinesiology (AK)

The original descriptive term used to explain the medical specialty that combines the best tenets of physical medicine and clinical nutrition with energy and environmental medicine — the updated name is Professional Applied Kinesiology (PAK™).

Aspartame

A synthetic sweetener that is a potent neurotoxin and needs to be banished from the food supply.

Associated Points

Points along the spine on the bladder meridian which can correlate with any meridian imbalance. Clinically, they are associated with spinal subluxations.

Atlas

The top cervical vertebra of the spine (also referred to as C1), upon which rests our head (the occipital bone). Below it articulates with the axis. The dens of the axis is a post that extends upwards from the axis that allows a great rotation for the atlas.

Auto-Immune Disease

An epidemic of one hundred fifty plus diseases affecting 23 million Americans, 10 to 1 more woman than men, shown to be caused by one chemical at 1/25,000th the amount considered safe by the EPA.

Autonomic Nervous System

Think of this as your automatic nervous system; it runs on its own. It is made-up of two divisions: the sympathetic and parasympathetic. Superficially, these may be likened to the accelerator and the brakes of your car, respectively. On a deeper level the parasympathetics run the life sustaining cellular activities 24/7 and the sympathetics interrupt them to get us out of danger.

Axis

The second cervical vertebra which sits under the atlas and provides its wide range of rotational motion with its pin, called the dens, around which the atlas rotates.

B.

Bile

The fluid made by the liver, stored in the gallbladder; a mixture containing: 90% cholesterol, phosphatidyl choline (lecithin), taurine and bile salts. This mixture helps to digest and absorb fats and the fat soluble vitamins, A, D, E, F and K.

Bio-Impedance Analysis (BIA)

Developed by NASA for monitoring the health of our astronauts, BIA provides a quick non-invasive measure of key body compartments including: total body water, both intra and extra-cellular, total fat, and body cell mass. It provides a reading known as the phase angle which is a quick indicator of your cell membrane health. Serial BIA readings are extremely useful in monitoring the body's physiological changes to lifestyle changes. It is, therefore, a key tool for creating a personalized health program.

Bis-phenol A

An endocrine disrupting chemical found in the lining of about 2/3 of canned goods and carbonless paper. Another harmful chemical that needs to be taken out of use.

Body Cell Mass

With aging, changes in function are primarily due to alterations in this compartment. This compartment is functionally the most important in determining energy expenditure, protein needs and metabolic response to physiologic stress. Numbers 40 or greater, are good. Less than 40 signifies a need to build muscle.

Butyrate

A short chain fat produced by the action of our intestinal bacteria on the fiber in our diet. It is the preferred fuel of the colonic epithelial cells; it prevents cancer and removes toxic substances from our bodies. It is what gives butter its yellow color, and is why ghee works, used in Ayurvedic medicine for centuries, for body cleansing (panchakarma).

Calcaneal Stress Tolerance Factor

The maximum degree of heel elevation that an individual can tolerate in their footwear prior to global muscle weakness.

Carpal Tunnel

The tunnel made by the two rows of four wrist bones that make up a "u-shaped" tunnel through which the median nerve traverses to give strength to our thumb and first two fingers.

Categories 0,1,2,3

These relate to the pelvic-spinal complex stress MAPs with increasing severity from very little (category 0) to a severe amount (category 3) which involves inter-vertebral disc compression and degeneration. (Refer to Stress MAPs illustrations.)

Cell Membrane

The skin of the cell that is actually its brain. The fluid-like membrane that consists of a bilipid membrane of phosphatidyl choline on the outer and inner cell membrane surfaces with essential fatty acids lying sideways. Built into the membrane are protein switches (receptor & effector) that extend through the membrane and provide awareness of the environment through a physical sensation.

Central Integrative State

The overall function of our central nervous system's ability to maintain conscious coherent activity necessary for higher brain function, such as learning and memorizing. This is the net excitatory or inhibitory state determined by the paraventricular nucleus in the hypothalamus.

Cerebrospinal Fluid (CSF)

The clear liquid made by ultra-filtration of the venous blood in the choroid plexus, secreted in the four hollow areas of the brain known as ventricles. This is pumped by cranial and spinal motion around the brain, down the spinal cord where it exits with the spinal nerves and then goes into the organs the nerves sub-serve. This fluid carries oxygen and glucose to feed the neurons and removes wastes. There is both an outward (prodromic) and inward (antidromic) flow of cerebral spinal fluid.

Cervical Compression Test

A test designed to stress potentially injured areas of the soft tissue of the neck. The patient is seated with the head rotated, the examiner gently compresses the head on the neck to see if pain is elicited.

Cervical Spine

The upper part of the spine formed by the seven neck vertebrae that form a forward curve (cervical lordosis). They allow the exit of the nerves that form the brachial plexus, giving strength to the muscles of the shoulders, arms and hands. They also give rise to the sensory nerves to our head and house the lower brain stem with its various neurological structures associated with coordination of the autonomic nervous system. The top six vertebrae contain openings for the vertebral artery that feeds the middle part of the brain.

Challenge

The manual application of a vector of force into a physiological area while simultaneously testing an intact muscle to see if a change in the nerve outflow occurs, usually resulting in the inhibition of a muscle to fire. It thus provides a reproducible methodology for bridging the conscious and the sub-conscious.

Chelation

From the word "claw" referring to the removal of heavy metals from the body. Abundant published evidence builds a convincing case that toxins like lead and mercury are adversely affecting the outcome of most treatment today for virtually all health problems. There are over 7,000 references on Ethylenediaminetetraacetic acid (EDTA) and lead removal.

Cholesterol

An important sterol (wax) that is a component of our cell's membranes—both outer and inner. A precursor to sex steroids in the ovaries and testes as well as adrenal cortical hormones—80% is converted in the liver into bile salts for the digestion and absorption of fats; another large area of use is the corneum of the skin for protective purposes. Cholesterol in our cell membranes controls the rate of cellular reproduction. Total cholesterol levels below 180 are associated with increased cancers and infections.

Chronobiology

Referring to the science of the circadian rhythms of the body. It is postulated that over one hundred physiological functions depend on these rhythms for their set point. Some of these include: body temperature, clotting, pain perception and blood pressure.

Circadian Rhythm

The 24 hour sleep-wakefulness cycle.

Cobbs Angle

A radiographic measurement of the degree of scoliosis or lateral spinal curvature. Used to define the degree of scoliosis progression. Monitoring a scoliosis is considered to be of low significance if the Cobb's Angle is 20° or less.

Collagen

The most abundant protein built in our bodies and the major component of connective tissue. It occurs in larger amounts than all other proteins put together, and is dependent on adequate Vitamin C for formation. As a fibrous protein, it strengthens the skin, blood vessels, bones, teeth and is the intercellular 'cement' that holds the cells together in various organs and tissues.

Co-morbidities (also known as disease adjacencies)
The web-like effects of aberrant cell signaling that coincide with or arise in conjunction with distortions in intercellular connectivity. For example, increased pro-inflammatory chemical messengers (cytokines) similarly affect the gut, heart and brain.

Compressed Treatment
A term I coined to describe a new treatment paradigm of total body care where full body alignment, muscle balancing and electrical stimulation is done repetitively in a series to quickly reduce stress MAPs. Months and years of accumulated trauma and stress is thereby reduced in short order. Lifestyle counseling (diet, supplements, posture, exercise, etc) is key as well.

Cranial Bones
There are 22 in number and they articulate with each other by a joint known as a suture. Motion of these bones helps pump cerebrospinal fluid to feed and nourish the brain and nervous system, as well as to up-regulate our neuro-endocrine axis. This is the area just behind our eyes where our brain folds in upon itself and becomes our endocrine system. This aids our ability to handle stress, have normal endocrine and immune function, and sleep cycles. Research has also indicated that this mechanism is intimately involved in the control of the tone (strength) of the body's ligaments most likely by an increased intelligence of our electromagnetic field.

Cranial Sacral Respiratory Motion
The synchronous motion of the cranial bones, spine and sacrum due to the dural membrane attachment throughout the system. The physiological system that nourishes the nervous system, removes its waste and delivers chemical messages throughout the body.

Cranial Stress Complex
A term used to describe the adaptation of the cranial bones to stress, resulting in diminished function reflected in alterations of any of the physiological parameters of the neuro-endocrine axis.

Cruciate Suture
The suture at the roof of the mouth, between the two palatine bones.

D.

DHA
Docosahexaenoic acid—the essential fatty acid from cold water fish that
makes up half of the brain's fat.
DHEA
Dihydroepiandrosterone—an adrenal hormone that has a direct input on
healthy immunity and aging.
Diaphrams — 3 Types
1) Oral—the floor of the mouth.
2) Respiratory—the muscle function that fuels the breath and pumps
electricity (chi) through our meridians.
3) Pelvic—the muscular floor that holds our rectum and reproductive organs.
Double Crush Injury
Relates to two areas of compression creating abnormal neurological function.
For example, the nerve to the wrist muscles may be compromised at both
its exit from the neck as well as at the wrist (carpal tunnel). Creates an often
overlooked, but crucial component of structural dysfunction and pain.
Driver's Foot
A term coined by the author to describe the common posterior-medial
misalignment of the heel bone (calcaneus) caused by driving for long periods
of time with the right foot rotated externally instead of straight up.
Dura Mater
Literally, the "tough mother"—our brain sits in a hammock of ligaments that
separates the two cortices, and the cerebellum from the cortex. This dural
structure lines the inside of our cranium and forms a tube that the spinal cord
sits in.

E.

Emergence
How our genes are translated into our health and disease patterns.

Endocrine Disrupter or Endocrine Disrupting Chemical (EDC)
The U.S. Environmental Protection Agency (EPA) has defined this as "an exogenous agent that interferes with the production, release, transport, metabolism, binding, action, or elimination of natural hormones in the body responsible for the maintenance of homeostasis; and the regulation of developmental processes." This definition is not limited to endocrine disrupting effects exclusive of the estrogen system. Rather, endocrine disruption encompasses effects on the endocrine, immune and nervous system, such as: alterations in both male and female reproduction, changes in neuro-endocrinology, behavior, metabolism and obesity, prostate cancer, and thyroid and cardiovascular endocrinology. These consist of pesticides and industrial chemicals that have been released into the environment.

Endocrine System
The glandular system that is intimately connected to our nervous system; secretes chemicals called hormones that are manufactured in one area that travel to other areas where they have a distant physiological effect.

Endothelium
The single cell lining of our vascular system that needs to be protected with nutrients from whole foods to prevent heart disease. Research has shown that one serving of fast foods damages a rat's endothelium for six weeks.

Epigenetic
How our environment shapes our structure and function. Meaning above the gene. Epigenetics can be thought of as the software that directs the genomic hardware of a computer, deciding which genes are expressed. These epigenes that sit on our genes can be readily modified by our environment and this outdates the rigid view that genes cause disease. They act like 'the fine tuning knob on our genetics,' recently found to be transferrable over generations.

Epigenome
The software that runs the show.

Essential Fatty Acids (EFA's)
This refers to the omega 6 and omega 3 fatty acids that can't be made by our body, but need to be consumed daily, in an unadulterated form for health and vitality.

Excitotoxin
A class of chemicals known to excite brain cells to death. There is abundant evidence that these play a large role in neuro-degenerative diseases like,

Parkinson's, Alzheimer's and Amyotrophic Lateral Sclerosis. Common forms of excitotoxins include: glutamate (as in monosodium glutamate, MSG), Nutra Sweet or Equal and aspartate (as used in aspartame).

Exposome
A term used to describe all of the receptors in our body that interface with the environment; this is what picks up "the total load" (e.g., heavy metals, endocrine disruptors, etc.).

F.

Facet Joints
Also known as the pre and post-zygapophyseal joints. These are the gliding, sliding joints at the back part of our vertebrae that help to make the opening, or window, that the nerves exit from the spinal column to the outside.

Facilitation
The normal neurological firing of a nerve leading to muscle action.

Family Health Team (FHT)
A healthcare organization that includes a team of family physicians, nurse practitioners, registered nurses, social workers, dietitians, and other healthcare professionals who work together to provide healthcare for their community.

Fascia
The connective tissue matrix that lies underneath our skin that forms one continuous layer throughout our body.

First Line Therapy
Recommended by our National Institutes of Health (NIH), American Heart Association, American Cancer Society and many others as a "first line" treatment for conditions most doctors see every day. Examples of conditions include: high cholesterol, high blood pressure, high blood sugar/diabetes, heart disease, osteoarthritis, and many others.

Fixation
A group of three vertebrae that are stuck together ostensibly due to the intrinsic inter-vertebral musculature that results in a specific bilateral inhibited muscle pattern.

Four R Program
Refers to a program for gastrointestinal restoration consisting of: remove (pathogens, antigens, toxins), replace (stomach or pancreatic enzymes as

needed), re-innoculate (gut bacteria themselves with probiotics or their fertilizer or prebiotics), and repair (the addition of nutrients to heal the mucosa like: aloe vera polysaccharides, vitamin E, l-glutamine, l-arginine, EPA-DHA, zinc carnosine and pantothenic acid).

Frequency Specific Microcurrent (FSM)
A microcurrent (less than 1 millionth of an ampere) system that increases ATP production (healing energy) by 500%. Useful for a variety of situations including neuro-musculoskeletal pain syndromes. Slam dunks include: shingles (herpes), nerve pain, myofascial pain, concussion, post-op wound healing and pain reduction

Functional Medicine (FM)
A systems-based approach to the prevention and treatment of chronic complex disease.

G.

Gait
Refers to the pattern of cross-crawl motion used in walking. May either refer to this or may also refer to the fact that PAK™ has discovered that each of the six meridians that end on the foot may not fire normally and contribute to specific muscle imbalances.

Gallbladder
The organ under the liver that stores bile to emulsify fats and remove toxins from the body.

Generic
A term applied to a drug that has undergone the seven-year post marketing surveillance period by the FDA. This means it has been proven safe by tens of millions of patients who have taken it over seven years. Considered to be one of the primary requirements for taking a drug by Dr. Micozzi, MD, PhD., the past senior investigator in the Diet and Cancer Program at the National Cancer Institute.

Genomic
Pertaining to the 23 pairs of genes that carry our "book of life". Think of this as our hardware.

Genomic Stability
The ability of our genes to make exact copies of themselves—failure to do so

is the root cause of all disease; referred to as genomic instability. Minerals like iron, magnesium and zinc, and vitamins like B6 and B12 together are capable of enhancing genomic stability.

Golgi Tendon Organ (GTO)

The stretch-activated receptors located at the ends of a muscle that detect tension and fire to prevent damage to the muscle when overloaded.

H.

HBLU

Healing from the Body Level Up (HBLU.org). An innovative healing system developed by Dr. Judith Swack utilizing muscle testing. She's had "slam dunk" results with allergies, asthma, anxiety, PTSD, trauma, depression and phobias, as well as, happy marriages and successful careering.

Heal Helper

A tool invented by the author to measure the maximum amount of heel elevation an individual may tolerate in a shoe (calcaneal stress tolerance) prior to the creation of a global inhibition of muscular function, presumably from spinal cord stretching or tethering.

Heart Rate Variability (HRV)

A reflection of the function of the autonomic nervous system; a measure of the time gap between individual heart beats while your body is at rest. The heart speeds up when you inhale, and slows down when you exhale. The difference is known as the HRV. A healthy, well-rested body will produce a larger gap and higher HRV than a stressed out, over-trained body. Low heart rate variability is predictive of mortality from all causes. It has been shown to be improved with subluxation reduction.

Homeostasis

Neuro-endocrine immune balance

Hormesis

The concept that small things can have unexpectedly large consequences, both good and bad.

HPA Axis

An acronym for the hypothalamic-pituitary-adrenal endocrine relationship that is the core of our stress response; the literal set point involved in over 100 physiological baseline parameters. The HPA axis has been found to be up or down regulated in those suffering from various forms of depression.

Hiatal Hernia

A sliding of the stomach up through the opening in the diaphragm for the esophagus, as a direct result of the tightening of the psoas muscles, secondary to a bilateral sacroiliac sprain (Category II), weak abdominal muscles or a combination thereof. May give the symptoms of gastro-esophageal reflux disease (GERD) (see Appendix: Key Gastrointestinal and Immune Function Areas, p281).

Hippocampus

The area of our brain once believed responsible for memory storage, but more recently understood as a way-station that coordinates storage and retrieval of information.

Holographic Subluxation

A descriptive term used when a bone bends upon itself creating dissonance or direct dysfunction. A common example is the sacrum, which is composed of a fusion of five separate vertebrae. Prolonged sitting, like in an airplane seat, may bend the sacral segments apart, creating inhibition of the pelvic muscles contributing to chronic back pain. Bone is a crystalline emulsion and will bend, to some degree, according to the external forces applied to it.

Hydrochloric Acid (HCL)

The digestive enzyme produced by the stomach. This particular chemical takes six times more energy to make than any other one in the human body; due to the fact that hydrogen and chloride atoms that make it up have to be concentrated 100,000 times to go from a pH of 7.4 (blood) to a pH of 2 (stomach acid).

Hypochlorhydria

The state of not producing enough hydrochloric acid that comes with aging and stress—symptoms are bloating, less than one hour after eating and gas.

Hypothalamus

One of the three components of the neuro-endocrine axis. The hypothalamus links the nervous system to the pituitary gland. It is responsible for neuro-endocrine immune coordination, modulating such mechanisms as body temperature, hunger, thirst, hormone release and autonomic functions.

I.

ICAK

The International College of Applied Kinesiology-the organization of doctors practicing PAK™. There are chapters throughout world: Canada, USA, Europe and AustrailAsia.

Ileocecal

The true sphincter valve that separates the end of the small intestine (distal ileum) from the colon. This valve may become stuck open or closed and create symptoms of toxicity or constipation respectively. (see Appendix: Key Gastrointestinal and Immune Function Areas, p.281).

Ileocolic

The thickening of the lining of the descending colon at the point it enters the pelvic girdle and becomes the sigmoid. May spasm and cause bowel problems or abdominal pain (see Appendix: Key Gastrointestinal and Immune Function Areas, p.281).

Immune Complex

The name given to a white blood cell once it has ingested an undigested food or foreign substance. They create an inflammatory response wherever they settle in the body.

Immune System

The system in our body responsible for monitoring the presence of and eliminating foreign invaders. Half of our immune system is wrapped around the 23 feet of small intestine because in a lifetime 40-60 tons of food will pass through this tubing. Two forms of lymphatic tissue are present to protect us from foreign invaders called the GALT (gut-associated lymphatic tissue) and the MALT (mucous-associated lymphatic tissue).

Immuno-Excitotoxicity

A term coined by Dr. Russell Blaylock to describe the process by which inflammatory immune over-activity drives excitotoxicity, both known to play important roles in all neuro-degenerative diseases, especially Parkinson's disease and Alzheimer's dementia.

Inhibition

Opposite of facilitation or a neurological state in which the action potential is reduced creating no firing, such as a weak muscle or a lack of a neurological response.

Insertion

The point at which a tendon of a muscle is attached to the surface of a bone by rootlets known as Sharpey's Fibers. When a muscle contracts, it moves the insertion towards the origin.

Interferential Therapy (IF)

The superficial application of a medium-frequency, alternating current modulated to produce low frequencies up to 150Hz, it promotes the healing of soft tissue injuries by increasing the blood supply; and thus, simultaneously reducing the pro-inflammatory chemicals while delivering healing nutrients. It is considered more comfortable for the patients than transcutaneous electrical nerve stimulation.

Inter-Vertebral Discs (IVDs)

These are ligamentous shock absorbers that hold the vertebrae apart, and create space for the free flow of information throughout the nervous system. They consist of two parts. There is a central ball bearing called the nucleus pulposus that allows for flexion, extension, lateral bending and rotation. It is under a tremendous amount of pressure and is held in place by 15 to 25 concentric lamellae called the annulus fibrosus. The adult spine elongates by one inch at night as the nucleus pulposus sucks in water and rehydrates.

Intestinal Dysbiosis

An imbalance in the gut bioreactor (biome) consisting of 3 to 5 lbs of thousands of species of bacteria, molds, and viruses which live in a commensal relationship with our body, manufacturing various vitamins and short chain fats that provide crucial functions in our body.

Inter-Professional Education (IPE)

When two or more professions learn with, from and about each other to improve collaboration and the quality of care; recently added by the World Health Organization to its global health agenda.

K.

KISS

Kinematic Imbalances due to Suboccipital Strain—the concept that groups the symptoms and signs associated with functional disorders of the cervical spine into an entity linked to easily recognizable clinical situations. To be used as a tool to improve contact in communication with other caregivers of infants and children to improve the contact between pediatricians and specialists of Manual Therapy in Children (MTC)

Kyphotic

The middle curve of the three spinal curvatures, located in the thoracic spine, whose direction is posterior or towards the back of the body. An increase of this curve, or hyper-kyphosis, is associated with a decreased lung capacity. It is associated with significant increases of all causes of mortality.

L.

Lateral
Meaning towards the outside or outer part of the body.

Leaky Gut (Metabolic Endotoxemia)
A term used to describe a lack of integrity in the small intestine pores that are supposed to open to let digested food in and then close, much like a turn style. A downstream effect of chemicals (e.g., from antibiotics taken medically or in our food supply, non steroidal anti-inflammatory drugs, glyphosate and Bt toxin from GMO, other pesticides and herbicides) which creates a systemic inflammatory response and represents the cornerstone for many diseases.

Lean Muscle Mass
That part of our body that is not fat or water—levels greater than 40 are desirable.

Ligament
A fibrous band of connective tissue that typically surrounds a joint and limits its circumscribed range of motion. When injured there are three degrees of sprain: 1) minor stretch-slight tear 2) moderate stretch-moderate tear 3) frank rupture-surgical intervention.

Liver
The largest organ of our body; the engine that cleans our bloodstream, assembles nutrients into body parts, and helps store vitamins: A, D, B12, iron and blood substances used in coagulation.

Lordotic
The forward curves of the cervical and lumbar spines.

Low–level laser therapy
The superficial application of lasers at wave lengths between 632 and 904 nanometers into the skin in order to produce anti-inflammatory chemicals by electro-magnetic energy to the soft tissues.

Luo Points
Points in the acupuncture system that connect the flow of energy in one meridian to another.

Lymphatic System
A closed system of fluids that arise from fluids entering the tissues from the vascular system. There is twice as much lymph in the body as there is blood. The lymphatic system is propulsed by muscle contraction, and drains back into the vascular tree in the subclavian veins.

M.

Magnesium
"The stress mineral" responsible for 700 of the enzyme functions in the human body. Important for genomic stability, healthy heart and vascular function. The majority of people in today's world are deficient.

Magnesium Stretch Test
A quick functional test developed by the author to screen for a functional magnesium insufficiency. A muscle that is intact becomes inhibited after being stretched; and retested correlates with either a low normal or below normal RBC magnesium test or a low DEXA test.

Mechanoreceptor
The pressure and position-sensitive nerve endings. These are ubiquitous and are imbedded in all of the body's joints, muscles and organs to allow for autonomic nervous system function.

Medial
Meaning towards the midline or middle of the body.

Mediators
The name given to substances that are made in response to body functions.

Mercury
Considered to be the second most toxic element on the planet, after plutonium. Has been continuously used in medicine in a variety of ways to no avail. A known neurotoxin put into the environment by coal burning (fish), used in dental amalgams, and used in manufacturing of all vaccines, or used as a preservative in some.

Metallotheinase
One key enzyme the human body uses to remove heavy metals like lead, mercury, cadmium and arsenic.

Metallothioneins
Proteins composed of about 30% cysteine that are one of the most important

detoxification systems for all species.

Micronutrients

Those nutritional factors essential for our survival and longevity that do not contain calories.

Moist Cold

An exceptional healing modality used to both reduce pain and inflammation, while simultaneously promoting increased vascularity to enhance inflammatory waste removal (lymphatic drainage) and deliver nutrients to promote healing (see Appendix: Correct Use of Moist Cold, p.278).

MSG

Monosodium glutamate—the chemical of choice given to create obese rats and mice for scientific research. It works by destroying the hypothalamus' satiety center. Unknown pregnant mothers consuming foods containing MSG may create gross obesity in their children. Federal law allows food processors to use any name for MSG as long as the amount is less than 99% pure MSG. Masquerading by many names like: natural flavoring, textural vegetable protein and more. It is used in all fast food establishments. It is a known neurotoxin that must be eliminated from our food supply.

MSQ (Medical Symptoms Questionnaire)

A tool to assess the functional stress an individual is currently experiencing with respect to various areas of physiology including: head, eyes, ears, nose, mouth/throat, skin, heart lungs, digestive tract, joints/muscles, weight, energy/activity, mind, emotions and other. A score greater than 50 is cause for concern (see Appendix).

MTC

Manual therapy in children

Murphy's Sign

A simple test to check for gallbladder congestion using palpation. First, the patient lies supine with knees bent to relax the abdominal musculature. Then, the examiner gently probes under the liver in the right upper quadrant to elicit a response which may range from no pain to severe pain. Increased pain is associated with gallbladder dysfunction (e.g., congestion, stones or infection).

Muscle Spindle Cells

The neurological receptors located in the belly of a muscle that provide a continuous stretch signal to the brain. These receptors along with golgi tendon receptors, provide the largest input to the cerebellum, and provide a key non-invasive way to positively affect the brain.

Muscle Test

The isolation and testing of muscles to directly examine a person's nervous system function either locally or systemically. By observing/determining injury or lack of function in a specific muscle is a local use. Systemically, bilateral muscle inhibitions may serve to guide a clinician to an organ or glandular problem. Sometimes referred to in the literature as a manual muscle test (MMT).

Muscle Test Grades

Manual muscle tests are graded on a scale of 1 to 5. Grades 1 and 2 are pathologic with no discernable function, grades 3 and 4 are functionally very weak and weak respectively with grade 5 normal.

N.

Natural Selection

The 'coarse tuning' knob of Mother Nature on our genetics.

Neuro-Endocrine Axis

Our brains fold in upon themselves in the middle of our heads, just behind our eyes and they become the command/control organs of our Endocrine System which consists of our pineal, pituitary gland and hypothalamus. They control our sleep-wakefulness cycles, reproductive cycles, stress response, immunological surveillance and ligamentous tone.

Neuro-Lymphatic Reflex

Areas of lymphatic stasis; they are both muscle and organ specific which when firmly rubbed facilitate the lymphatic drainage for the specific related structures, resulting in improved muscle and organ function.

Neuro-Muscular Spindle

These are specialized nerves in the belly of a muscle that detect change of length and rate of change of length of muscle filaments. They can be manually treated to facilitate or inhibit the muscle's function. These receptors along with golgi tendons are the primary input into the brain.

Neuron

Cells of the nervous system that transmit information by becoming electrically charged.

Neuroscience

The study of the nervous system

Neurovascular Points

Points that exist primarily on the head, thought to be remnants of vascular tissue corresponding to various muscle groups; drawn high and tractioned for a period of time, they increase the vascular supply to the specific muscle.

Nervous System

The body's ultimate super system that controls and coordinates all of the body's functions including the endocrine and immune systems. The brain and spinal column make up the central nervous system or CNS and the peripheral nerves are everything outside of the CNS.

Nervous System—Parasympathetic

The autonomic or self-running nervous system is broken down into two parts for ease of understanding. The parasympathetic part is the let down and relax mode of your nervous system exiting from the cranium and sacrum to provide digestion, respiration, food assimilation and reproduction. In essence, it is this part of the autonomic nervous system that allows the cells to be open, sustaining life, allowing healing to take place.

Nervous System—Sympathetic

The second part of the autonomic nervous system. This system comes directly out of the thoracic spine to promote the acute and chronic responses to stress. This activates the fight or flight response to a threat, and is meant to act in short pulsations. The problem with today's world is that this part of people's nervous systems gets locked in a feed-forward pattern, promoting chronic complex disease.

Neurotransmitters

Chemicals that are used to relay, amplify and modulate signals between a neuron and another cell. They are classified as inhibitory or excitatory. They are made in the central nervous system in the brain. And they are made in the peripheral nervous system in the autonomic ganglia, GI tract, kidney, T-Cells, smooth muscle and organs and adrenal medula.

Nociceptor

Specialized nerve endings that create the sensation of pain when they are stretched.

Nutrarian

A person who chooses their food based on its nutrient density.

Nutrigenomics
How nutrition and phytochemicals 'speak to our genes.' The interface between nutrition and genomics. The science of nutrigenomics is the study of how naturally-occurring chemicals in foods alter molecular expression of genetic information in each individual.

O.

Obesogens
Chemicals that inappropriately alter lipid homeostasis to promote adipogenesis and lipid accumulation; substances that modulate bio-energetics and the conversion of food calories to stored lipids (e.g., pesticides).

Origin
The term used as a point of reference to denote the fixed point at which a muscle is attached to a bone, which when it contracts, pulls the opposite end—the insertion—towards it. Consisting of a group of tendonous fibers called Sharpey's Fibers that insert into the outer shell or periosteum of the bone. These fibers can be torn from the bone, inhibiting the muscle function.

Origin-Insertion Technique
A PAK™ muscle technique used to normalize avulsion injuries at the beginning and end points of a muscle. Deep transverse friction massage is applied to recreate normal muscle function.

Orthomolecular Therapy
The use of "the right molecules" coined by Dr. Linus Pauling and Dr. Abram Hoffer.

P.

Pain
An unpleasant sensory and emotional experience associated with actual or potential tissue damage, or described in terms of such damage (statement from the International Association for the study of pain).

Pelvic-Spinal Complex
A term coined by the author to describe the kinematic chain involving the pelvis and spine for the purpose of clarifying their inherent functional inter-relationships for ease of understanding.

Pelvis

A collection of three bones at the bottom of our spine that forms the foundation of our spine. A triangular bone called the sacrum is wedged between two other bones called innominates (or unnamed because no one could figure out what they looked like). Singly termed ilium; the joint between the two is called the sacroiliac joint (SI). These two joints move gyroscopically in a small figure eight pattern when we walk or run.

Persistent Organic Pollutants (POPs)

These are endocrine-disrupting chemicals associated with the development of the metabolic syndrome and type II diabetes. Pthalates, bisphenol A, PCB's, polybrominated diphenyl ethers, perfluoro-compounds and organotin compounds are some examples.

Phase Angle

A bio-impedance measurement, ranging from 0 to 20 degrees, that is age and sex adjusted. This measurement gives a 'snapshot' of an individual's overall health, with increased angles associated with improved outcomes and vice versa.

Phytochemicals (plant derived chemicals)

A term coined to represent the thousands of plant-sourced compounds that have functional effects in animal tissues; optimal immune function in humans has recently discovered to be dependant on these as well as longevity.

Posture

The upright alignment of a person's body that serves as a direct indicator of brain function.

PPOD Syndrome

Mechanically induced pelvic pain and organ dysfunction syndrome (pronounced 'pea-pod'). The link between compressive injuries to the lumbo-sacral plexus resulting in a wide array of pelvic pain, bladder dysfunction, bowel dysfunction, gyn/sexual dysfunction.

Pthalates (also known as plasticizers)

A class of diverse chemicals that make up plastics; they are virtually inescapable because they are present in everything—foods, toiletries, clothes, cosmetics, medications, devices, home and office construction materials, machines, industrial and auto exhaust, etc. They damage our body by poisoning the peroxisome proliferator activated receptors (PPARS)—in essence they destroy the cellular machinery that controls how we metabolize fats, starches, sugars and proteins and are therefore implicated in obesity, metabolic syndrome X, diabetes, cancer, atherosclerosis and joint pain. Carcinogenic substances from plastics that are 10,000 more present by molecular weight than any other carcinogen today. They mimic estrogen, act as environmental endocrine disrupters, deplete body stores of zinc and need to be sweated out (as in a Far InfraRed Sauna) to be removed.

Professional Applied Kinesiology (PAK™)

Over 100 muscle testing approaches have evolved. Since the term Applied Kinesiology had been in general use for a long time, the International College of Applied Kinesiology, USA Chapter, created this term to differentiate the official professional application endorsed by the founder, Dr. George Goodheart.

Pronation

To turn or rotate inwards towards the midline of the body.

R.

Respiratory Adjustment

A painless, non-forceful method of body realignment that utilizes inspiration coupled with manual correction to accomplish the task. This is very subtle and relaxing while at the same time effective and painless.

Risk to Benefit Ratio

The considerations one must make before considering the appropriateness of a therapy. For example, are the possible side effects of a medication worse than the condition itself?

S.

Sacroiliac Joint

A diarthrodial joint with hyaline cartilage on the sacral side and fibro cartilage on the iliac side. It has numerous ridges and depressions indicative of its function for stability more than motion.

Sacroiliac Sprain/Strain

The two sacroiliac joints move in a small gyroscopic figure "8" during the normal walking gait. Superimposed on this motion, which is termed rotation and counter-rotation, is flexion and extension. Injury to the sacroiliac ligaments (sacroiliac sprain) creates up-stream affects due to a loss of any one, or a combination, of the following functions. The top of the sacrum is known as the sacral base due to its function as the foundation for the entire spine, so once the sacral base becomes unlevel, the entire spine above it is affected. For ease of understanding, we will discuss them individually even though in reality a combined effect takes place. The most common occurrence is that of a bilateral sacroiliac sprain/strain. Typically, the right sacroiliac joint is rotated back, and the left forward. This creates a low sacral base on the right with a chain of upstream compensatory changes above it.

Sclerotome

The pattern of referred pain from a ligament/joint that is sprained or injured.

Scoliosis

Any lateral curvature of the spine; a scoliosis may be "functional" which means it straightens on forward bending without any rib cage deformity, this is not considered to be of any consequence or functional. When there is deformity of the rib cage that does not go away with forward bending it is called a "structural" scoliosis. It is considered to be serious due to the fact that this is more likely to effect cardio-pulmonary function.

Second Brain

The term applied to the small intestine for the following reasons: the nerve plexus inside the small intestine (the enteric nervous system) has 100 million neurons, equal to the number in the spinal column. It is only connected to the central nervous system by one to two thousand of those 100 million neurons. It is very capable of its own reflexogenic activity.

Shock Absorber Test

The term in PAK™ used to describe an intact muscle becoming inhibited while a non-related joint is simultaneously percussed. This is used to screen for potential trace mineral insufficiencies (e.g., zinc, copper and manganese) linked to ligamentous instability.

Skin Receptors

In the symphony that is human movement, the conductor is made of stretch reflexes in the skin over the muscle, which fire when the skin is stretched allowing the underlying muscle to hear the message (through a local spinal cord pathway) telling the team "we're moving, and you relax." When abrasion occurs, it disorganizes the communication and creates a feed-forward muscle inhibition that needs to be manually corrected by moving the skin in all directions of the muscle to reset it.

Small Intestine

The 23 feet of tubing from the stomach to the large intestine (named the duodenum, jejunum and ileum from proximal to distal). If spread out, consists of one tennis court of absorptive surface area, having 70%-80% of the entire immune system intrinsically connected to it. Responsible for 50% of the body's detoxification—now called the second brain.

Soft Tissue Injury Clinics (STICs)

The organized team approach to the diagnosis and treatment of soft tissue injuries consisting of chiropractic, deep muscle therapy, acupuncture, First Line Therapy and functional medicine.

Spinal Dysarthrias

A term synonymous with subluxation, or vertebral subluxation complex, to denote an altered physiological state of a vertebral motor segment.

Spinal Stenosis

This refers to a decreased width in the diameter of the canal inside the spine that the spinal cord is in. It usually occurs in the lumbar spine secondary to degenerative changes in the spinal tissues. If it is caused by soft tissue (bulging discs) this is amenable to conservative treatment (traction, adjustment, core body building). If due to boney encroachment (vertebral lipping, spurring) surgery may be indicated.

Spine

Also called the spinal or vertebral column. Part of the central nervous system (neuro) axis of the body. The organ consisting of 24 vertebrae connected by inter-vertebral discs and longitudinal ligaments that has three curves and that make it a spring-loaded organ giving it 16 times more strength and stability.

Spondylogenic reflex syndrome (SRS)

Empirical clinical observations have shown relationships between the axial skeleton and the peripheral soft tissues. Mediated through the reflexogenic pathway of the central nervous system, the SRS is the reproducible, causative relationship between the reciprocal functionally abnormal position (segmented dysfunction) of skeleton parts of the axial skeleton and the local, anatomically determined non–inflammatory rheumatic soft tissue changes.

Spondylolisthesis

A bilateral pars interarticularis defect with forward translation of one vertebra on the next below it. Graded on the percentage of a forward slippage of one vertebral body on the vertebral body below it.

Spondylolysis

A defect in the pars interarticularis, most commonly affecting the fifth and fourth lumbar vertebrae due to a fatigue or stress fracture.

Sprain

A stretch and/or tear of a ligament (a band of fibrous tissue that connects two or more bones at a joint).

Strain

An injury to either a muscle or a tendon (fibrous cords of tissue that connect muscle to bone).

Sprain-Strain Severity Grade

In general, a Grade I or mild sprain/strain is caused by over-stretching or slight tearing of the ligament/muscle/tendon with no instability, and a person with a mild sprain usually experiences minimal pain, swelling, and little or no loss of functional ability. Although the injured muscle is tender and painful, it has normal strength. A Grade II sprain/strain is caused by incomplete tearing of the ligament/muscle/tendon and is characterized by bruising, moderate pain, and swelling. A Grade III sprain/strain means complete tear or rupture of a ligament/muscle/tendon.

Stress Receptor

Specific areas of fascial contraction on the head, sacrum, hands and feet that relate to specific muscles throughout the body. One may consider them to be like a "circuit breaker" that inhibits normal muscle function.

Subluxation

A term used by the chiropractic profession to designate misaligned vertebrae.

Supination

To turn or rotate outwards away from the midline of the body.

Surrogate Testing

A unique testing pattern to PAK™ where the nervous system of one person is utilized to evaluate/test the nervous system of another. It is only used for special circumstances where either a person is too young or incapacitated to use their own muscles volitionally.

Systems Biology

The approach that seeks to understand how biological circuits involving genes and metabolic pathways interact to regulate biological activities in normal and pathological states.

T.

Tarsal Tunnel

Each foot has 26 bones that make up three arches: the medial and lateral longitudinal arches and the metatarsal arch. Just medial to the heel bone (calcaneus) is a fibro-osseous tunnel, the tarsal tunnel, through which passes the tibial nerve, two terminal branches and their corresponding arteries and veins (see Appendix: Understanding the Tarsal Tunnel Complex and Tarsal Complex Stress MAPs, p.250-252).

Tarsal Tunnel Syndrome

When the heel bone (calcaneus) is sprained posteriorly this compresses the posterior tibial nerve where it passes on the inner side of the heel bone on its way to innervate the four layers of plantar muscles. This may result in heel pain, medial arch/foot pain or lateral foot pain (see Appendix: Understanding the Tarsal Tunnel Complex and Tarsal Complex Stress MAPs, p.250-252).

Therapy Localization

The term used to describe the change in a muscle's state when a person simultaneously touches an area of their body. Used in PAK™ to determine areas of dysfunction.

Tinel's Test

An orthopedic test designed to elicit nerve compression symptoms at the wrist with forced extension.

Total Body Fat

The measure of fat in a person. The range is sex adjusted with the normal range for a man (15%-20%), and a woman (20%-25%). We know that excess fat mass is associated with heart disease, stroke, diabetes, cancer, osteoarthritis, sleep apnea, gout, infection, gall stones, and many other conditions. Job performance, mobility and appearance are also affected.

Total Body Water

The average range is 55%-65%. Proper hydration is very important. Checking athletes before playing may save many lives. The total body water may be divided into intra-cellular and extra-cellular compartments. An elevated extra-cellular water is suggestive of a toxic state.

Total Load

The sum total in the body of toxins from the environment (exotoxins) and from bacterial action in the gut (endotoxins).

Triggers
Anything that initiates an acute illness or the emergence of symptoms.

V.

Vertebra
Bone located in the spine. The human spine is composed of 24 vertebrae: 7 in the neck (cervical spine), 12 in the mid-back (thoracic spine), and 5 in the low back (lumbar spine). Each vertebra (except the atlas) has a body, two transverse processes, and a spinous process (see Appendix: Normal Vertebral Complex, p.249).

Vertebral Subluxation Complex
A term applied to the resulting altered physiology from vertebral misalignment including: altered motion (pathomechanics), tissue changes (histopathology), muscle changes (myopathology), and altered nervous system function (pathophysiology).

Web of Wellness
The eight underlying fundamental biological processes which form a web, which implies that each part affects every other part. These include: body-mind (attitude or spirit), alignment, diet, digestive, liver detoxification, immune, endocrine, cellular communication and oxidative reduction balance.

X.

Xenobiotics
Foreign chemicals that may mimic the body's hormones, blocking receptors and altering normal physiology.

References—Introduction—Healthy Stories

1. Nimgade, Ashok MD, et al. (2010) Increased Expenditures for Other Health Conditions After an Incident of Low Back Pain, *Spine*; 35:769-777.
2. Provinciali, L. et al. (1996) Multimodel treatment to prevent the late whiplash syndrome. *Scandinavian Journal of Rehab Medicine*; 28:105-111.
3. Hass, M. et al. (2004) Dose-response for chiropractic care of chronic low back pain. *Spine* ; 4: 574-583.
4. Song Xing Hug, et al. (2007, May 14) A preliminary study of neck-stomach syndrome. *World Journal of Gastroenterology* ;13 (18): 2575-2580.
5. National Safety Council, *Injury Facts,* (2011 ed.),p.10.
6. Ibid, p.31.
7. Ibid, p.2
8. Norris S, et al. (1983, Nov) The prognosis of neck injuries resulting from rear-end vehicle collisions. *Journal of Bone and Joint Surgery* (British), vol 65-B, no. 5
9. Berglund, Anita et al. (2001, Aug) The association between exposure to a rear-end collision and future health complaints. *Journal of Clinical Epidemiology,* 54; 851-856.
10. Squires B, et al. (1996, Nov) Soft-tissue Injuries of the Cervical Spine, 15-year follow up, *Journal of Bone and Joint Surgery* (British), vol 78-B, no 6, pp. 955-7.
11. Ibid, p.65
12. Ibid, p.4
13. Langevin HM. (2006) "Connective tissue: a body-wise signaling network?" *Medical Hypothesis* :66(6):1074-1077.
14. Veljkovic M., Dopsaj V., Stringer WW., et al. (2010) "Aerobic exercise training as a potential source of natural antibodies protective against human immunodeficiency virus-1. *Scandinavian Journal Medical Science Sports,* 20:469-74.
15. Suhr F., Rosenwick C., Vasiliadis A., et al. (2010) "Regulation of extracellular matrix compounds involved in angiogenic processes in short and long-track elite runners. *Scandinavian Journal Medical Science Sports,* 20:441-8.
16. Banes AJ, Lee G, Graff R, et al. (2001) "Mechanical forces and signaling in connective tissue cells: cellular mechanisms of detection, transduction, and responses to mechanical deformation. *Current Opinion Orthopedics,* ;12:389-96

17. Langevin, HM., Bouffard, NA., Badger, GJ, et al. (2005) "Dynamic fibroblast cytoskeletal response to subcutaneous tissue stretch ex vivo and in vivo." *American Journal of Physiology Cell Physiology*; 288: C747-56.

18. Hammer, W. (2010, Aug,12) "The Science Behind the Laying on of Hands," *Dynamic Chiropractic*, Vol28, Issue 17.

19. Gant, Charles MD, PhD. (2008) Drug Free Solutions to Mental Health Disorder: Treating Mental Health Disorders Through Nutrition, Mindfulness, and Detoxification, p.29.

20. Yoshimizu, Nabuhiro MD,PhD. (2009) *The Fourth Treatment for Medical Refugees, Richway International*, p.65.

21. Roof, N. (2010) Editorial for Kosmos, *The Journal for World Citizens:* Creating the New Civilization, Spring-Summer.

22. Korten, D. (2010, November) *Agenda for a New Economy—From Phantom Wealth to Real Wealth*, p.104.

References: Chapter 1

1. Crinnion, Walter ND. (2010) *Clean, Green and Lean*, p. 20.

2. Shabecoff, Philip and Alice. (2010) *Poisoned for Profit—How Toxins are Making Our Children Chronically Ill*, p.40.

3. Lim L, et al. (April 2009) "Chronic Exposure to the Herbicide, Atrazine Causes Mitochondrial Dysfunction and Insulin Resistance: PLOS ONE: 4(4), 5186.

4. Nakazawa, DJ. (2008) *The Autoimmune Epidemic*, pp. 70,150.

5. IBID, p194.

6. Shabecoff, Philip and Alice.(2010) *Poisoned for Profit—How Toxins are Making Our Children Chronically Ill*, p35.

7. Broussard, CS., et al. (2011, April) Maternal treatment with opiod analgesics and risk for birth defects, *American Journal of OB GYN*, ;204 (4).

8. Shabecoff, Philip and Alice. (2010) *Poisoned for Profit—How Toxins are Making Our Children Chronically Ill*, p 21.

9. Li De-Kun, et al. (2012, July 27) A Prospective Study of In-utero Exposure to Magnetic Fields and the Risk of Childhood Obesity; *Scientific Reports*, e-pub.

10. Brown, Lester. (2011) *World on the Edge*, p 186.

11. Slaughter, Anne-Marie, Director of Policy Planning, *US Dept of State* 2009-11; preface to the report, p2.

12. Marvasti, Farshad Fani M.D.,M.P.H. et al. (2012) *New England Journal of Medicine:* 367: pp 889-891.

13. Life Extension Foundation (2010). FDA , *Failure, Deception and Abuse— The Story of an Out-of -Control Government Agency and What it Means for Your Health,* p X.

14. CD reference—CCHR.org (Citizens Commission on Human Rights)

15. http:/www.rd.com/your-america-inspiring-people-and-stories/lobbyings-long-arm/Article108833.ht

16. Davis K., Schoen C., Stremikis K. (2010 Update) *Mirror, Mirror on the Wall —How the Performance of the U.S. Health Care System Compares Internationally,* the Commonwealth Fund.

17. Lessig L. (2010, Spring) "Institutional Corruption: When Purpose and Trust are Misplaced." *Kosmos.*

18. Holman, H. MD. (2010, June) *Functional Medicine Update.*

19. Wright, J.MD, Lenard, L, PhD.(2001, August 20) *Why Stomach Acid is Good for You,* p31.

20. www.kaiseredu.org (topics)

21. www.stanford.wellsphere.com/aging-senior-health-article/RX-costs/707895

22. IBID

23. Reyes, AJ. (1983) Pathogenesis of arrhythmogenic changes due to magnesium depletion, *SA Medical Journal,* 311-312.

24. Eisenberg, M J. (1992) Magnesium deficiency and sudden death; *American Heart Journal,*124;2: 544-49.

25. Rasmusson, H. S., (1989) Clinical intervention studies on magnesium in myocardial infarction; *Magnesium,*8:316-25.

26. Canon, L A et al.(1987) Magnesium levels in cardiac arrest victims: relationship between magnesium levels and successful resuscitation; *Annals of Emergency Medicine,* 16, 532

27. Almonznino, Sarafiam, D. et al. (2007) Magnesium and C-Reactive protein in heart failure: and anti– inflammatory effect of magnesium administration? *European Journal of Nutrition;* 46:230-37.

28. Hoyes, J V. (July 1994) Effect of Magnesium sulfate on the ventricular rate control in atrial fibrillation. *Annals of Emergency Medicine,* 24; 1: 61-64.

29. Gottlieb, SS. (1994, May) I V Magnesium: a cost effective anti-arrhythmia; *Emergency Medicine* :53.

30. Gullestad, Al, et al., (1993) The effect of magnesium versus verapramil on superventricular arrythmias. *Clinical Cardiology*: 16: 429-434.

31. Nielson, F. H., (2007) Dietary magnesium deficiency induces heart rhythm changes, impairs glucose tolerance and decreases serum cholesterol in post menopausal women. *Journal of American College of Nutrition*, 26;2:121-132.

32. Morgan, KJ et al.(1985) Magnesium and Calcium Dietary Intakes of the US Population. *Journal of American College of Nutrition*. 1895; 4: 195-206.

33. Clark, Michael R.: (2010, February) "Health After 50." *Johns Hopkins Medical Letter.*

34. Robinovitch, Stephen PhD et al.(2013, Jan 5) Video capture of the circumstances of falls in elderly people residing in long-term care: an observational study. *The Lancet*; vol.381; issue 9860, p47-54.

35. Leveille, SG. et al. (2009) Chronic musculoskeletal pain and the occurrence of falls in an older population. *JAMA*, 302 (2) 2214-2221.

36. Schieppati, M et al. (2003,October) Neck muscle fatigue affects postural control in man. *Neuroscience*, Vol 121, Issue 2, pp. 277-285.

37. Galm, R., et al. (1998) Vertigo in patients with cervical spine dysfunction. *European Spine Journal*, number 7, pp.55-58.

38. Giles, Linton G F., et al. (2003, July 15) Chronic Spinal Pain: A Randomized Clinical Trial Comparing Medication, Acupuncture and Spinal Manipulation. *Spine*, 28 (14):1490-1502.

39. Muller, Reinhold ,et al. (2005, Jan) Long-Term Follow-up of a Randomized Clinical Trail Assessing the Efficacy of Medication, Acupuncture and Spinal Manipulation for Chronic Mechanical Spine Pain Syndromes, *JMPT*. Journal manipulation and physical therapy, vol28, number 1.

40. Seaman, David. (2011,June 6) Pain– Basic Mechanisms. *International College of Applied Kinesiology Proceedings.*

41. Macfarlane, Gary et al. (2011, September 22) Widespread body pain and mortality: a prospective population based study. *British Medical Journal BMJ* 323:66s.

42. Kivoja, J., et al. (2001, July) Chemokines and their receptors in Whiplash injury:Elevated RANTES and CCR-5; *Journal of Clinical Immunology*; 21(4):272-7.

43. Kivoja, J., et al. (2001,October) Systemic Immune Response in Whiplash injury and ankle sprain; elevated IL-6 and IL-10; *Journal of Clinical Immunology*;101 (1):106-112.

44. Takeda, N., et al. (2010, July) Circadian clock and vascular disease. *Hypertension Research* :33 (7):645-651.

45. Robera, R., et al. (2008,January) Melatonin—insulin interactions in patients with metabolic syndrome. *Journal of Pineal Research*; 44 (1): 52-56.

46. Bron, R., et al. (2009, October) Rhythm of digestion: keeping time in the gastrointestinal tract. *Clinical Experiments in Pharmacology and Physiology*, 36 (10): 1041-1048.

47. Lewy, A J. (2009,December) Circadian misalignment in mood disturbances. *Current Psychiatry Reports*, 11 (6): 459-465.

48. Tatsuhiko, Kupo et al. (2006, September 15) Prospective cohort study of the risk of prostate cancer among rotating shift workers: findings from the Japan collaborative cohort study. *American Journal of Epidemiology* ;164(6): 549-555.

49. Blask, D. E., et al. (2009, December) Circadian stage-dependent inhibition of human breast cancer metabolism and growth by the nocturnal melatonin signal: consequences of its disruption by light at night in rats and women. *International Cancer Therapy*; 8 (4): 347-353.

50. Peres, SMP, et al., (2001, December) Hypothalamic involvement in chronic migraine. *Journal of Neurosurgery and Psychiatry* ; 71 (6): 747-751.

51. Garstand, Susan B., et al. (2006, November) "Osteoarthritis: Epidemiology Risk Factors and Pathophysiology" *American Journal of Physical Medicine and Rehabilitation*; Vol 85, No11, pp. S2-S11.

52. National Safety Council- 2011, *Injury Facts*

53. *British Journal of Bone and Joint Surgery*, (Nov 1996) "Soft Tissue Injuries of the Cervical Spine 15 Year Follow up", Vol 78-B, No 6: pp955-7, 535

54. Ingrid, Sitte, et al. (2009, January 15) Intervertebral Disc Cell Death in the Porcine and Human Injured Cervical Spine After Trauma: A Histological and Ultrasound Study. *Spine*, Vol 34: issue 2: pp131-140.

55. Bogduk, N., et al. *The Pathomechanics of Back Pain*. p.63.

56. IBID

57. Jones, David, et al. *The Textbook of Functional Medicine*. The Core Clinical Imbalances p.9.

58. www.chinapost.com.tw/health/allergien/... /allergies-cost.htm.

59. Greenberg, Paul, et al. (2003,December) The Economic Burden of Depression in the United States: How Did It Change Between 1990 and 2000?, *Journal of Clinical Psychiatry* 64:12,p.1465.

60. Farzaneh - For Ramin, et al. (2010,January 20) Association of Marine Omega 3 Fatty Acid Levels With Telomeric Aging in Patients with Coronary Heart Disease, *JAMA*, Vol 303, no 3.

61. Xu Qun, et al. (2009, June) Multivitamin use and telomere length in women. *American Journal of Clinical Nutrition*; vol 89, No 6, 1857-1863, pp1857-1863.

62. Espel, Elissa S., et al. (2004,December 7) Accelerated telomere shortening in response to life stress. *Proceeding of the National Academy of Sciences of the United States of America. (PNAS)* vol 101, no 49,17312-17315.

63. Janda, David H, MD. (2003) *The Awakening of the Surgeon, (A Family Guide to Preventing Sports Injuries and Death.)*

64. www.macinac.org

Chapter II - Functional Medicine References

1. Jones, David, et al. (2005) What is Functional Medicine? *The Textbook of Functional Medicine*; p5.

2. Scharz, B., et al. (1999) Intestinal ischemic repurfusion syndrome: pathophysiology, clinical significance, therapy: *Weinklin Wochenschr* ; 111 (14); 539-48.

3. Fasano, Alessio, et al. (2008, November) The Auto-immune process can be arrested if the interplay between genes and environmental triggers is prevented by re-establishing intestinal barrier competency. *American Journal of Clinical Pathology* :173(5); p.1243-52.

4. Maes, M., et al. (2007) "Increased serum IGA and IGM against LPS of enterobacteria in chronic fatigue syndrome (CFS): Indication for the involvement of gram negative intestinal permeability". *Journal of Affective Disorders* :99;237-240.

5. Cani, Patrice, et al. (2007) "Metabolic Endotoxemia Initiates Obesity and Insulin Resistance" *Diabetes* ;56:1761-1762.

6. Felton, C. V. et al. (1994) "Dietary polyunsaturated fatty acids and compositions of human aortic plaque" *Lancet*, 344:1195-1196.

7. Peskin, Brian, et al. (2008, January 1) *The Hidden Story of Cancers*. p277. Houston, Texas: Pinnacle Press.

8. Vasquez, Alex. (2009, September 1) *Chiropractic and Naturopathic Mastery of Common Clinical Disorders— Concepts, Perspectives, Algorithms and*

Protocols, p80. Austin, Texas: Functional Integrated Medicine for Chronic Hypertension.

9. Baker, Sidney (2003, August 27) *Detoxification and Healing—the Key to Optimal Health*; p71. New York, NY: McGraw-Hill

10. *Human Genetics*, (2008, May);123(4):321-32

11. Bland, J. S., et al. (1995; November 1) *Alternative Therapies for Health and Medicine*. 1 (5); p62-71

12. Lerman, RH., et al. (2008, November 9) Enhancement of a modified Mediterranean-style, low glycemic load diet with specific phytochemicals improves cardiometabolic risk factors in subjects with metabolic syndrome and hypercholesterolemia in a randomized trial. *Nutrition and Metabolism.*

13. Lerman, RH., et al.(2010) Subjects with elevated LDL cholesterol and metabolic syndrome benefit from supplementation with soy protein, phytosterols, hops rho iso-alpha acids and acacia milotica proanthocyanidins. *Journal of Clinical Lipidology* 4, p.59-68.

14. Lerman, Robert M.D., PhD, et al. (2006) Double—Blind, Placebo—Controlled Trial Examining the Effects of TIAA/Acacia Supplementation on Insulin Homeostasis. *Functional Medical Research Center.*

15. Patterson, C et al. (1991,September) Natural Skeletal levels of lead in Homo Sapiens, sapiens uncontaminated by technological lead. *Science of the Total Environment*; 107:205-236.

16. Weisskopf, M. G., et al.(2009) A prospective study of bone lead concentration and death from all causes, cardiovascular diseases, and cancer in Department of Veterans Affairs Normative Aging Study. *Circulation*; 120:1056-1064.

17. Valera B, et al. (2009) Environmental mercury exposure and blood pressure among Nunavik Inuit adults. *Hypertension*; 54:981-86.

18. Gardnor, et al., (2009) Mercury induces an unopposed inflammatory response human peripheral mononuclear cell in utero. *Environmental Health Prospective*,117:1932-38.

19. Galland, Leo MD., et al. (2006,July) Patient-Centered Care: Antecedents, Triggers and Modulators; Chap 8, *Textbook of Functional Medicine*, p 87. Gig Harbor, Washington: Institute for Functional Medicine.

Chapter III References—Professional Applied Kinesiology - PAK™

1. Rosner, Anthony L PhD, Cuthbert, Scott DC. *Technique Summary: Applied Kinesiology.* www.chiroaccess.com/articles/technique-summary-applied-kinesiology.pc

2. ICAK—USA and ICAK - international websites: AK Research Compendium. Dr. Scott Cuthbert; www.icak.com/college/research/publishedarticles.shtml.

3. Kendall, FP and Kendall, (1950) *Muscles—Testing and Function.*

4. Dvorak, Jiri, et al. (1990) Manual Medicine Diagnostics, *Georg Thieme Verlag* , p42.

5. Winsor, Henry MD. (1921,November) Sympathetic Segmental Disturbances—The Evidences of the Association, in Dissected Cadavers, of Viseral Disease with Vertebral Deformities of the Same Sympathetic Segments. *Medical Times*, pp. 1-7.

6. Wannamothee, S Goya, et al. (2006) Height Loss in Older Men—Associations with Total Mortality and Incidence of Cardiovascular Disease. *Archives of Internal Medicine* ;166: 2546-2552.

7. Martin, Michael, et al. (2002,August) Pathophysiology of lumbar disc degeneration: a review of the literature. *Neurosurgery Focus* ,13 (2).

8. Manchi, Kanti, Laxmaiah, et al. (2004, May 28) Prevalence of facet joint pain in chronic spinal pain of cervical, thoracic and lumbar regions. *Bio Medical Central Musculoskeletal Disorders*, Vol 5.

9. Langevin, Helen. (2006, June) Connective tissue: A body wide signaling network?: *Medical Hypothesis*; Vol 66, Issue 6, pp 1074-1077.

10. Pert, Candace MD. (2004, September) *Your Body Is Your Subconscious Mind.*

11. Zhang, J et al.(2006) Effect of chiropractic care on heart rate variability and pain in a multisite clinical study. *Journal of Manipulative Physiologic Therapeutics.* 29 (4): 267.

12. Dekker, JM, et al. (1997) Heart rate variability from short electrocardiographic recordings predicts mortality from all causes in middle-aged and elderly men. *American Journal of Epidemiology* ; 145 (10):899

13. Shoemaker, Richie MD.(2010) Surviving Mold—*Life in the Era of Dangerous Buildings*; p. XI.

14. Schmitt, WH Jr, Leisman G., (1998, December) Correlation of applied kinesiology muscle testing findings with serum immunoglobulin levels for

food allergies. *International Journal of Neuroscience* ;96 (3-4):237-44v.

15. Melillo, Robert. (2010, January 5) Disconnected kids - *Th e Ground Breaking Brain Balance Program for Children with Autism, ADHD, Dyslexia and other Neurological Disorders:* p230.

16. Jin, L, Qi M, Chen DZ, et al. (1999) Indole-3-carbinol prevents cervical cancer in human papilloma virus type 16 (HPV16) transgenic mice. *Cancer Research* ;59:3991-3997.

17. Bell MC, Crowley-Nowick P, Bradlow HL, et al.(2000) Placebo-controlled trial of indole-3-carbinol in the treatment of CIN. *Gynecologic Oncology* ; 78:123-129.

18. Bradfield C A, Bjeldanes LF. (1987) High–performance liquid chromatographic analysis of anticarcinogenic indoles in Brassica oleracea. *Journal of A griculture and Food Chemistry* ; 35:46-49.

19. van Niekerk ,W A. (1966) Cervical cytological abnormalities caused by folic acid deficiency. *Acta Cytologica* ; 10:67-73

20. Agarwal S, Mali S, Kishore N, (1976) Cervical cytology in folic acid deficiency of pregnancy. *Journal Obstetrics and Gynecology*, India ; 25 : 258-261, 541

21. Kitay DZ, Wentz WB. (1969) Cervical cytological abnormalities caused by folic acid deficiency. *American Journal Obstetrics and Gynecology* ; 104:931-938.

22. Whitehead N, Reyner F, Lindenbaum J. (1973) Megaloblastic changes in cervical epithelium: association with oral contraceptive therapy and reversal with folic acid. *JAMA* ; 226: 1421-1424.

23. Lindenbaum J, Whitehead N, Reyner F. (1975) Oral contraceptive hormones, folate metabolism, and the cervical epithelium. *American Journal of Clinical Nutrition* ;28:346-353

24. Butterworth CE Jr, Hatch KD, Macaluso M, et al. (1992) Folate deficiency and cervical dysplasia. *JAMA* ; 267:528-533.

25. Ahn WS, Yoo J, Huh SW, et al. (2003) Protective effects of green tea extracts (polyphenon E and EGCG) on human cervical lesions. *European Journal of Cancer Prevention* ;12:383-390

26. Romney SL, Palan PR, Duttagupta, C, et al. (1981) Retinoids and the prevention of cervical dysplasias. *American Journal of Obstetrics and Gynecology*;141: 890-894

27. Wylie-Rosett JA, Romney SL, Slagle NS, et al. (1984) Influence of vitamin A

on cervical dysplasia and carcinoma in situ. *Nutrition and Cancer* ; 6 (1): 49-57

28. Dawson EB, Nosobitch JT, Hannigan EV.(1984) Serum vitamin A and selenium changes in cervical dysplasia. *Federation Proceedings*; 42:612.

29. Harris RWC, Forman D, Doll R, et al. (1986) Cancer of the cervix uteri and vitamin A. *British Journal of Cancer* ;53:653-359. 542

30. Yehuda S, Carasso RL. (1993) Modulation of learning pain thresholds, and thermo- regulation in the rat: determination of the optimal omega 3 to omega 6 ratio. *Proceedings of National Academy of Science USA* ;90: p10345–10349.

31. Yehuda S., Brandys Y., Blumenfeld A, Mostofsky DI. (1996, September) Essential fatty acid preparation reduces cholesterol and fatty acids in rat cortex. *International Journal of Neuroscience*. 86 (3-4), p249-56.

32. Papakostas, GI., et al. (2010, August) S-adenosylmethionine (SAMe) augmentation of serotonin reuptake inhibitors for antidepressant non-responders with major depressive disorder: a double-blind, randomized clinical trial. *American Journal of Psychiatry;* 167 (8), p 942-8.

33. Ingber, Donald MD, PhD. (2003) Mechanobiology and Diseases of Mechanotransduction: *Annals of Medicine* ;35: (8), pp564-77.

34. Ibid

35. Pick, Marc. (1999) *Cranial Sutures, Analysis, Morphology and Manipulative Strategie*s., p.V. Eastland Press.

36. Goab, Jens et al. (2005, December 15) Reduced reactivity and enhanced negative feedback sensitivity of the hypothalamus-pituitary-adrenal axis in chronic whiplash-associated disorder. *Pain*, vol 119, Issues 1-3, pp219-224.

37. Salford, Leif et al. (2003, June) Nerve Cell Damage in Mammalian After Exposure to Microwaves from GSM Mobile Phones; Environmental Health Perspectives. Vol 111, No7, pp881-883.

38. Lonn, Strefan, et al. (2004, November) Mobile Phone Use and the Risk of Acoustic Neuroma. *Epidemiology*: Vol 15 (6), pp653-659.

39. Hardell, Lennert, et al. (2006, February) Case-control study of the association between the use of cellular and cordless telephones and malignant brain tumors diagnosed during 2000-2003. *Environmental Research*; Vol 100. Issue 2, pp232-241.

40. Freidman, Joseph, et al. (2007, August 1) Mechanism of short-term ERK activation by electromagnetic fields at mobile phone frequencies.

Biochemistry Journal (405), pp559-568.

41. Meikle, MC, et al. (1980) Effect of tensile mechanical stress on the synthesis of metalloproteinases by rabbit coronal sutures in vitro. *Calcified Tissue International* ;30 (1):77-82.

42. Morques, Andrea, et al. (2010) Evaluation of Stress Systems by Applying Non-invasive Methodologies: Measurements of Neuroimmune Biomarkers in the Sweat, Heart Rate Variability and Salivary Cortisol. *Neuroimmunomodulation* ; 17: p205-208.

43. Teodorczyk-Injeyan, Julita PhD et al. (2011) Elevated Production of Inflammatory Mediators Including Nociceptive Chemokines in Patients with Neck Pain: A Cross- Sectional Evaluation. ;34: pp 498-505.

44. Frigerio, A.(1974) *Essential Aspects of Mass Spectrometry* , John Wiley and Sons Inc.

Failure to Thrive References

1. Beidermann, Heirir M.D. (2005) Manual Therapy in Children: Proposals for An Etiologic Model, *Journal of Manipulative Physiology and Therapy*;28:211.el-211.el5.

2. Poritsky, Raphael PhD, (1984) *Neuroanatomical Pathways*, Case Western Reserve University, Dept of Anatomy, Cleveland, Oh. WB Sauellers

3. Beidermann, H. (1992, June) Kinematic Imbalances Due to Suboccipital Strain in Newborns, *Journal of Manual Medicine*, (no.6), pp151-156.

4. Ibid.

5. Taubin, A. (1969) Latent spinal cord and brain stem injuries in newborn infants. *Developmental Medicine and Child Neurology* ;11, p54-68.

6. Murphy, Donald DC, et al. (2009) Outcome of Pregnancy-Related Lumbopelvic Pain Treated According to a Diagnosis-Based Decision Rule: A Prospective Observational Cohort Study, *Journal of Manipulative Physiology and Therapy* ; 32; p616-624.

7. Hurwitz, El, et al. (2006) Epidemiology of low back syndromes. In Morriss CE, editor. *Low back syndromes: integrated clinical management*. New York:McGraw-Hill; p83-118.

Neonatal Bloody Stools References

1. Landauer, MR., et al. (2003, November-December) Genistein treatment protects mice from ionizing radiation injury. *Journal of Applied Toxicology*, 23(6):p379-85.
2. Dittmank, et al. (1995, February) Bowman-Birk protein as inhibitor (BBI) modulates radio-sensitivity and radiation-induced differentiation of human fibroblasts in culture. *Radiotherapy and Oncology*, 34(2):p137-43.
3. Jagetia, GC. (2007) Radioprotection and radio-sensitization by curcumin. *Advances in Experimental Medicine and Biology*; 595:p301-20.
4. Lee, TK., et al. (2009, June) Allylmethylsulfide down-regulates X-ray irradiation-induced nucleus factor-kappa b signaling in C57/BL6 mouse kidney. *Journal of Medicinal Food*, 12 (3): p542-5.
5. Alaoui-Youssefi A., et al. (1999, September 15) Anticlastogenic effects of ginkgo biloba extract (EGb 761) and some of its constituents in irradiated rats. *Mutation Research*; 445 (1); p99-104.
6. Lee, TK., et al. (2004, January 10) Ginseng reduces the micronuclei yield in lymphocytes after irradiation. *Mutation Research*, 557(1): p75-84.
7. Lee, TK., et al. (2010, May 16) Radioprotective effect of american ginseng on human lymphocytes at 90 minutes post-irradiation; a study of 40 cases. *Journal of Alternative and Complementary Medicine*, (5): p561-7.
8. Kropacova, K et al. (1998, May-June) Protective and therapeutic effect of silymarin on the development of latent liver damage. *Radiats Biol Radioecol.*, ;38(3):411-415.
9. Selig, C et al. (1993) Radio-protective effect of N-acetylcysteine on granulocyte/ macrophage colony-forming cells of human bone marrow. *Journal of Cancer Research and Clinical Oncology.* 119 (6): 346-9.
10. Uchida, S, et al. (1992) Radioprotective effects of epigallocatechin 3-0-gallate (green tea tannin) in mice. Life Science, 50(2):147-52.
11. Velioglu-Ogunc A, et al. (2009, August) Reseveratrol protects against irradiation-induced hepatic and ileal damage via its anti-oxidative activity. *Free Radical Research.*,25:1-12
12. Chawlaa, R., et al. (2005, September-October) 3-0-beta-D-galactopyranoside of quercetin as an active principle from high altitude podophyllum hexandrum and evaluation of its radioprotective properties. *ZNaturforsch* C, 60(9-10);728-38.

13. Zhang, R et al. (2006, May) Alterations in gene expression in rat skin exposed to 5g Fe ions and dietary vitamin A acetate. *Radiation Research*, 165(5):570-8).

14. Vorotnikova, E et al. (2004, February) Retinoids and TIMP1 prevent radiation-induced apoptosis of capillary endothelial cells. *Radiation Research*, 161(2):174-84.

15. Wittenborg, B et al. (1999, November) Ascorbic acid inhibits apoptosis induced by xradiation in HLEO myeloid leukemia cells. *Radiation Research*, ;152(5):468-78.

16. Prasad, KN et al. (2003, April) Alpha tocopheryl succinate, the most effective form of vitamin E for adjuvant cancer treatment a review. *Journal of the American College of Nutrition.*, 22(2):108-17.

17. Floersheim, Gl., et al. (1988, June) Differential radioprotection of bone marrow and tumor cells by zinc aspartate. *British Journal Radiology*, 61(26):501-8.

18. Takahashi, M et al. (1992, January) Fatty acids on transformation of cultured cells by irradiation and transfection. *Cancer Research*, vol 52, :134-162.

Autism References

1. Kagen MD, et al. (2009, October) "Prevalence of Parent-Reported Diagnosis of Autism Spectrum Disorder Among Children in the US," 2007 *Pediatrics.* Volume 124, Number 4.

2. O'Shea, Tim DC.5 (2010) *Vaccination Is Not Immunization.* Available from http://www.thedoctorwithin.com.

3. Geier, M. (2005) "A Two-Phased Population, Epidemiological Study of the Safety of Thimerosal-Containing Vaccines: a Follow Up Analysis." *Medical Science Monitor*, 11(4), pp 160-170.

4. Saputo, L., et al. (2010, February) "The Infection Deception: Unanswered Questions about the Swine Flu Controversy Part 1," *The Townsend Letter*, p 73.

5. Landrigan, Philip, MD. (2010, January 16) What Causes Autism? Exploring the Environmental Contribution, Current Opinion in Pediatrics.

6. Dufault, Renee, et al. (2009, Jan 26) "Mercury from Chlor-Alkali Plants Measured Concentrations in Food Product Sugar." *Environmental Health.* 8:2.

7. Cannell, John. (2008) "Autism and Vitamin D." *Medical Hypothesis*, Vol 70, Issue 4, p. 750-759.

8. Yehuda S, et al. (1998) "Fatty Acids and Brain Peptides." *Peptides*, 19(2):407-419.

9. Cutler, R G, et al. (2002, October) "Evidence that Accumulation of Ceramides and Cholesterol Esters Mediates Oxidative Stress–Induced Death of Motor Neurons in Amyotrophic Lateral Sclerosis." *Annals of Neurology*, 52:4:448– 457.

10. Moser, A B, et al. (1999, January) "Plasma Very Long Chain Fatty Acids in 3000 Peroxisomal Disease Patients and 29,000 controls." *Annals of Neurology*, 45(1):100-10.

11. Kane, P C. (1997,August) Peroxisomal Disturbances in Children with Epilepsy, Hypoxia and Autism. *Prostaglandins, Leukotrienes and Essential Fatty Acids* . 57:2:265.

Drug-Resistant Clostridium Difficile Infection, Severe Abdominal Pain and Diarrhea References

1. Csoka, AB., et al. (2009, November) 'Epigenetic side-effect caused by a drug may persist after the drug is discontinued.' Epigenetic side effects of common pharmaceuticals: a potential new field in medicine and pharmacology. *Medical Hypotheses*. 73(5):770-80.

2. Schmidt, WH Jr., et al.(1998) Correlation of applied kinesiology muscle testing with serum immunoglobulin levels for food allergies. International J *Neuroscience*, 96 (3-4); 237-244.

Severe Asthma References

1. Engel Roger M, DC,DO et al. (2007) The Effect of Combining Manual Therapy with Exercise on the Respiratory Function of Normal Individuals: A Randomized Control Trial. *Journal of Manipulative Physical Therapies* ;30. p.509-513.

2. *Asthma Action America*, a national asthma education program supported by the GlaxoSmithKline Respiratory Institute.

3. Saglani S, Bush A. (2007 February) "The early life origins of asthma." *Current Opinion in Allergy and Clinical Immunology*, 7(1)83-90.

4. aafa.org (asthma and allergy foundation of America), page 2.

5. *Dr. Perlmutter's Heads Up Newsletter*, (2007, November) Volume 7, Number 7.

6. Gvozdjakova A, et al. (2005) "Coenzyme Q10 supplementation reduces corticosteroids dosage in patients with bronchial asthma." *Biofactors*, 25(1-4):235-40.

7. Castro-Rodriquez JA, et al. (2008, June) "Mediterranean diet as a protective factor for wheezing in preschool children." *Journal of Pediatrics*, 152(6):823-8, 828-e1-2.

8. Mickleborough TD. (2008,Jul) "A nutritional approach to managing exercise-induced asthma." *Exercise and Sport Sciences Review*, 36(3):135-44.

9. Contijo-Amoral C, et al. (2007) "Oral magnesium supplementation in asthmatic children: a double-blind, randomized placebo-controlled trial." *European Journal of Clinical Nutrition*, 61:54-60.

10. Blitz M, et al. (2005,October 19) "Inhaled magnesium sulfate in the treatment of acute asthma." *Cochrane Database of Systemic Reviews*, (4):CD003898.

11. Shaheen SO, et al.(2007,June) "Randomized, double-blind, placebo-controlled trial of selenium supplementation in adult asthma." *Thorax*, *BMJ*;62(6):483-90. 551

12. Lau, BH, et al. (2004) Pycnogenol as an adjunct in the management of childhood asthma. *Journal of Asthma*, 41:825-32.

13. Pearson, PJ, et al. (2004,August) Vitamin E supplements in asthma: a parallel, group-randomized, placebo-controlled trial. *Thorax*, 59(8):652-6.

14. Tecklenburg, SL, et al. (2007,August) Ascorbic acid supplementation attenuates exercise- induced bronchoconstriction in patients with asthma. *Respiratory Medicine*, 10: (8):1770-8.

15. Choi, IS, et al. (2008, December) Effects of dehydroepiandrosterone on the cytokine production in peripheral blood mononuclear cells from asthmatics. *Korean Journal of Internal Medicine*, 23(4):176-81.

16. MacRedmond, et al. (2010, July) Conjugated linoleic acid improves airway hyper reactivity in overweight mild asthmatics. *Clinical and Experimental Allergy*; vol 40,pp1071-8.

17. Urashima M, et al.(2010) Randomized trial of vitamin D supplementation to prevent seasonal influenza A schoolchildren. *American Journal of Clinical Nutrition* ;92 (5) 1255-60.

18. Toohey L. (2010) Vitamin D: The versatile nutrient. *American Journal of Clinical Chiropractic*: 20 (1) 4 and 21.

19. Murphy, DJ. (2009) Our schools, Autism and Vitamin D. *American Journal of Clinical Chiropractic*; 19 (2).

20. Johnson, Christine Cole PhD, et al. (2005,June) Antibiotic exposure in early infancy and risk for childhood atopy. *Journal of Allergy and Clinical Immunology*, vol 115, issue 6, p 1218-1224.

21. Barr, R Graham, MD. "The Secret Cause of Asthma?" *Bottom Line's Hushed Up* 100, p78-9.

22. Kozyrskyl, Al., et al. (2007, June) Increased risk of childhood asthma from antibiotic use in early life. *Chest*, 131 (6): 1753-9.

23. Engel, Roger M., DC, DO, et al. (2007) The effect of combining Manual Therapy with Exercise on the Respiratory Function of Normal Individuals: A Randomized Control Trial. *Journal of Manipulative and Physical Therapies*; 30. 509–513.

24. Guiney PA, et al. (2005,January) Effects of osteopathic manipulative treatment on pediatric patients with asthma: a randomized—controlled trial. *Journal American Osteopathic Association.*, 105 (1): 7-12.

Recurrent Otitis Media References

1. Ouwehand, A., et al. (2008) Probiotics Reduce Incidence and Duration of Respiratory Tract Infection Symptoms in 3-5 year old Children. *Pediatrics*, 121:S115.

2. Hegerma, R., et al. (1987) An association between recurrent otitis media in infancy and later hyperactivity. *Clinical Pediatrics* :26(5)253-57.

3. Adesman, A. R., et al.(1990) Otitis media in children with learning disabilities and in children with attention deficit disorder with hyperactivity. *Pediatrics*, 85(3):442-6.

Attention Deficit Disorder (ADD) and Attention Deficit Hyperactivity Disorder (ADHD) References

1. Gould, MS., Wash T., Munfakh, JL., et al. (2009, June 15) ADHD, Sudden death and use of stimulant medications in youth. *American Journal of Psychiatry.*

2. Morse, N. (2009) A Meta-Analysis of blood fatty acids in people with learning disorders with particular interest in Archidonic Acid. *Prostaglandins, Leukotrienes, and Essential Fatty Acids.*

3. Bouchard, M F, et al. (2010, June) Attention-Deficit/Hyperactivity Disorder and Urinary Metabolites of Organophosophate Pesticides. *Pediatrics,* Vol 125, Number 6.

4. Cuthbert, SC, Barras, M. (2009, October) Developmental delay syndromes: psychometric testing before and after chiropractic treatment of 157 children. *Journal Manipulative and Physiological Therapeutics,* 32(8)660-9.

Fainting References

1. Khosla, Sundeep MD, et al. (2003, Sept 17) Childhood Distal Forearm Fractures Over Thirty Years—A Population-Based Study. JAMA, :290:1479-1485.

Chronic Drug-Resistant Throat Infection Reference

1. Nance, Dwight, et al. (2007, August) Autonomic innervations and regulation of the immune system (1987- 2007). *Brain, Behavior, and Immunity.* Vol 21, Issue 6, p 736-745.

Allergies and Asthma Reference

1. Takeda, Yasuhiko, et al. (2004) Relationship between vertebral deformities and allergic diseases. *Th e International Journal of Orthopedic Surgery,* vol 2; number 1.

Chronic Juvenile Migraines References

1. Bigal, Marcelo, et al. (2008, August 19) Chronic migraine in the population: burden, diagnosis and satisfaction with treatment. *Neurology,* 71; 559-566.

2. Bogduk, Nikolai, MD, PhD. (1995) *Anatomy and Physiology of Headache, Biomedicine and Pharmacotherapy,* vol 49, no.10, 435-445.

Arm Paralysis—Post Cervical Fracture References

1. Brantingham JW, et al. (2011 June) Manipulative therapy for shoulder pain and disorders: expansion of a systemic review. *Journal Manipulative*

Physiological Therapeutics ; 34 (5):314-46.

2. Charles, Eugene DC. (2011) Chiropractic management of a 30 year old patient with parsonage-turner syndrome, *Journal of Chiropractic Med.* 10, 301-305.

Recurrent Sinus Infection, Drug-Resistant References

1. Maloney, Beth Alison. (2009) Saving Sammy: *A Mothers Fight to Cure Her Son's OCD*, p. 124. New York, NY: Crown Publishers (division of Random House).
2. Wen, L., et al. (2008,October 23) Innate immunity and intestinal microbiota in the development of Type I diabetes. *Nature*, 455(7216):1109-13.
3. Turnbaugh, PJ., et al. (2009, January 22) A core gut microbiome in obese and lean twins. *Nature*, 457 (7228): 480-4.
4. Yaddanapudi, K., et al. (2010,July) Passive transfer of streptococcus-induced antibodies reproduces behavioral disturbances in a mouse modal of pediatric autoimmune neuropsychiatric disorders associated with streptococcal infection. *Molecular Psychiatry*, 15 (7):712-26.
5. Lin, H., et al. (2010,April) Streptococcal upper respiratory tract infection and psychosocial stress predict future tic and obsessive-compulsive symptom severity in children and adolescents with Tourette Syndrome and obsessive-compulsive disorder. *Biological Psychiatry*, 67(7):684-91.

Severe Mercury Poisoning References

1. Blaylock, Russell MD. (1997) *Excitotoxins: The Taste That Kills*, p. 38. Santa Fe, New Mexico: Health Press.
2. Hightower, Jane MD. (2009) *Diagnosis: Mercury—Money, Politics and Poison.* p.241; Washington, DC: Island Press.
3. Trasande, L. 2005.
4. Hightower, Jane, MD. (2009) *Diagnosis: Mercury—Money, Politics and Poison.* p.208: Washington, DC: Island Press.
5. Fukuda. 1999, *Verada*, 1995, 2005.
6. Hightower, Jane, MD. (2009) *Diagnosis: Mercury—Money, Politics and Poison.* p.244: Washington, DC: Island Press.

7. Virtanen 2005, Sorensen 1999, Salonen 1995, 2000; Rissanen 2000, Guallar 2002; Frustacia 1999; Stern 2005.

8. Hightower, Jane, MD. (2009) *Diagnosis: Mercury- Money, Politics and Poison*. p.250: Washington, DC: Island Press.

9. Ibid, p.251, 252.

10. Ibid.

Post Extraction Trismus—Lockjaw References

1. Dvorak, J. and Dvorak, V. (1984) *Manual Medicine Diagnostics*. New York: Thieme-Stratton, Inc.

2. Riva, John J., et al. (2010) Inter-professional education through shadowing experiences in multi-disciplinary settings. *Chiropractic and Osteopathy*,18:31.

Amennorhea References

1. Murphy, Donald R., et al. (2009) Outcome of pregnancy-related lumbo-pelvic pain treated according to a diagnosis-based decision rule: a prospective observational cohort study. *Journal of Manipulative and Physiological Therapeutics*, :32:616-624.

2. Oschman, James (2003) *Energy Medicine in Therapeutics and Human Performance*. Edinburgh:Butterworth Heineman, p 93.

3. Ibid, p93.

4. Pickup, A. (1978) Collagen and behavior: A model for progressive debilitation. *Medical Science,* p 6, p 499.

5. Church, Dawson (2009) *The Genie in Your Genes*, Santa Rosa, Ca: Energy Psychology Press, p 198.

24. (GERD) Gastro-Esophageal Reflux Disease References

6. Wright J, Leland L. *Why Stomach Acid is Good for You—Natural Relief from Heartburn, Indigestion, Reflux and GERD*, M. Evens and Cer, 2001, p 10.

7. Peura D, et al. Achlorhydria and enteric bacterial infections. In: Hott p, Russell R,eds. Chronic Gastritis and Hypochlorhydria in the Elderly, pp127-142. Boca Raton, F: CRC Press 1993.

8. Wright J, Leland L. *Why Stomach Acid is Good for You—Natural Relief from Heartburn, Indigestion, Reflux and GERD,* M Evens and Cer, 2001, p11.

9. Ibid, p 40.

5. Young Martin F. et al. Chiropractic Manual Intervention in Chronic Adult Dyspepsia. *Eur J of Gastroenterology and Hepatology* April 2009, 21:482-486.

Cervical Herniated Nerve Plexus (HNP) and Left Arm Pain References

1. Hurwitz, et al. (1996) Manipulation and mobilization at the cervical spine. A systematic review of the literature. *Spine*, 21:1746-60.

Rheumatoid Arthritis/Electric Blankets– Reference

1. Ober C., Sinatra S., Zucker M. (2010) *Earthing—the Most Important Health Discovery Ever?* Laguna Beach, Ca.: Basic Health Publications Inc. ISBN-978-1-59120 2837.

Chronic Insomnia and Tension Headaches- Reference

1. Cuthbert, Scott DC, Rosner, Anthony PhD. (2011) Physical causes of Anxiety and Sleep Disorders. *Alternative Therapies in Health Medicine*; 17(4): 54-57.

Alopecia Arreata References

1. Jaffee, Russell. (Nov, 2010) The Alkaline Way: Integrative Management of Autoimmune Conditions. *Townsend Letter*, p44.
2. Nakazawa, DJ. (2008) *The Autoimmune Epidemic.* page 164. New York, NY: Touchstone (division of Simon and Schuster) ISBN 978 074327 7754
3. ibid, page 165.
4. ibid, page 159.
5. ibid, page 230.
6. Fasano, A MD. (2008, November) Physiological, pathological, and therapeutic implications of zonulin-mediated intestinal barrier modulation-living life on the edge of the wall. *American Journal of Pathology*, 173:1243-52.

Bell's Palsy References

1. Morris, AM. (2002) Annualized incidence and spectrum of illness from an outbreak investigation of Bell's palsy. *Neuroepidemiology*; 21 (5) 255-261.
2. Campbell, K E et al. (2002) Effects of climate, latitude, and season on the incidence of Bell's palsy in the US armed forces. October 1997 to September 1999. *American Journal of Epidemiology*. 156 (1);32-39.
3. Sullivan, FM et al. (2007) Early treatment with prednizolone or acyclovir in Bell's palsy. *New England Journal of Medicine* ;367 (16); 1598-1607.

Gallstones—Right Upper Abdominal Pain—References

1. Tsai, CJ. et al. (2006,November 27) Weight, Cycling and risk of gallstone disease in men. *Archives of Internal Medicine*;166 (21): 2, 369-74.
2. Jeons, SU., et al. (2012,January) Obesity and gallbladder diseases. *Korean Journal Gastroenteralogy* ; 59 (1): 27-34.

Incontinence References

1. Cuthbert, Scott, et al. (2012) Conservative chiropractic management of urinary incontinence using applied kinesiology: a retrospective case-series report. *Journal of Chiropractic Medicine*: 11, 49-57.
2. Browning, James E. DC (2008,September 30) *Pelvic Pain and Organic Dysfunction - The PPOD Syndrome.* preface p 5, Denver, Colorado:Outskirts Press.
3. IBID.

Severe Epicondylitis with Two Torn Rotator Cuffs References

1. Brantingham, JLN, (2011, June) *Journal of Manipulative and Physiologic Therapeutics.*
2. newchoice.com.

A Twenty-Year Cluster Headache References

1. Maykel, W. (2001-2002) Case History-Cluster Headache. *International College of Applied Kinesiology –USA*. Proceedings of the Annual Meeting; p. 135-138.

2. Headache Classification Committee of the International Headache Society. (1988) Classification and diagnostic criteria for headache disorders, cranial neuralgias and facial pain. *Cephalgia* :8 (Suppl. 7):35-7:cited in Walling, AD., Cluster Headache *American Family Physical* (1993); 47(6): 1457-63.

3. Walling, AD., ibid.

4. Mathew, Nt. (November 1990) Advances in Cluster Headache. *Neurologic Clinics* ;8(4): 867-90.

5. Hardebo, JE. (1984) The involvement of trigeminal substance P neurons in cluster headache. Headache ; 24:294 cited in Mathew, op. cit.

6. Cited in Mathew, ibid.

7. Cited in Mathew, ibid.

8. Cited in Mathew, ibid.

9. Tfelt-Hansen P., et al. (2013, January) Sumatriptan: a review of it's pharmacokinetics, pharmaco dynamics and efficacy in the acute treatment of migraine. *Expert Opinions on Drug Metabolism and Toxicology.* 9(1) 91-103.

10. IBID.

11. Ekbom, K, et. (1991) AI. Treatment of acute cluster headache with sumatriptan. *New England Journal of Medicine*; 325:322-26 cited in Ferrari MD, Saxena PRS, Clinical effects and mechanism of action of sumatriptin in migraine. *Clinical Neurology and Neurosurgery*, 1992; 94 (Suppl.):S73-77.

12. Drummond PD, Lance JW.(1984) Thermographic Changes in Cluster Headache. *Neurology*, 34:1292, cited in Mathew, op. cit.

13. Drummond PD, Anthony M. (1985) Extracranial vascular responses to sublingual nitroglycerin and oxygen inhalation in cluster headache patients. *Headache* 25:70, cited in Mathews, NT, op. cit.

14. Sandy, R. (1992) The Influence of Pineal Gland on Migraine and Cluster Headaches and the effects of treatment with Pico Tesla magnetic fields. *International Journal of Neuroscience* : 67(1-4); 145-171.

15. Lance, JW., (1982) *Mechanism and Management of Headaches*, ed. 4. London, Butterworth Scientific, p. 205, cited in Mathews NT op. cit.

16. Reik, L. (1987) Cluster headache after head injury. *Headache* 27: 509. cited in Mathew NT op cit.

17. Mathew, NT., Rueveni, U. (1983) Cluster-like headaches following head trauma. *Headache* 28: 297.

18. Headache Classification Committee of the International Headache Society: (1988) Classification and diagnostic criteria for headache disorders, cranial

neuralgia, and facial pain. *Cephalgia*; (suppl. 7).

19. Walling AD, op. cit.

Vocal Cord Paralysis—Spasmodic Dysphonia-Reference

1. Swack, Judith PhD . She is the founder of HBLU, Healing from the Body Level Up. Her work focuses on the conscious alignment of body, unconscious and Spirit to achieve better harmony and improved health.

Understanding Normal Pelvic Spinal Complex Motion -References:

1. Martin, Michael MD, et al. (2002,August) Pathophysiology of lumbar disc degeneration:a review of the Literature. *Neurosurgery*—Focus 13 (2).

Stay Well Adjusted References: Stay Tuned Up

1. Masarsky, CS., Todres-Masarsky, M. (2010) Effects of a single chiropractic adjustment on divergent thinking and creative output: a pilot study Part 1; *Chiropractic Journal of Australia*, 40;57-62.

2. Smith, DL et al. (2006) The effect of chiropractic adjustments on movement time: A pilot study using Fitt's Law. *Journal of Manipulative and Physiological Therapeutics*, 29 (4);257-266.

3. Zhang, et al.(2006) Effect of chiropractic care on heart rate variability and pain in a multisite study. *Journal of Manipulative and Physiological Th erapeutics*, 29(40):267.

4. Dekker, JM., et al. (1997) Heart rate variability from short electrocardiographic recordings predicts mortality from all causes in middle-aged elderly men. *American Journal of Epidemiology*, 145(10):899.

5. Giles, Linton G., et al. (2003, July 15) Chronic Spinal Pain: A Randomized clinical trial Compare Medication, Acupuncture and Spinal Manipulation. *Spine*; 28(14): 1490-1502.

6. Muller, Reinhold, et al. (2005, January) Long-term follow-up of Randomized Clinical Trial Assessing the Efficacy of Medication, Acupuncture and Spinal Manipulation for Chronic Mechanical Spine Pain Syndromes, *Journal of Manipulative and Physiological Therapeutics*, vol. 28; no 1.

7. Stasson, WB., et al. Report to Congress on the Evaluation of the

Demonstration of Coverage of Chiropractic Services under Medicare, Waltham Mass: Brandeis University, Schneider Institutes for Health Policy.

8. Hurwith, EL., et al. (2008,February 15) Treatment of Neck Pain: Noninvasive Interventions: results of the Bone and Joint Decade 2000-2010 Task Force on Neck Pain and Its Associated Disorders. *Spine*, Vol.33, No 4S, pp.S123-S152.

9. Young, Martin, et al. (2009, April) Chiropractic Manual Intervention in Chronic Adult Dyspepsia. *European Journal of Gastroenterology and Hepatology*, 21: 482-486.

Mattress Matters References

1. Ghaly, M, et al. (2004) The biologic effects of grounding the human body during sleep as measured by cortisol levels and subjective reporting of sleep, pain and stress. *Journal of Alternative and Complementary Medicine*, 10 (5): 767-776.

2. Sinatra, Stephen MD, et al.(2010, April 9) *Earthing*, p.176, Laguna Beach, California:Basic Health Publications.

Tricks to Keeping a Positive Magnesium Status References:

1. Morgan, KJ, et al.(1985) Magnesium and Calcium Dietary Intakes of the US Population. *Journal of the American College of Nutrition.* 4:195-206.

2. Slutsky I, Abumaria N, Wu LJ, et al. Enhancement of learning and memory by elevating brain magnesium. *Neuron*, 2010 Jan 28;65(2):165-77.

A Short List of Technologies to Be Wary Of References

1. Seralini, Giles-Eric, et al. (2012) Long term toxicity of a Roundup herbicide and a round-up tolerant genetically modified maize. *Food and Chemical Toxicology*.

2. Samsel, A., Seneff, S. (2013, April 18) Glyphosate's Suppression of Cytochrome P450 Enzymes and Amino Acid Biosynthesis by the Gut Microbiome: Pathways to Modern Diseases. *Entropy*, 15, pp1416-1463.

CPSIA information can be obtained
at www.ICGtesting.com
Printed in the USA
BVOW08*1043190817
492485BV00016B/72/P